Reconsidering Dementia Narratives

Reconsidering Dementia Narratives explores the role of narrative in developing new ways of understanding, interacting with, and caring for people with dementia. It asks how the stories we tell about dementia—in fiction, life writing, and film—both reflect and shape the way we think about this important condition.

Highlighting the need to attend to embodied and relational aspects of identity in dementia, the study further outlines ways in which narratives may contribute to dementia care, while disputing the idea that the modes of empathy fostered by narrative necessarily bring about more humane care practices. This cross-medial analysis represents an interdisciplinary approach to dementia narratives which range across auto/biography, graphic narrative, novel, film, documentary, and collaborative storytelling practices. The book aims to clarify the limits and affordances of narrative, and narrative studies, in relation to an ethically driven medical humanities agenda through the use of case studies.

Answering the key question of whether dementia narratives align with or run counter to the dominant discourse of dementia as 'loss of self,' this innovative book will be of interest to anyone interested in dementia studies, ageing studies, narrative studies in health care, and critical medical humanities.

Rebecca A. Bitenc completed her PhD on 'Dementia Narratives in Contemporary Literature, Life-Writing and Film' at Durham University, UK. Her research interests include critical medical humanities, narratology, and narrative ethics. She is a member of the Dementia and Cultural Narratives Network and the Northern Network for Medical Humanities Research. She has an M.A. in English, French, and Psychology from Albert-Ludwigs-Universität, Germany.

Routledge Advances in the Medical Humanities

Thinking with Metaphors in Medicine
The State of the Art
Alan Bleakley

Medicine, Health and Being Human
Edited by Lesa Scholl

Meaning-making Methods for Coping with Serious Illness
Fereshteh Ahmadi and Nader Ahmadi

A Visual History of HIV/AIDS
Exploring the Face of AIDS Film Archive
Edited by Elisabet Björklund and Mariah Larsson

Communicating Pain
Exploring Suffering Through Language, Literature and Creative Writing
Stephanie de Montalk

Reconsidering Dementia Narratives
Empathy, Identity and Care
Rebecca A. Bitenc

Moments of Rupture and the Importance of Affect in Professional Learning and Practice
Research Perspectives from Surgical Training and Medical Education
Arunthathi Mahendran

For more information about this series visit: https://www.routledge.com/Routledge-Advances-in-Disability-Studies/book-series/RADS

Reconsidering Dementia Narratives
Empathy, Identity and Care

Rebecca A. Bitenc

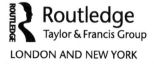

LONDON AND NEW YORK

First published 2020
by Routledge
4 Park Square, Milton Park, Abingdon, Oxon OX14 4RN
605 Third Avenue, New York, NY 10017

First issued in paperback 2023

Routledge is an imprint of the Taylor & Francis Group, an informa business

© 2020 Rebecca A. Bitenc

The right of Rebecca A. Bitenc to be identified as author of this work has been asserted by her in accordance with sections 77 and 78 of the Copyright, Designs and Patents Act 1988.

All rights reserved. No part of this book may be reprinted or reproduced or utilised in any form or by any electronic, mechanical, or other means, now known or hereafter invented, including photocopying and recording, or in any information storage or retrieval system, without permission in writing from the publishers.

Trademark notice: Product or corporate names may be trademarks or registered trademarks, and are used only for identification and explanation without intent to infringe.

British Library Cataloguing-in-Publication Data
A catalogue record for this book is available from the British Library

Library of Congress Cataloging-in-Publication Data
A catalog record has been requested for this book

ISBN: 978-1-03-257062-4 (pbk)
ISBN: 978-0-367-15134-8 (hbk)
ISBN: 978-0-429-05526-3 (ebk)

DOI: 10.4324/9780429055263

Typeset in Times New Roman
by codeMantra

Publisher's Note
The publisher has gone to great lengths to ensure the quality of this reprint but points out that some imperfections in the original copies may be apparent.

To Clara Maria

Contents

List of figures xi
Preface xiii
Acknowledgements xv

Introduction: reconsidering dementia narratives 1
Two starting points 1
Why narrative? 4
Biomedicine and the cultural meaning of dementia 8
   A brief history of dementia 9
   Demography and demonisation 10
   Reconsidering dementia: reparative moves 11
   The Alzheimer's 'epidemic': care, cost, and social justice 12
Literary dementia studies and the medical humanities 14
   Illness narratives: countering master narratives and
      exploring the experience of illness 16
Outline of chapters 17

PART I
Storytelling, experience, and empathy 23

1 **Narrating experiences of dementia: embodied selves, embodied communication** 25
 Embodied selves, embodied communication 26
 Inside views: life writing by people with early-onset dementia 30
    Memory 32
    Language 36
    Perception, movement, and the senses 38
    Emotions and cognition 40
    Time 43
    The social world: intimate relationships and strangers 45
    The experience of flow in dementia 47

    From the caregiver's perspective: intersubjectivity in David
      Sieveking's documentary Vergiss Mein Nicht *50*
      Viewing symptoms of dementia *51*
      The communicating body in film *53*
      Embodied selves and relational selves *56*
    Conclusion 58

2   **From the outside in? Experience and empathy in fictional dementia narratives**   63
    Still Alice: *from fiction to film 65*
    Experiencing dementia/experimenting with the novel 71
      Out of Mind *72*
      House Mother Normal *76*
      The Unconsoled *83*
    Concluding reflections on narrative empathy 88

PART II
Life writing, self-writing, and creating identities   97

3   **Life writing at the limits: narrative identity and counter-narratives in dementia**   99
    Narrative identity in dementia: friend or foe? 100
    Reconsidering master and counter-narratives 103
    The problem of counter-narratives in dementia: reading
      first-person accounts 105
    Coherence in 'broken' counter-narratives: 'Mrs Mill'
      and other stories 114
      Janet's story: confabulation, continuity, and agency *120*
      Counter-narratives in context: the editor's role *121*
    Conclusion 122

4   **Relational identity in (filial) caregivers' memoirs**   128
    The aesthetics, ethics, and politics of caregivers' memoirs 128
    Gender, genre, and the self: rethinking relational identity
      in dementia 137
      My Father's Brain *138*
      Do You Remember Me? A Father, a Daughter,
        and a Search for the Self *142*
      Tangles: A Story about Alzheimer's, My Mother, and Me *148*
    Conclusion 154

PART III
Narrating dementia/rethinking care   159

5   **Care-writing reconsidered: towards a new practice of dementia care**   161
  Exploring caregivers' dilemmas 162
    Care or coercion? Autonomy in dementia 163
    'Bad grooming': intimate care in dementia 168
    'No good choices': institutionalisation in dementia 171
  Imagining alternative approaches in dementia care 174
    Reconsidering confabulation 175
    The power of music 178
    From control to letting go: being with vs. symptom management 180
  Challenging care practice 183
  Conclusion 185

6   **Making readers care: bioethics and the novel**   190
  Ethics and the novel: countering, stereotyping, and disturbing 192
    Scar Tissue: biomedicine and the hermeneutics of selfhood 193
    Narrative and neuroimaging: raising epistemological questions 197
    House Mother Normal: disturbing care 201
  Exploring bioethics: 'living through' as 'thinking through' 205
    Still Alice: (precedent) autonomy and suicide in dementia 207
    Mode, medium, and the suicide plot 208
    Have the Men Had Enough? Gender and the economies of care 213
  Conclusion 219

Dementia narratives and beyond   225

Bibliography   231
Index   249

List of figures

4.1 The problem of inverted child-parent relations in Haugse (1998: 31) by permission of the author illustrator John Haugse — 151
4.2 Facial expression and gesture indicate emotional distress in Leavitt (2010: 102). Image courtesy of Sarah Leavitt — 153
5.1 (a, b) 'Good grooming': Ethical issues in personal care in Leavitt (2010: 110). Images courtesy of Sarah Leavitt — 169
5.2 Care as connection in Leavitt (2010: 111). Image courtesy of Sarah Leavitt — 170
5.3 (a, b, c) Figuring the effects of caregiver stress in Leavitt (2010: 116–7). Images courtesy of Sarah Leavitt — 172
5.4 Drawing style as part of narrative rhetoric in Leavitt (2010: 116). Image courtesy of Sarah Leavitt — 173
5.5 Letting go and being with in Leavitt (2010: 78). Image courtesy of Sarah Leavitt — 182

Preface

A few years ago, I was out with my 'mummy friends'—women I had met through baby groups after the birth of my daughter Clara. At one point, my research, and by implication dementia became the topic of conversation. From the other end of the table one of my friends called, 'Shoot me if I ever get that way!' Her comment has stuck with me. Not because it was entirely out of the ordinary. When I tell people about my research, I get one of several reactions: People will tell me about a family member with dementia, who is 'no longer there' or 'no longer herself.' They will talk about how hard it was (for themselves or someone else in the family) to look after a 'loved one' with dementia. Or I might get a comment like the one above, suggesting that life with dementia is not worth living and that the person I am talking to would rather die than lose her cognitive capacity. What struck me was that in 2016, nearly twenty years after Tom Kitwood's seminal *Dementia Reconsidered* thoroughly challenged the way people with dementia are perceived and treated, negative preconceptions about dementia still prevail.

This book is about the stories we tell about dementia—the ones told by novelists and film-makers, but also by family care partners and by people with dementia themselves. It is also about how these stories interact and become entangled with wider cultural narratives, with the stories we tell about identity, selfhood, ethics, empathy, and care. Dementia, as these narratives demonstrate, is tied up with our value systems—with our notion of who and what matters.

People want to know what drew me to this topic. They ask me whether I have had a 'case of dementia' in the family. The simple answer would be 'No,' if the question is understood as whether a personal experience has made me so passionate about this topic. The more complex and truthful answer is 'Yes, but….' I was drawn to this topic initially by my interest in language—and specifically my interest in what happens when language breaks down. While pursuing a joint degree in literature, linguistics, and psychology, I spent a substantial amount of my time working alongside speech therapists, doing EEG experiments in a neurolinguistic laboratory on speech and language disorders, or completing course work in neuropsychology. Frustrated with the epistemological uncertainties of EEG experiments—as well as, to be honest, the lack of a handy MRI machine to conduct my own study on language pathology—I chose to pursue my interest in neurolinguistics through an entirely different field: literary studies.

This project has morphed many times over the years. Initially concerned with how fictional dementia narratives represent the disease syndrome and what narrative techniques are used to evoke a sense of 'what it's like' to be living with dementia, I later became more interested in the ethics, aesthetics, and politics of dementia life writing. I soon realised that dementia raises a host of philosophical questions (Who am I without my memories?), ethical conundrums (Am I obliged to force my family member with dementia to eat when she no longer wants to?), and political issues (How much money do we allocate to dementia care? And significantly, *who* cares for people with dementia and under what conditions?). Reading widely across media and genres (including theatre, opera, and poetry), I finally returned to my home base—narrative studies—as a lens to approach questions of experience, empathy, ethics, identity, and care.

But like most people I know, I have also had 'dementia in the family.' Both my maternal grandparents lived with dementia towards the end of their lives. My grandad's language became more poetical—but we still tried to make sense of what he said and, I think, even enjoyed the beauty and evocativeness of his language. When I visited, he seemed contented in the nursing home to which he finally moved. Nor—despite his previous intellectual prowess—did his life to me seem tragic, a 'death before death.' His death, when it came was absolute and it was then that we grieved.

My grandmother was diagnosed with dementia when she was in her late 80s. She was by then living in Shetland, to where she had removed herself after my grandfather's death. I never got to visit her at the time. But I got a sense, from other family members, that visiting her and interacting with her actually became easier as the condition progressed. (And this, despite such 'problem behaviour,' as the professional jargon has it, as undressing in front of others.) So, yes, professionally and within the context of my own family, I have first-hand experience of dementia—although it goes without saying that this experience is not at all comparable to being a family care partner. But, in any case, my interest was foremost spiked by academic questions: what does it mean to lose language—for the person, her sense of self, and her relationships? And how can one, paradoxically, represent a condition considered beyond language through language? Crucially, too, my own experience departs from dominant narratives about dementia as 'tragedy,' 'death before death,' and 'loss of self.' As this book aims to demonstrate, the stories we tell about dementia are enmeshed with this predominantly dehumanising discourse, but they are also more complex. They tell of relationships improved, of humour, of love, as well as of despair, ethical conundrums, and systemic failings. They explore what it means to be human. They spin yarns in which dementia is the plot-device through which family heritage is unearthed and (murder) mysteries unfold. Others present calls to action to change dementia care. Stories about dementia may solidify stereotypical views of people with the condition, but they may also challenge or surprise. Most importantly, the stories told by people with dementia, I believe, exert an ethical call for those of us not (yet) affected to engage and to listen.

Acknowledgements

First and foremost, I would like to thank David Herman, for his inspiring intellectual curiosity, constant encouragement, and extraordinary generosity of spirit.

Research for this book was supported by the Arts and Humanities Research Council, UK, and I am indebted to the Faculty of Arts and Humanities, Department of English Studies, Ustinov College, and what is now the Institute—and used to be the Centre—for Medical Humanities at Durham University for financial as well as for non-material but important intellectual support and inspiration.

I would like to thank Sarah Leavitt and John Haugse for their generous permission to reproduce artwork from their graphic memoirs. A big thank you also to David Clegg from the Trebus Project for the permission to use the stories collected in *Tell Mrs Mill Her Husband Is Still Dead*, as well as for his insightful comments on the production, editing process, and initial reception of these stories. Parts of my work on this collection discussed in Chapter 3 have previously been published in an article entitled '"No Narrative, No Self"? Reconsidering Dementia Counter-Narratives in *Tell Mrs Mill Her Husband Is Still Dead.*' *Subjectivity* (2018) 11: 128–43.

I am furthermore indebted to the anonymous reviewers for their valuable comments and encouraging feedback, as well as to the editing team at Routledge.

Many colleagues, friends, and family members have contributed in their own unique ways to the process by which this research has evolved. While too numerous to list, none are forgotten. Special mention is due, though, to my parents, Karl and Deborah Reichl, for being there from start to finish.

And finally, thank you to my daughter Clara for keeping me in the here and now and an enormous thank you to my husband Urban: for sharing your life with me and for your steadfast support throughout this entire venture—despite not ever reading a single line from this book!

Introduction
Reconsidering dementia narratives

Two starting points

Consider these extracts from two contemporary dementia narratives:

> Mum says ... that she feels lucky and glad and relieved now Grandma is dead. But she says she also feels a coward too because now Grandma is dead she can ignore the problem of all the other Grandmas and she shouldn't, she should be inspired to do something and she knows she isn't going to. She is going to dodge the issue now. She doesn't want to think about senile dementia or hear about it or read about it ever again. She isn't an activist and she can't help it. But somebody, somewhere, will have to do something soon. They'll have to. We've tinkered around enough with the start of life, we've interfered with all kinds of natural sequences, and now we'll have to tinker with the end. Mum says, "Your generation, Hannah, will have to have pro-death marches, you'll have to stop being scared to kill the old." Will we?
> (Margaret Forster *Have the Men Had Enough?* 1989: 250)

> I've been thinking about myself. Some time back, we used to be, I hesitate to say the word, 'human beings.' We worked, we made money, we had kids, and a lot of things we did not like to do and a lot of things we enjoyed. We were part of the economy. We had clubs that we went to, like Kiwanis Club and Food Bank. I was a busy little bee. I was into all sorts of things, things that had to do with music. Just a lot of things I did back then when I was, I was about to say – alive – that may be an exaggeration, but I must say this really is, it's living, it's living halfway.
> (Cary Henderson, *Partial View: An Alzheimer's Journal* 1998: 35)

The first extract is taken from Margaret Forster's novel *Have the Men Had Enough?* (1989) and the second from Cary Henderson's *Partial View* (1998), a collaboratively created first-person account about living with Alzheimer's. Forster's novel explores the difficulties of providing home care for an ageing relative with dementia. Henderson, by contrast, explores what it's like to be living with dementia for the person affected. Both narratives address the uneasy question of what makes us human and when a meaningful life ends. Both position dementia as a problem case: dementia is seen to threaten the very humanity of the person with dementia, and as the quotation from Forster highlights, may put that person's life at risk.

In the following, I want to use these two examples as entry points into my study of (more or less) contemporary dementia narratives.[1] I ask what questions these narratives raise, and what they tell us about how we conceive dementia, a condition that has increasingly come to the fore of public awareness. I begin with Forster's novel.

Dementia represents a major public health concern. As our societies age, more and more people are affected by dementia. Accordingly, the number of people involved in providing care—from family members to professional caregivers—is rising. Social science research suggests that family caregivers experience ill health, depression and social alienation due to their caregiving duties. Increasing incidence rates of dementia, coupled with restricted financial and human resources raise moral questions about solidarity and caregiving. Forster's novel explores the 'burden' of family caregiving and, as early as 1989, it asks how much future generations will be prepared to invest—emotionally as well as financially—in older and increasingly incapacitated generations.

At the same time, international reports and local scandals show that dementia care frequently falls short of what may be called adequate or indeed humane care (see also Burke 2016). People with dementia[2] are disadvantaged, neglected, or even abused. Indeed, their life may no longer be considered worth protecting, as the debate about euthanasia in dementia exemplifies (Johnstone 2011, 2013). Rectifying abusive situations and creating sustainable and humane dementia care, in which both caregivers and people with dementia can thrive, represents one of the global challenges of the present century. In Forster's novel, the major conflict revolves around the problems of providing home care while balancing the needs of all family members involved.

Significantly, the story is not told from the perspective of the person with dementia but from two familial caregivers: Jenny, the daughter-in-law of the character with dementia, and her granddaughter, Hannah. Neither of these women is Grandma's primary caregiver; rather, that role falls to her daughter Bridget. The main conflict in the novel arises from Bridget's desire to keep her mother at home—and her inability to sustain home care without the help from other family members. The extract quoted above must be situated in the larger context of the novel's plot; rather than being a description of dementia, it is a description of the daughter-in-law's reaction to her mother-in-law's death. More precisely, it represents Jenny's reaction as mediated through her own daughter's perspective and includes a discussion about the responsibility and the limits of responsibility when it comes to caring for people with dementia. Jenny's call for urgent action—at first seemingly similar in nature to the advocacy story Alzheimer's Associations tell—in fact represents a call for political action towards legitimizing euthanasia. However, as is typical of the novel, Hannah's narrative critically reflects on her mother's perspective and ethical stance. 'Will we?' she writes, in response to her mother's injunction that her generation will 'have to stop being scared to kill the old' (250). The novel then, within its narrative plot, opens up for discussion the process of decision-making regarding end-of-life care and the (il)legitimacy of life-ending measures, such as voluntary euthanasia or physician-assisted suicide.

Have the Men Had Enough represents dementia care as a downward spiralling nightmare, impossible to sustain for familial caregivers. As Lucy Burke notes about this novel, Grandma's death represents a resolution of the care crisis without actually offering a solution to the problem of how to live with dementia or care for people with this condition (Burke 2015: 39). Heike Hartung (2016: 202–3) goes so far as to suggest that the novel advocates suicide and euthanasia in dementia. While I disagree with the latter analysis, the novel clearly does raise questions about the value and quality of life in dementia and about intergenerational justice. In particular, it frames these questions through a feminist enquiry into why dementia care is still predominantly carried out by women. It taps into one of the most prominent storylines about dementia propounded through public media—that is, of Alzheimer's as an 'epidemic' that will lead to an insurmountable global 'care crisis.' As a novel, though, Forster's text offers its own vision of this situation and invites its readers to think through some of the complex ethical issues dementia raises.

This narrative then both reflects the sociopolitical context of dementia care in the late 20th/early 21st century while raising a number of questions relating to the role of fictional narratives in current ethico-political debates about dementia: How do the rhetoric and aesthetics of a fictional text interact with the ethics of dementia care? How are readers invited to think and feel about the character with dementia, the problem of dementia care, and the question of euthanasia? What role does the mode of representation (narrator, focalisation), the medium (print text vs. visual media), and the genre (novel, autobiography, or documentary) play in structuring the reader's response? What effects might narrative empathy either for the character with dementia or for caregivers have on readers' attitudes and actions towards people with dementia or their caregivers in 'real life'? This study aims to address these questions relating to the role of fictional dementia narratives in the current social and political context of dementia care and thereby contribute to ongoing debates about the role of narratives both in first-wave and second-wave (or critical) medical humanities.[3]

Despite addressing a broad band of my research questions, Forster's text does not, however, exhaust the possible issues that dementia narratives both raise and attempt to answer. Cary Henderson's autobiographical writing speaks to another dominant storyline about dementia: that is, of dementia as a tragic 'loss of self' and 'death before death.' It is one of a growing number of first-person accounts or autopathographies[4] written by people with dementia about what it is like to live with this disease syndrome. Like other illness narratives, Henderson's *Partial View* (1998) writes against the dominant storyline in Western popular and biomedical culture (Swinnen and Sweda 2015), which denies people with dementia continuing subjectivity.

Henderson's journal evokes in a lively fashion how the world of a person with dementia changes—mentally, physically, and socially. Henderson writes about no longer being considered a 'human being' because of his inability to be a 'productive' member of society. He details how Alzheimer's interferes not only with his working life and recreational activities but also with his ability to interact with others and feel part of his family and wider social circle. Yet in doing so Henderson seems also to have internalised the values of the society he lives in. In describing himself as only partially 'alive,' as 'living halfway,' he both expresses his subjective experience of living with Alzheimer's and also confirms stereotypical views of the disease as a kind of 'living death.' As such, the text problematizes the view that illness narratives act as unilateral counter-narratives to the dominant dehumanising view of a given disease.

If Henderson's journal deals with the experience of living with dementia and the stigma attached to the disease, it also feeds directly into debates about narrative identity and the politics, ethics, and aesthetics of life writing. Henderson's journal represents a collaborative project: between Henderson and the photographer Nancy Andrews, but also between Henderson and his wife and daughter, who transcribed, organised, and edited his many tape recordings. Using a tape recorder allowed Henderson to tell readers about his experience long after he had lost the ability to write. His journal thus expands but also highlights the limits to life writing in dementia. The episodic nature of his 'musings' also raises the question of how coherent a narrative need be in order to function as an identity narrative—as a means of claiming selfhood in the social sphere. Critically reflecting on his work therefore draws attention to both the potential enabling and pernicious effects of narrative as a tool for claiming identity or identities in dementia. More generally, Henderson's autopathography highlights several important roles narrative plays in current discourses about dementia. Problematizing and clarifying the role of narrative in dementia studies and in the medical humanities more generally constitutes the primary aim of the present study.

Why narrative?

Despite recent calls to curtail the role narrative plays in medical humanities research (Woods 2011), narrative remains both an important target of analysis and crucial research tool. In particular, narrative is intimately connected to the debates around dementia. This is not to say that other forms of self-expression, such as music, art, photography, or other literary genres, such as poetry or drama,[5] do not represent illuminating areas of study in relation to contemporary representations of dementia. However, including these genres would have made this study scientifically unmanageable. Furthermore, this monograph is based on the premise that narrative and narrative studies have something particular to contribute to public discourse on dementia, to the growing field of literary dementia studies, and to medical humanities research more generally. I present in short my working hypotheses here. The remainder of the introduction will contextualise these claims by providing the background to biomedical and cultural understandings of dementia, literary dementia studies, and the medical humanities. Developing and testing the hypotheses outlined here constitutes the body of this study.

First, narrative functions as a sense-making device (Herman 2013, Hutto 2007a, 2007b). I contend that in order to make sense of dementia we need to consider it at the person level rather than at (or at least in addition to) a sub-personal level, where phenomena such as neurotransmitters, neurons, and fibrillary tangles are situated (see also Sabat and Harré 1994: 147). Dementia narratives open up the possibility of exploring dementia (and indeed, other aspects of what it means to be human) at the person level. In dealing with persons and their life worlds, narratives provide a privileged site for addressing the complex effects of dementia on the person. Narratives deal primarily in the 'medium-sized, human-scale world of everyday experience' (Herman 2013: x). In evoking a rich experiential account, similarly to the argument put forth by Havi Carel (2008) for phenomenology, narratives may counter and complement biomedical understandings of dementia as a pathology of cognition. Further, collaborative life writing projects (Clegg 2010) and conversational storytelling in dementia highlight that narrative remains an important tool for people with dementia to make sense of their environment and of their place in it (Hydén 2018). While I do not mean to suggest that neurological research into the disease does not have its place, given the personal and societal effects of dementia there is also an urgent need to consider this condition holistically and within the domain of human action and meaning.

Second, both fictional and non-fictional illness narratives may contribute to a better understanding of the phenomenology of dementia. However, narratives, too frequently seen as affording 'insight' into a given disease, also need to be scrutinised for the ways they construct and represent the experience of a given disease (Woods 2011). By drawing on the tools of cross-medial narratology, I aim to reflect on how the experience of living with dementia is aesthetically mediated and how the representation of people or characters with dementia is harnessed to the rhetorical aims and affective structures of a given storyworld. I explore the possibilities but also the *limitations* of narratives of dementia to further our understanding of the lived experience of the disease—especially vis-à-vis narratives told 'from the inside'—and their ability, or indeed inability, to counter negative stereotypes of people with dementia as 'living dead.'

Third, narrative identity is relevant to the discourse about selfhood in dementia. Narrative identity has come to the fore in discussions about what constitutes a 'self'[6] and how we claim identity for ourselves. A whole range of scholars from different disciplines have probed the extent to which selfhood or identity is constituted through narrative (see Bruner 1991, 2003, 2004, Dennett 1993, Eakin 1999, 2008, Ricœur 1991a, 1991b)—some arguing that identity is always narratively constructed. However, such views have not gone unchallenged (see, for instance, Sartwell 2000, Strawson 2004). Galen Strawson (2004), in particular, provides a damning critique of the narrativist approach. Most importantly for my argument, he highlights how according to strong narrativist views of identity he and with him many others risk not being considered as persons at all (447).

Without going into the particulars of the debate here, the narrative identity hypothesis is clearly relevant to the discourse about people with dementia in which 'selfhood' becomes a contested terrain. People with dementia will eventually struggle to tell a coherent life story and may risk no longer being considered persons on that ground. At the same time, the concept of narrative identity has also been employed to draw attention to how people with dementia continue to claim identities for themselves (Hydén 2018), or how caregivers and others who interact with the person with dementia may contribute to the social construction of identity—perhaps by telling that person's story for them. Narrative identity also becomes relevant, then, when considering the extent to which identities are constituted and held in relationships. Relational identity, especially as it has been explored in life writing studies (Eakin 1998, Friedman 1988, Mason 1980, Miller 1994), plays an important role in understanding how identity, both of the person with dementia and of family caregivers, is constructed and reconstructed in familial life writing about the disease.

The present study explores the implications of narrativist accounts of selfhood for people with dementia. I outline both the strengths and limits of the narrative account when it comes to capturing the processes by which identity is constituted in the context of dementia. In this way, I adopt a position within the debate that can be characterised as a moderate or qualified narrativist approach. Narrative is a crucial vehicle for performing and communicating identity. Nonetheless, certain aspects of selfhood—understood in phenomenological terms as a persistent point of view and an engaged creation of a life world—are better understood through the lens of embodiment and embodied experience. Narrative can be a means of communicating this changing sense of being-in-the-world—as in the case of narratives told by people with dementia—but it is not constitutive of selfhood as such. The ontological question of whether selfhood persists in dementia cannot easily be answered, and certainly not by me. I therefore propose, with Stephan Millett (2011), that we bracket or even disregard the question of whether selfhood is 'lost' and instead concentrate on how narrative is used to claim identities or communicate the experience of living with dementia.

Determining the limits of the narrative identity hypothesis as well as suggesting the importance of considering the embodied and relational aspects of identity in dementia (and in stories about dementia) therefore constitutes another important strand of my research.

And finally, narrative is at the heart of a number of debates within the medical humanities about insight or understanding, empathy, and ethics (Woods 2011). These concerns about the role and function of narrative are equally central to my discussion about dementia narratives. At issue is whether narrative, and the novel in particular, provides an inroad into understanding the life world of others (Bitenc 2012, Felski 2008, Waugh 2013), whether narrative empathy leads to prosocial action or more caring healthcare professionals (Charon 2006, Keen 2007, Whitehead 2017), and how narrative ethics play out more generally in the context of our social being as moral agents (Meretoja 2018, Morris 2002, Nussbaum 1990, 1995, 1997).

While I do not doubt that storytelling plays an important role in shaping the moral imagination and in developing the capacity for intersubjectivity (see also Hutto 2007b), it is equally important to acknowledge the embodied nature of intersubjective experience (Ratcliffe 2007, Zahavi 2007). Different medial representations of dementia—across film, graphic narratives, and print texts—might be able to draw on and exploit such embodied intersubjectivity, and not just the resources afforded by storytelling, to further an understanding of others. More importantly, the causal link that has been proposed between the reader's experience of narrative empathy and consequent ethical, moral, or altruistic action must be questioned (see Keen 2007). Indeed, although empathy has long been heralded as a good to be cultivated, more recently scholars have drawn attention to the nefarious use of empathy as a form of appropriation or as a tool for managing patients (Garden 2007, Hester 2016). Drawing on feminist affect theory, Anne Whitehead (2017) shows how the effects of empathy can divide rather than unite 'us' in a common humanity, or might be damaging to the object of empathy. It is important, then, to determine what literature can and cannot do when it comes to enhancing the moral and empathetic capacities of readers. Further, my study goes beyond questions of empathy to explore other ways in which narrative fiction may be relevant for dementia care: namely, by opening up, and *keeping open* (see Whitehead 2011: 59), important debates about specific dilemmas relating to the care of people with dementia.

The aim of this books is not to provide a *comprehensive* analysis of the ways dementia is represented in contemporary film, fiction, and life writing. Nor does it trace the literary history of this condition by providing a *diachronic* exploration of the medical and cultural attitudes to dementia, old age and age-related decline—a history which, as other authors have shown, is long and complex (see, among others, Ballenger 2006, Thane 2005, Wetzstein 2005). Instead, I consider dementia principally as a contemporary problem—as it is currently construed in medical, socio-economic, and demographic terms—and examine the way this problem of dementia is constructed in the cultural imaginary in Western, industrialised societies. This focus on issues of identity, empathy, and ethics as they surface and interact with hypercognitive, productivity-demanding capitalist value systems, and specific health-care, political, and academic institutions in the Western world entails that this study also does not offer a *cross-cultural comparative* approach to dementia narratives. Even within the range of countries included (Australia, Canada, US, UK, and Europe) there is huge variability between social care and political systems. To have included dementia narratives from Asian, Middle Eastern, and African cultures alongside the current case studies would have meant disregarding important cultural and economic differences; ignoring different concepts of identity, family, or honour; and neglecting the differences in healing systems and other sociocultural practices that constitute the context for such narratives. A truly comparative approach would necessitate a thorough engagement with the context and culture of 'non-Western' dementia narratives.[7] Both a diachronic exploration and cross-cultural comparisons of attitudes towards people with dementia are certainly worth exploring in their own right, and I hope this study will provide a point of departure for future research.

Instead, by engaging with a range of case studies across genres, media, and modes,[8] I outline ways of understanding the cultural significance of dementia within a loosely related value system in which dementia is construed as disease syndrome and in which identity is constructed around cognitive functioning, with a view to developing a more nuanced understanding of how 'we' (in the global North) construct and consequently live with this condition. My aim is to raise awareness for a strand of literature that is only slowly receiving critical attention—that is, fictional and non-fictional dementia narratives across a range of media—to situate this literature in contemporary discourses about dementia and selfhood, empathy, and ethics, and to mine its potential for an as yet imperfectly understood and certainly underfunded area of healthcare: dementia care. To contextualise my discussion of dementia narratives, I turn, first, to a brief sketch of the biomedical and cultural meanings dementia has accrued, before situating my approach in current literary dementia studies and the medical humanities.

Biomedicine and the cultural meaning of dementia

Dementia is a progressive neurodegenerative syndrome, that is, a clinical term which describes a constellation of symptoms that may be caused by a number of underlying diseases, such as Alzheimer's disease, vascular dementia, frontotemporal dementia, Lewy body dementia, and others. Common symptoms include a range of impairments to cognitive functions, among them memory and language, as well as behavioural changes. Since Alzheimer's disease currently constitutes the most common form of dementia, the term is frequently used for the whole disease syndrome in cultural discourses. I prefer predominantly to use the umbrella term 'dementia' as both the more accurate and more inclusive term, unless where Alzheimer's has been diagnosed or is specifically the topic of a given narrative. For ease of reading, however, I at times use the term 'disease,' even though strictly speaking dementia is not a disease but a syndrome.

Despite difficulties in determining the factors that cause dementia, as well as difficulties in distinguishing 'normal' from 'pathological' ageing,[9][10] neurobiological disease models of dementia currently underpin our understanding of the condition. Rather than delving into state-of-the-art neurobiological explanations of the disorder, I here want to trace the biomedical history and the biocultural meanings attached to dementia, in order to suggest some reasons why dementia narratives—the stories we tell each other about dementia across different media and in different contexts—need to be considered or perhaps reconsidered.

A brief history of dementia

In the 'age of Alzheimer's' it may be difficult to imagine that cognitive decline in old age was not always considered pathological.[11] The conceptual history of dementia is well documented.[12] Although Alois Alzheimer presented his famous case study of Auguste D. in 1906, it was only in the late 1970s and early 1980s, due to a complex set of socio-economic, technological, and political developments, that dementia emerged as disease category (Ballenger 2006, Fox 1989, Gubrium 1986, Holstein 2000, Lyman 1989). Alzheimer's became the dread 'disease of the century' (Thomas 1983). It is worth keeping in mind the complex social history of the biomedicalisation of dementia when approaching this disease syndrome as a contemporary problem. Tracing the history of Alzheimer's highlights the degree to which diseases, in general, are always at least partially socially constructed (Hacking 1999a, 1999b) and accrue meaning in their biocultural context (Morris 1998).

In short, the representation of people with dementia is not 'neutral.' Biomedicine has created a discourse of 'facts' about the disease syndrome, but even this purportedly scientific description is an interpretation of the condition that impacts on the way it is treated and experienced. Biomedical approaches to dementia do not pay due attention to the way diseases of all sorts are, in part, socially constructed; nor do they consider the potentially harmful or iatrogenic[13] effects of biomedical practice itself. However, my focus here is not on biomedicine but on the way a biomedical category like dementia is wedded to cultural meanings. The damaging effect of disease labels lies not in the labels themselves but in the cultural meaning that, because of these practices of naming and categorisation, certain illnesses accrue (Couser 1997, Sontag 1979, 1989).

There are, as Lucy Burke underscores, ethical consequences that follow from the 'particular "descriptive" categories' used to evoke Alzheimer's 'and the ways of seeing that they prescribe' (Burke 2007b: 64). Accordingly, the present study reconsiders the interpretive aspects of the purportedly descriptive categories we have developed: not just the biomedical model of Alzheimer's disease but the metaphors we use and stories we tell to conceptualise dementia in the present age. As David Morris suggests, 'The stories we tell ... are not just entertainment. They are the material with which a culture redefines its own image and self-understanding' (1998: 277). Examining the images and stories that have grown around dementia may thus provide an insight into how contemporary Western societies construct human identity. At the same time, understanding 'how Alzheimer's is perceived and represented' will, hopefully, lead to benefits for those living with this disease syndrome (Basting 2003a: 88).

Demography and demonisation

While demographic changes clearly play an important role in the contemporary 'rise' of Alzheimer's, the particular fear generated by dementia is due to this condition threatening core values in contemporary Western societies, such as youth, productivity, autonomy, capability, and rationality (Basting 2003a, Snyder 1999). Importantly, the worth of a person, or indeed the status of personhood itself, is determined on the basis of whether or not a person conforms to these values (Post 2000). Ethicist Stephen Post calls attention to the risks inherent in current 'hypercognitive' value systems, in that people with dementia may be removed from the sphere of moral concern. In the worst case, their lives might no longer be considered worth protecting and they may be under pressure to consent to physician-assisted suicide or may become the victims of euthanasia or murder. Indeed, as Megan-Jane Johnstone reveals, the way media coverage constructs dementia and thereby influences public understanding of the disease has contributed to what she perceives as a subtle but noticeable shift towards euthanasia as a 'solution' for people with dementia at any stage in the disease (Johnstone 2011, 2013).

If people with dementia are dehumanised, the core element of this dehumanisation lies in the fact that dementia is commonly understood to be synonymous with 'losing one's self.' This notion long remained unquestioned and formed the basis of both popular and scientific understandings of the disease syndrome (see Millett 2011). Indeed, as Herskovits (1995) argues, scientific literature on dementia tended to enforce the notion that the self is lost, by using such disturbing metaphors as 'death before death' and a 'funeral without end' (Cohen and Eisdorfer 1986, qtd. in Herskovits 1995: 148). Popular discourse too is rife with images that characterise people with dementia as 'shells,' 'husks,' 'ghosts of their former selves,' or even 'zombies' (Behuniak 2011). Frequently family members will state of a person with dementia that he or she is 'long gone.' Although such descriptions speak to the loss that family members go through, such statements deny the continuing subjectivity of the person with dementia. Indeed, Herskovits characterises the current construction of Alzheimer's disease as a '*monsterizing of senility*' (Herskovits 1995: 153, original emphasis), and Wetzstein speaks of a 'demonisation' of dementia in public discourse (Wetzstein 2005). Such metaphors as *shell, husk*, or *vegetable* are deeply troubling since they risk removing people with dementia from the sphere of personhood and hence moral concern.

Reconsidering dementia: reparative moves

Since the 1980s a growing body of research on dementia, especially from a social constructivist perspective, has engaged in what Herskovits identifies as 'reparative work' (Herskovits 1995: 159). This work aims to reconstitute the humanity and dignity of people with dementia and challenges the notion that selfhood is simply 'lost.' Karen Lyman discusses how disease labelling and seeing all aspects of behaviour as pathological facilitates social and medical control (1989: 599). The biomedicalisation of dementia may result in a self-fulfilling prophecy of impairment (Lyman 1989: 599). In short, the conjunction of labelling and stigma results in the 'spoilt identity' of the person to whom a disease label is attached (Goffman 1963). Sabat and Harré (1992) reveal how the social positioning of people with dementia as confused, and of their behaviour as meaningless, threatens the recognition of their discursive acts as displays of selfhood. In other words, we need to listen to people with dementia in order to recognise them as semiotic subjects (Sabat and Harré 1994). If we fail to do so people with dementia lose their selfhood—not due to the dementing illness but because of the way they are socially positioned.

Tom Kitwood, a pioneer in dementia studies, similarly, draws attention to the way social-psychological factors contribute to the process of dementia and may thereby undermine the personhood of those living with the condition. By highlighting the 'malignant social psychology' pervasive in care settings, Kitwood explores the dynamic interplay between neurological processes of degeneration and psychological factors such as disempowerment, infantilisation, labelling, and objectification in the progression of dementia (Kitwood 1990, 1997: 45–9). His exhaustive description of the factors which contribute to the dehumanisation of people with dementia in care settings is followed by practical guidance on how to prevent these processes from occurring: his dementia care mapping system has since been implemented in numerous care environments with the aim of developing more person-centred care in dementia.

A growing literature explores the question of what may actually *constitute* personhood or selfhood in dementia. This question has been addressed in, for instance, philosophical and psychiatric practice-based investigations of the disease syndrome (Hughes, Louw, and Sabat 2006). As I suggest in Chapter 1, the vexed ontological question of the persistence of selfhood in dementia may perhaps best be understood if we view selfhood in phenomenological terms as the 'first-personal perspectival givenness' of the world (Zahavi 2007). This subjective perspective on the world, I argue, persists until the very end, as people with dementia continue to experience their being-in-the-world as long as they are alive. By contrast, the social identities or personae of a person with dementia may indeed be eroded, both by disease processes and social interactions, relatively early on.

One of the reparative moves within dementia studies, with particular relevance for this study, has been to see selfhood as narratively constructed. Research on how selfhood is constructed in dementia has been crucial in drawing attention to the narratives people with dementia tell (Hydén 2011, 2018, Hydén and Örulv 2009, Lyman 1998, MacRae 2010, Phinney 2002, Ryan, Bannister, and Anas 2009, Usita 1998) and also in emphasising the degree to which identity construction relies on the collaboration of others (Sabat and Harré 1992, 1994, Small et al. 1998). However, some risks attach to positing identity as constituted by narrative in the context of neurodegenerative diseases such as Alzheimer's. People with dementia do experience significant decline in their linguistic capacities and in their ability to remember aspects of their life. Both of these symptoms clearly affect the ability to 'tell a life story' and thereby reclaim social identity for oneself. The present study explores this very tension, both in the context of fictional writing and in the context of life writing by and about people with dementia. In particular, I investigate how these narratives position themselves in relation to the dominant master narrative of dementia as loss of self, and to what extent narratives by and about people with dementia may act as counter-narratives to the current Alzheimer's construct (Chapter 3).

The Alzheimer's 'epidemic': care, cost, and social justice

Dementia has become a major public health concern. Demographic prognoses of 'graying' societies have led analysts to cast dementia as an 'epidemic,' 'plague,' 'rising tide,' 'wave,' or even 'silent tsunami' (Zeilig 2013: 260). Such apocalyptic rhetoric is motivated by statistical estimates presented in the World Alzheimer's Report 2009, according to which the number of people with dementia will nearly double every twenty years: to 65.7 million in 2030 and 115.4 million in 2050 (Alzheimer's Disease International 2009: 8). Dementia is cited as the leading cause of dependency and disability among older people, and in 2010 the global economic cost of dementia was estimated at over 604 billion US dollars (Alzheimer's Disease International 2010: 5). Dementia, on these accounts, represents one of the greatest social, health, and economic challenges of the 21st century.

Alzheimer's Disease International and related associations have been instrumental in raising awareness about dementia and improving the lives of those affected. Nonetheless, there are some negative implications inherent in the plot lines that the association employs in order to justify the urgent need for action. For one, the alarmist notion of an Alzheimer's 'epidemic,' fed by demographic statistics, is likely to increase fear and dread of the disease. Such imagery dehumanises people with dementia by turning them into an indistinguishable mass that will 'swallow' the resources of more able-bodied and able-minded sectors of society. We must therefore question the metaphors used to conceptualise dementia and ask how they make us see, understand, and feel about this disease. On a different plane, as a number of scholars have pointed out (Ballenger 2006, Fox 1989), the association's lobbying strategy to increase funding for *research* into the disease is usually based on the projected costs dementia will incur if it is not cured. The advocacy movement uses statistics to support their claim for urgent action, but this use of statistics unwittingly undermines claims for more money to be invested in dementia *care*: supporting people with dementia and their caregivers, or investing resources in developing better insurance care plans and therapeutic interventions is not (yet) a top priority.

Although health-care provisions differ greatly between different Western countries, dementia emerges as a problem across the board. It is evident that dementia challenges these systems, or rather that health-care systems fail people with dementia. In the US, for instance, middle-class families affected by dementia frequently fall through the net of insurance policies until they have spent all savings and assets and qualify for state benefits. Furthermore, policies such as Medicaid and Medicare often do not cover the type of care a person with dementia still living at home needs. In the UK, an ailing NHS struggles to offer the kind of care suitable for a person with dementia. Agencies send different carers to people with dementia daily, undermining the possibility for a care relationship to form. Government cuts to the care budget of local councils mean that people with dementia cannot be adequately cared for at home, resulting in increasing numbers of people with dementia in hospital beds. However, hospital visits have been noted to cause rapid decline in the functioning of people with dementia. Further, limited visiting hours for family caregivers deprive people with dementia in institutions of the familiar faces and support that would help orientate them and make them feel safe. In sum, institutions are not set up to cater for the needs of the deeply forgetful. Importantly, besides these local problems, changes to the basic principles of the welfare state over the last decades present major challenges for dementia care. As Lucy Burke (2015) notes, the spread of neo-liberal economic tendencies adversely affects dementia care by turning it into a commodity—one that will not be available to everyone who may need it in the future.

The growing prevalence of dementia together with declining welfare state systems then raises a number of questions. On the one hand, how do we as a society rise to the ethico-political dilemmas dementia raises in terms of social justice? What duty do we have to care for growing segments of dependent people in society? How do we conceptualise people with dementia and what effect does this have on their treatment in society? Are we moving towards political recognition of people with dementia or will euthanasia of the cognitively impaired become the norm in the next decades (Johnstone 2011, 2013, Kaufman 2006)? As Wetzstein (2005) argues, the combination of the biomedical concept of dementia with reductionist notions of personhood has serious implications for how we treat people with dementia. No longer considered a person due to the loss of cognitive functions, a 'non-person' may no longer seem to have a life worth protecting. At the same time, the loss of cognitive functions inevitably leads to a loss of autonomy, which raises a different set of questions concerning coercion and paternalism. How can the need to protect people with dementia be balanced with the need to respect their autonomy? And what autonomy do people with dementia retain when it comes to making end-of-life decisions and to planning ahead through the use of advance directives or the nomination of a proxy?

Fictional and non-fictional dementia narratives, I suggest, provide a means to address, or at least articulate more precisely, questions of this sort. Of course, literature does not provide answers or solutions to all the challenges of dementia care, but it does complement other modes of enquiry and offer a critical contribution to current debates. Dementia narratives might then function as moral laboratory to explore dementia care, an idea I develop more fully in Chapter 6.

Literary dementia studies and the medical humanities

Dementia has become ubiquitous in our times. It features not only in news reports, but in TV series, films, novels, plays,[14] short stories, autobiographies, graphic memoirs, and documentaries. It has become a major theme in poetry and even a topic deemed suitable for operatic exploration (see Maxwell and Langer 2010). Dementia is discussed on radio programmes via personal blogs and during coffee breaks. But what can a literary exploration of dementia contribute to our understanding of dementia and of its place in our society?

In recent years, a growing number of literary and cultural scholars, as well as academics working in fields such as gerontology, have analysed the way dementia is represented in contemporary literature, film, and life writing. Apart from a number of dispersed articles, three essay collections (Maginess 2018, Ringkamp et al. 2017, Swinnen and Schweda 2015) and by now three monographs (Falcus and Sako 2019, Medina 2018, Zimmermann 2017) attest to the fact that the representation of dementia across literary genres and cultural artefacts is of increasing interest. Many of these essays pursue an ethically driven agenda in suggesting that dementia narratives further our understanding of the phenomenology of dementia and thereby counter reductionist biomedical approaches to the disease syndrome. They also challenge stereotypical representations of people with dementia across different genres, including film, and argue that these representations have serious implications for how we think and feel about, and therefore act towards, people with dementia. Others are concerned with how dementia functions as a metaphor itself to reflect on complex ethical issues of postmodern Western societies. Unfortunately, not all contributions are equally circumspect as to the language they use to discuss dementia, or the ways their own analysis might at times confirm dominant stereotypes about dementia.

Foremost among the scholars to critically explore cultural representations of dementia, disability scholar Lucy Burke has challenged the representation of dementia in film-poetry (Burke 2007b), life writing (Burke 2007a, 2008), and fictional narratives (Burke 2015, 2016, 2017, 2018). Burke specifically questions the notion that selfhood is lost in dementia and explores how personhood is constructed (or fails to be constructed) in illness narratives (Burke 2014). Her analysis stresses the sociopolitical relevance of dementia discourses and the need to challenge cognitivist notions of personhood in the context of neo-liberal politics. Burke's exploration of how dementia is represented in contemporary media represents an ethico-political analysis geared towards acknowledging the personhood of people with dementia. Her aim is the recognition of the basic human rights of people with dementia to dignity and care.

Although I agree with Burke's aim, my work is slightly different in both focus and method. Like Burke, I am interested in how narratives contribute to current debates about dementia. In a second step, however, I am interested in how narrative studies may inform current debates about the role of narrative in the medical humanities more generally. Given my concern with the tools of narrative studies, I pay more attention to how genre, medium, and mode shape the representation of dementia. So, while Burke, in an article on narrative identity in dementia life writing (2014), somewhat incongruously discusses Michael Ignatieff's novel *Scar Tissue* as primary case study, my aim is to explore how genre conventions (e.g. autobiography vs. novel) govern and shape the way we understand narrative identity and other aspects of living with dementia.

As literary dementia scholars demonstrate, attending to the way dementia is constructed in the cultural imaginary is crucial, since it informs the way dementia is lived, experienced, and treated. My study therefore follows in these footsteps, while according more attention to first-person accounts as well as to generic and medial differences between dementia narratives than has, but for some exceptions, so far been the case. However, my argument is also more specific than simply deconstructing the way dementia has been represented in literature in the last thirty odd years. I suggest that dementia narratives provide key insights into the dilemmas of dementia care outlined above—dilemmas having to do with resource allocation, best care practice, questions of autonomy and coercion, and end-of-life decisions. Indeed, novels, films, and life writing about dementia may function as a form of 'social phenomenology' (Felski 2008: 89) or 'practical counterpart of phenomenology' (Waugh 2013), offering a means to 'live through' (Rosenblatt [1938] 1995) and think through dementia care dilemmas. In short, dementia narratives can work as a moral laboratory for considering the dilemmas of dementia care, with critical readings of these texts contributing to a new ethics and practice of dementia care. Although the Alzheimer's disease movement since the 1980s has garnered increased research funds in an effort to 'defeat' dementia (Fox 1989)—in the popular militaristic parlance of contemporary illness discourse—a cure for the multifactorial disease processes that cause dementia remains elusive. Since there is no cure in sight, the primary question remains how people with dementia can best be cared for and, also, how those who provide this care—professional and familial caregivers alike—can best be supported.

Illness narratives: countering master narratives and exploring the experience of illness

Literary dementia studies must also be situated in the context of earlier and ongoing research on illness narratives. In recent decades there has been both a surge in the publication of illness narratives and a growing scholarly interest in these stories about illness and disability—from Arthur Kleinman's seminal *The Illness Narratives* (1988) and Arthur Frank's *The Wounded Storyteller* (1995), across literary studies of pathography (Bolaki 2016, Hawkins 1993, Wiltshire 2000), to Rita Charon's practice-based *Narrative Medicine* (2006, 2017). While the focus was initially on doctors' narratives of illness (Montgomery Hunter 1993, Whitehead 2014), illness narratives soon became the prerogative of the ill person herself (Vickers 2016). Indeed, illness narratives may be considered paradigmatic counter-narratives which allow the ill person to reclaim her subjectivity in the face of reductionist biomedical (Frank 1995) and culturally stigmatising constructions of diseases (Avrahami 2007, Couser 1997).

There are, of course, problems in defining what constitutes the master narrative of dementia and what may constitute a counter-narrative—as I discuss in more detail in Chapter 3. In general, however, counter-narratives become active when one group of society is unduly marginalised or stigmatised (Bamberg and Andrews 2004). While stigma invariably attaches to diseases (Goffman 1963), it seems particularly salient in those conditions that are in some form culturally significant (Couser 1997). I argue that dementia is one such culturally significant condition. As a 'disease of memory,' it taps into contemporary Western societies' obsession with the capacity to remember. More importantly, it attacks those aspects of human cognition that are considered to distinguish humans from other animals—language, higher-order thought, and memory. Dementia therefore goes to the heart of discussions of what it means to be human. Like other illness narratives, dementia autopathographies challenge cultural and biomedical constructions of the condition while exploring what it's like to live with a given disease and how this experience affects one's sense of identity.

These two elements of illness narratives—(1) 'countering' and (2) exploring the experience of a given illness with the object of elucidating both health-care professionals and the general public—have been central to the development of the medical humanities. In first-wave or mainstream medical humanities, such narratives were accordingly integrated into medical training with the aim of broadening health-care professionals' understanding of a disease as more than a set of biomarkers and symptoms. Recently, the critical medical humanities and health humanities alike (Crawford et al. 2010) aim to widen the scope of the field beyond the focus on doctor-patient encounters, on illness experience, and/or on health-care education (Whitehead and Woods 2016: 3). Due to the underlying assumption that engagement with literature promotes more empathic doctors, which may be seen to underpin certain models of health-care education, proponents of the medical humanities have, perhaps rightly, been accused of 'retrograde rhetoric regarding the "humanizing humanities"' (Spiegel 2012: 205). From other sides, the role of the humanities as 'supportive friend' (Brody 2011: 6), in the service of medicine, has equally been challenged (Viney et al. 2015: 3).

In contrast to the supportive role, medical humanities scholars frequently position themselves as opposed to the structures and institutional power of biomedicine. Mobilising the notion of 'critique,' Therese Jones stresses that humanities research methods 'enable and promote fearless questioning of representations, challenges to the abuses of authority and a steadfast refusal to accept as the limits of enquiry the boundaries that medicine sets between biology and culture' (Jones 2014: 27–8). Jones' optimistic evaluation of the almost 'revolutionary' potential of the humanities might, however, be challenged in turn. Medical humanities scholars may be criticised for assuming a merely oppositional stance to biomedicine—providing an endless 'critique' without being able to go beyond that critique. As Viney and his collaborator suggest, 'the arts, humanities and social sciences are best viewed not as in service or in opposition to the clinical and life sciences, but as productively entangled with a "biomedical culture"' (Viney et al. 2015: 2). This monograph problematizes the different ways in which dementia narratives are in opposition, complicit, and entangled with biomedical discourses on dementia. While engaging with themes that have been relevant to both first-wave and second-wave medical humanities, I aim to move beyond dualistic possibilities which set biomedicine up as the main target of criticism. I focus instead on the subversive and problematic empathetic potential of literature, but also on the positive contributions critical literary scholarship may be able to make in the context of rethinking current dementia care, as well as in the context of rethinking the role of narrative and narrative identity in the medical humanities more generally.

Outline of chapters

The chief aim of the present study is to delineate the potential and limitations of narrative, and narrative studies, when it comes to challenging the current dementia construct and developing new ways of understanding, interacting with, and caring for people with dementia. Narrative is examined in its many permutations and with regard to its different functions: as representational tool, as tool for meaning-making, and as tool for identity construction. But it also emerges as central to two concepts that are at the heart of debates in narrative medicine and the critical medical humanities: (narrative) empathy and (narrative) ethics. To explore these concepts and different functions of narrative, the study moves back and forth between fictional and non-fictional narratives as well as between different media and subgenres within these two categories. The two opening chapters in Part I are concerned with exploring the experience of living with dementia as well as the relationship between techniques of representation, narrative empathy, and understanding. Part II moves on to explore the aesthetic, ethical, and political implications of the emerging genre(s) of dementia life writing. A final pair of chapters in Part III engages with how fictional and non-fictional narratives may inform the development of dementia care and thereby contribute to ongoing debates about the role of narrative and narrative ethics in the medical humanities.

Chapter 1 explores how life writing might contribute to a better understanding of how dementia transforms self-experience as well as one's relationships to the physical and sociocultural world. To develop this question, I draw, first, on a range of autopathographies, that is, illness narratives by people with dementia themselves. Second, and as a point of contrast, I explore issues of intersubjective understanding in David Sieveking's documentary film *Vergiss Mein Nicht* (2012). On the one hand, I argue that attending to the embodied nature of selfhood can redress the simplistic or reductive notion that the self is 'lost' in dementia. On the other hand, I explore how different storytelling media (especially documentary film and photography) foreground aspects of embodied selfhood and provide means of exploring the potential of embodied communication in dementia. While Chapter 1 introduces the important notion of embodiment and relatedly, embodied communication, it is the least theoretical of all chapters, intended to introduce readers to the field of dementia studies, and particularly to the life world of dementia. My aim is to allow the words of people with dementia within the context of this chapter to 'speak for themselves' as entry point into this study. Later chapters more explicitly take up the issue how genre, medium, and the larger discursive culture of a given dementia narrative shape its meaning, as well as its ethical and political impact.

Chapter 2 addresses two fields of enquiry: First, to what extent do fictional narratives (in particular the novel and film) act as a 'practical counterpart of theoretical phenomenology' (Waugh 2013: 24)—or, to put the question another way, how (using what techniques) may they be able to simulate what it's like to be living with dementia? Second, does simulating the experience of dementia lead to an empathetic engagement with the dementing protagonist, and if so, is it reasonable to assume that narrative empathy translates to prosocial action towards real people with dementia? By exploring these questions across a range of case studies (Lisa Genova's novel *Still Alice* and its film adaptation, J. Bernlef's *Out of Mind*, B.S. Johnson's *House Mother*

Normal, and Kazuo Ishiguro's *The Unconsoled*) I aim to suggest how these fictional dementia narratives may contribute to the current theory of narrative empathy while also highlighting the importance of questioning the 'empathy-altruism hypothesis' (Keen 2007), which is commonly invoked in first-wave medical humanities contexts as a reason for incorporating the arts into medical training.

Part II turns to questions of identity, self-presentation, and representation in the emerging genre(s) of dementia life writing. My focus here shifts more squarely to the ethics, aesthetics, and politics of dementia life writing. Chapter 3 addresses the possibilities and limitations of the notion of narrative identity and narrative coherence in the context of neurodegenerative diseases such as Alzheimer's. I ask to what extent dementia life narratives, like other illness narratives, may function as counter-narratives to the dominant cultural construction of dementia as 'loss of self' and 'death before death' and how genre conventions affect the construction of counter-narratives. To explore these questions, I consider two types of case studies: first, I return to autopathographies by people with early-onset dementia, and second, I consider collaborative life history projects in nursing homes, in particular the collection *Tell Mrs Mill Her Husband Is Still Dead* (Clegg 2010). Autopathographies emerge as entangled in popular discourses and genre conventions in ways which complicate the notion of counter-narrative. Collaborative life story work in turn stresses the collaborative nature of meaning-making in conversational storytelling while also challenging and redrafting notions of narrative coherence.

Chapter 4 shifts the focus to the genre of caregivers' memoirs. My intention is to highlight the particular political force of as well as the ethical issues raised by dementia life writing—in particular the problem of representing 'vulnerable subjects' (Couser 2004). At the same time, caregivers' memoirs represent ideal case studies to consider the role relational identity plays in dementia. I therefore develop a close analysis of select examples of filial caregivers' memoirs to address the impact of gender, genre, and medium on current understandings of relational identity: primarily, Jonathan Franzen's autobiographical essay 'My Father's Brain' (2002), Judith Levine's memoir *Do You Remember Me?* (2004), and Sarah Leavitt's graphic memoir *Tangles* (2010).

Part III centres on questions that arise in the context of dementia care. Chapter 5 argues that 'care-writing' (that is, caregivers' memoirs) may be considered a valuable source of evidence when it comes to theorising and developing dementia care. Caregivers' memoirs explore the dilemmas involved in supporting someone with progressive cognitive impairment. They thereby provide a means for readers to 'live through' (Rosenblatt 1995)— and think through—these difficult dilemmas. The authors of these memoirs imagine and develop alternative treatment and care options that can potentially be adapted to other contexts. Indeed, because they have lived alongside the person with dementia, familial care partners are ideally placed to identify that person's evolving needs and to advocate for them when those needs are no longer met—whether in the community or in institutional care. These authors can therefore articulate strategies for addressing the needs of people with dementia, and of their care partners, holistically. Extrapolating from these texts, readers gain awareness of key caregiving dilemmas, but may also take away ideas for implementing ways of being with or caring for a person with dementia, based on more open and creative attitudes to communication and care.

Lastly, Chapter 6 aims to develop new avenues for thinking about how literary fiction may intervene in medical humanities contexts by going beyond some commonly accepted notions about narrative as 'humanising' medical practice. While Chapter 2 problematized that there is a link between literature and the provision of empathetic care, Chapter 6 seeks to develop a critical view of fictional dementia narratives that does not simply slot into ethical agenda pursued by the medical humanities. Given the dominant view of the field as driven by an 'ethical imperative,' (Rees 2010, qtd. in Jones 2014), I ask whether fictional dementia narratives themselves are necessarily tools for 'the good,' or whether they may instead compound the stigma attached to dementia. That is, I investigate to what extent specific fictional dementia narratives live up to, or fail to live up to, the ethico-political standard that the term counter-narrative suggests, using Michael Ignatieff's *Scar Tissue* (1993) and B.S. Johnson's *House Mother Normal* ([1971] 2013) as case studies. Second, I aim to explore what other role (beyond supposedly creating empathetic individuals) narrative may play in the medical humanities. Returning to an old idea that literature acts as tool for ethical thinking, I suggest some ways in which dementia novels may prompt their readers to engage with bioethical questions that arise in contemporary Western care culture(s). To explore how different media and means of narrative presentation affect the process of bioethical decision-making, I discuss the film and book version of *Still Alice* as well as Margaret Forster's novel *Have the Men Had Enough?* (1989). I contend that these narratives offer insights into the bioethical dilemmas bound up with dementia care, developing care-oriented thought experiments more fully than would be possible in non-fictional accounts of dementia.

Notes

1 Since I discuss dementia as it has been constituted in the rise of the Alzheimer's movement in the 1970s and 1980s, I consider narratives from that time period until roughly 2018.
2 A note on terminology: First, talking about 'people with dementia' may seem to suggest a homogeneous group and clear-cut, stable disease category. However, dementia is a progressive disease syndrome with variable patterns of symptom progression. Second, throughout this study I prefer the term 'person with dementia' over the terms 'victim,' 'afflicted person,' or 'patient' that already constitute the person in a reductive way.

3 For a critical medical humanities approach see Viney, Callard, and Woods (2015) and Whitehead and Woods (2016). At the same time, the limitations inherent in the disciplinary label 'medical' are challenged by the emerging field of health humanities (Crawford et al. 2010). See also http://healthhumanities.org/. Note that this disciplinary label is also misleading in that the medical and health *humanities* include and are even driven by social science disciplines such as (medical) anthropology, psychology, and sociology.
4 Autopathography is defined as life writing about the progression of an illness and written by the person affected (Couser 1991, 1997, Graham 1997). Avrahami (2007) uses the term illness autobiography. Hawkins' study (1993) deals with both autopathography and pathography—illness narratives written by carers—under the heading of pathography.
5 Although there are strong arguments for categorising plays as narratives (Richardson 2007), I do not consider drama in this study.
6 The terms 'self,' 'identity,' 'person,' and 'life' are frequently used interchangeably. I acknowledge the contested nature of all these terms, but for ease of reading refrain from placing them in quotation marks.
7 For some cross-cultural or non-Western perspectives across anthropology and literary studies see Asai, Sato, and Fukuyama (2009), Cohen (1998), Holstein (2000), Hussein (2018), Leibing (2002), Nayar (2018), and Traphagan (2006).
8 Usage of the term 'mode' differs but a broad distinction can be drawn between uses of the term in local and global senses (Ryan 2005: 315). In the local sense, mode refers to types of representation within a narrative text (such as perspective or focalisation) as well as types of representation across narrative media (such as audio-visual in film but not print texts). In the global sense, mode is used as a term for what might be called macro-genres or higher-level text types, such as lyric, epic, and drama. Since the focus of this study is on narrative, my chief concern is with mode taken in the local sense.
9 See the famous 'Nun Study' in which the brains of elderly nuns who manifested symptoms of dementia while alive did not show the characteristic plaques and tangles of Alzheimer's on autopsy, while conversely, some of the brains that manifested plaques and tangles belonged to individuals who had not shown any symptoms of dementia when living (Snowdon 1997). The study has recently been explored in the stage drama *27* (Morgan 2011).
10 Compare Whitehouse (2008) who questions the validity of the Alzheimer's disease category. For other dissenting voices see Holstein (2000: 171).
11 See Leibing and Cohen (2006) on the pathologisation of senility.
12 See among others Ballenger (2006), Fox (1989), Gubrium (1986), Holstein (1997, 2000), Leibing and Cohen (2006), Shenk (2001), Wetzstein (2005), and Whitehouse, Maurer, and Ballenger (2000).
13 The term 'iatrogenic' relates to illness caused by medical examination or treatment.
14 See, among others, Tom Murphy's *Bailegangaire* (2009), Abi Morgan's *27* (2011), and Fiona Evans's *Geordie Sinatra* (2012).

Part I
Storytelling, experience, and empathy

1 Narrating experiences of dementia
Embodied selves, embodied communication

In illness our bodies change. Biomedicine attempts to reverse, halt, or alleviate the effects of bodily dysfunction. In pursuing this aim, biomedicine treats the body like an object to be fixed, rather than the locus of subjective experience. Accordingly, it has been criticised for paying too little attention to the *person* with disease and to the way the identity and life world of the person are changed through the experience of illness (Carel 2008, Frank 1995, Kleinman 1988). Using contemporary phenomenology, Havi Carel (2008) describes how bodily changes in illness radically transform our experience of ourselves as well as our relationships to the physical and sociocultural world. Paying attention to the multiple ways illness transforms subjective experience will not only provide a fuller understanding of a given illness, she argues, but will allow us to develop interventions that go beyond treating the physical body alone (Carel 2008: 73). I argue that life writing facilitates a phenomenological[1] approach to illness. These texts provide rich accounts of particular people in a specific context and can therefore contribute to a better understanding of how subjective experience changes in illness. In a second step such knowledge may be used to adapt and develop therapeutic and social interventions.

In this chapter, I explore the experience of living with dementia through autobiographical accounts both by people with dementia and through a documentary by a family care partner. I focus on embodied aspects of the disease as they are communicated by a range of narrative media, arguing that these embodied aspects shed a more nuanced light on what is lost, what changes, and what remains. To ground my discussion, I review how contemporary phenomenology, and particularly the notion of 'embodied selfhood' (Kontos 2005) and 'embodied' (or nonverbal) communication (Killick and Allan 2001) have been productively employed in dementia studies. I then turn to a close reading of contemporary first-person accounts— or autopathographies—by people with dementia, and conclude the chapter by exploring the potential for intersubjective understanding in David Sieveking's documentary *Vergiss Mein Nicht* (Forget-Me-Not) (2012).[2]

There are two different aspects to the relationship between embodiment and selfhood that I address. On the one hand, autobiographical narratives across different media highlight the extent to which embodied (self-) experience changes in this disease. That is, they show or describe how consciousness, emotions, cognition as well as body control are all affected by dementia. Yet these changes to self-experience also extend beyond the boundaries of the body. So, for instance, due to both the symptoms themselves and the stigma attached to the disease, relationships also undergo significant changes. The pernicious effect of illness on social interaction, in turn, has serious repercussions on the ill person's sense of self.

On the other hand, attending to the embodied nature of selfhood can redress the simplified notion that the self is 'lost' in dementia. Equating selfhood with high-level cognitive functioning or narrative identity can obscure (a) the extent to which memories are embodied (consider, for instance, examples of procedural memory such as the capacity to ride a bike, dance, or knit) and may thus persist even when verbal communication disintegrates, and (b) the extent to which selfhood can be understood as an embodied *perspective* that remains in dementia. This 'first-personal givenness of experience' (Zahavi 2007) may, furthermore, be communicated by drawing on nonverbal 'embodied' forms of communication. A key question is therefore how aspects of 'embodied selfhood' (see Kontos 2003, 2004, 2005) and embodied communication feature in various storytelling environments, including documentary film. Recognising embodied selfhood in dementia has important implications for dementia care, as it might lead to a more sensitive understanding of what is actually lost in the disease while allowing us to recognise and value the person who remains.

Embodied selves, embodied communication

In dementia studies, embodiment has been used to argue both for and against the notion that selfhood is lost (see Davis 2004 and Kontos 2003, 2004, 2005 respectively).[3] Embodiment has also been cited as a means to circumvent the equivocal question of selfhood in dementia altogether (Millett 2011). In this section, I do not intend to arbitrate between these opposing views and provide a definitive answer to what selfhood (or embodied selfhood) *is* or how it is constituted, nor to discriminate among terms such as self, identity, or personhood (see Millett 2011: 511).[4] Instead, I investigate how the notion of embodiment—and relatedly, embodied selfhood and embodied communication—can be productively used to engage with the subjective experience of dementia and, potentially, ground the moral standing of people with dementia not on a cognitive model of personhood but on our embodied nature as human beings.

The neurodegenerative nature of dementia impacts on memory, language, thinking, and reasoning, all of which are traditionally seen to define our personhood. However, less cognitively orientated parameters of personhood, such as emotion[5] and relationality,[6] are also impacted by the condition. Applying the notion of embodiment in dementia allows us to ask a number of questions: What do the changes on a neurological level entail for people with dementia and their experience of their own cognition, as well as their experience of self-efficacy in physical and social environments? How do these changes speak to and elucidate the common understanding that the person with dementia is in some sense 'losing herself'? And can embodiment perhaps provide a means of sustaining selfhood in dementia?

Pia C. Kontos develops the notion of 'embodied selfhood' (2003, 2004, 2005) to capture the idea that 'fundamental aspects of selfhood are manifested in the way the body moves and behaves' (2005: 556). Kontos's ethnographic study in a Jewish care home provides numerous rich examples to counter the dominant cultural conception that people with dementia experience a 'steady erosion of selfhood' (2005: 553). Kontos makes a substantial contribution to dementia studies by bringing to light the continued purpose and meaning with which people with dementia engage with the world (2004: 836). The strength of her analysis lies in attending to aspects of behaviour that are pre-reflective, or at least not overly reliant on higher-order cognition, as well as highlighting a multitude of nonverbal elements of communication, such as eye movement, eye contact, gesture, facial expressions, and posture. Yet Kontos perhaps does not sufficiently acknowledge that the brain is part of the body. She argues against cognitivist definitions of selfhood, but in the meantime does not pay due attention to how aspects of bodily behaviour are orchestrated by the brain and therefore also have a neurological substrate (even if some aspects rely on older brain structures and less on the neo-cortex). As such, the aspects of embodied selfhood, she describes, are equally at risk of being affected by dementia, and therefore of being eroded eventually—again making people with more advanced dementia open to the risk of being construed as non-selves.

Stephan Millett's (2011) proposal to ground an understanding of dementia in bio-phenomenology offers an illuminating alternative to Kontos's account. Millett proposes to leave aside the question of selfhood or personhood in dementia and instead focus on the experience of living with the disease, the continuity over time of an embodied individual, and our attitude towards that individual (Millett 2011: 515). The 'bracketing' of the question of personhood, Millett suggests, allows us to 'focus on the idea that there is a being with an inner life confronting us, a being with value simply because he or she has a "life-world"—a constructed meaningful world revealed to him or her through their senses' (515). Drawing on Jakob von Uexküll's biologically grounded phenomenology, Millett emphasises the role of the lived body through which each of us creates a meaningful world (510). This view allows us to recognise that

> there is a life-world – or directly experienced world – for people with dementia, who continue to experience the world and create meaning, even in the presence of severe cognitive degradation. It is clear that people with dementia have an *affective* response to certain stimuli: they laugh,

cry, express frustration and disappointment, engage playfully with others, and so on. Affective or emotional responses – signs of happiness, sadness, frustration, anger and the like – are indicators of an interior life the extent of which may not be determinable using cognitive criteria alone. From the affective responses we can infer that people with even late-stage dementia still react to, engage with, and co-create a life-world.

(510)

Drawing on bio-phenomenology, Millett argues that people with dementia continue to create a meaningful world and continue to be of value to others (517). His analysis widens the scope of subjectivity and meaningful interaction with the world beyond the examples of bodily intentionality provided by Kontos, to include 'bodily reactions of all sorts, to inputs from a range of external sources such as reactions to heat and cold, to smells, sounds and sights' (517). Millett's approach thereby suggests that there is a continuing inner world even in the most advanced stages of dementia. His approach is a rare example of research that disallows positing some kind of 'cut-off' point in the progression of dementia, at which stage the person no longer has an inner world and may therefore be considered valueless. Many reparative moves within dementia studies often, inadvertently, serve to enforce stigmatising and dehumanising accounts of the later stages of the disease, while 'recuperating' people with less severe symptoms into the sphere of the fully human. By contrast, as Millett states, 'by employing the concept of bio-semiosis we can acknowledge, with Sabat ... that people with dementia are semiotic subjects—that is, they are "driven by meaning"—but without committing to cognition-reliant definitions of selfhood and intentionality' (2011: 520).

However, despite Millett's assertions, it is difficult to see how the very basic sense of meaning-making (what he terms semiotic niche value)—such as reacting to hot or cold—differs from his example of a tick that reacts to warmth and butyric acid (516). Clearly, the moral standing of people with dementia is more closely related to what he terms ecological niche value—'which is a statement of their value to other organisms,' that is, 'their social interactions with other humans'—as well as to ontological niche value—'that is, the [pre-existing] capacity or potential of an organism to interact with its environment' (517). 'People with dementia—even severe dementia,' Millett writes, 'continue to have the capacity to interact with their environment and, simply because they have a body and the capacity to interact, they clearly occupy an ontological niche' (517). By highlighting ecological and ontological niche value—terms he borrows from Jakob von Uexküll's ecological studies—Millett moves closer to a social constructivist position that focuses on the importance of social interaction and relationships in maintaining the dignity of people with dementia. Furthermore, Millett turns to philosophers such as Aristotle, Jonas, and Lévinas in order to argue that 'each living thing has a unique non-instrumental value-for-itself' and 'each human being announces an ought-to-care to the world that places each of us under an obligation to help that being' (519)—an argument I fully agree with, but that does not follow from bio-semiosis alone.

Importantly, Millett's account acknowledges the effects that dementia has, especially on cognition, while productively circumventing the problem of making value-judgments based on aspects of cognition or on the notion of personhood. At the same time, he engages with Davis's suggestion that 'Kitwood's view that it is possible to maintain personhood at the extremes of this condition' may be 'damaging to those relatives forced to take on the role of primary carer' (Davis 2004: 369). Millett emphasises that 'if we take the view that people with dementia maintain a self we may place an unnecessarily high burden on the untrained family carers who do most of the work of care.' Such a view, he argues, denies carers 'a proper mourning for the loss of their loved one as the dementia progresses,' and induces feelings of 'guilt or shame at their changed feelings toward the obviously changing "person"' (Millett 2011: 509–10). Millett's account indicates how attitudes about people with dementia can shift towards a more sympathetic understanding without having to rely on notions of selfhood. Nonetheless, in the following discussion I retain the notion of embodied selfhood as a shorthand expression both for embodied aspects of identity and for the way each human being experiences the world—what phenomenologists refer to as the first-personal perspectival givenness of experiential life (Gallagher and Zahavi 2008, Zahavi 2007), which I claim persists in dementia.

Attending to the body in dementia also opens up the possibility of finding avenues for communication that do not rely heavily on coherent verbalisation. Speaking of 'embodied communication' as opposite to 'verbal' communication is of course misleading, since verbal communication is embodied. However, I use this term to draw attention to other ways that bodies and behaviour may speak. As Lisa Snyder (1999) highlights in her collection of interviews with people with dementia, because of the way the disease affects cognition, many individuals may not be able to maintain the same insight and verbal abilities as previously. 'But throughout the course of Alzheimer,' she writes, 'each person continues to convey messages through action, gesture, expression and behavior. The disease does not result in a complete inability to communicate. But it can require our time, energy, receptivity, and ingenuity to observe, listen, and comprehend effectively' (1999: 32–3). I agree with Snyder that the ability to communicate persists, although some forms of life writing may not be able to adequately capture this capacity for communication. Documentary film (and perhaps also graphic memoir, as I discuss in later chapters) offers a mediated opportunity to engage with these 'embodied' forms of communication and to train one's receptivity to channels of communication outside language (see also Killick and Allan 2001).

Inside views: life writing by people with early-onset dementia

> This is my attempt to leave a record of what is going on between my ears.
> (Taylor 2007: 3)

If severe illness generally threatens the production of a life narrative (Couser 1997: 5), then dementia, in particular, seems to threaten all aspects central to the autobiographical project: the *auto*/self in that it is seemingly eroded, the *bios*/life in that memory loss threatens the ability to remember and coherently narrate life events, and finally the *graphein*/writing is threatened by the erosion of higher-order cognitive functions. And yet, as the epigraph above taken from Richard Taylor's *Alzheimer's from the Inside Out* (2007) demonstrates, a steadily growing number of first-person accounts are being published, mainly by people with early-onset Alzheimer's disease.[7] Despite the challenges dementia poses, they present very successful 'attempts' to 'record' what it means to be living with a progressive neurodegenerative brain disease. These accounts have taken the form of articles in Alzheimer's care journals—such as Marilyn Truscott's articles of testimony and advice (Truscott 2003, 2004a, 2004b)—blogs,[8] and also book-length memoirs or autopathographies.[9] Many of the authors also appeared on radio programmes and TV shows, spoke at conferences, acted as board members for the Alzheimer's Association, or participated in documentaries about their experience (Pratchett and Russell 2009) as part of their fight to alleviate the stigma attached to dementia. As such, these autobiographical acts have played a crucial role in patient advocacy in the Alzheimer's movement.

In what follows, I draw on a range of autobiographical texts by people with early-onset dementia to explore what these accounts suggest about the changing nature of self-experience. Engaging with these narratives elucidates the range of changes across cognitive, bodily, and social spheres, suggesting in turn common themes that can be found across individual experiences of living with this condition. However, this is not to suggest that there is only *one* type of 'dementia experience.' On the contrary, these autobiographical accounts highlight the extent to which the experience of the condition and the progression of symptoms vary significantly from one individual to the next. Furthermore, while their authors differ in gender and nationality, these texts cannot be seen as representative for the entire population with dementia—across age, ethnicity, race, class, sexuality, debility, or geographical location. The autopathographers discussed in the following were all diagnosed with younger-onset dementia and come from largely white, educated, middle class backgrounds and share a heteronormative sexual orientation.[10] Before turning to aspects of the experience of dementia discussed in the case studies as such, therefore, I shall provide a brief review of some of the issues that a more truly cross-sectional sample may raise.

In contrast to autopathographies by one author, story collections offer the opportunity to represent a more diverse range of voices, including those who would not have the means or cognitive resources to tell and publish their stories without editorial, emotional, and financial support. Both Lisa Snyder's early collection *Speaking Our Minds* (1999) and Lucy Whitman's recent volume *People with Dementia Speak Out* (2016) fill this gap. Although dementia activists with early-onset forms of dementia still dominate Whitman's collection, her storytellers range across more diverse backgrounds in terms of age, class, ethnicity, and linguistic background; that is, non-standard regional or world English variants of English. A cursory view of these stories suggests that the challenge of getting—and later accepting—a diagnosis of dementia is indeed greater for people with young-onset dementia. Further, they face specific challenges to do with losing employment and lack of financial security when forced into early retirement. And yet, there are also many commonalities. In all cases, the response of the social world—whether positive or negative—seems to have the greatest impact on well-being and the ability to accommodate and adapt to the symptoms of dementia. Attitudinal changes, too, often inspired by being with others with the condition, or receiving the right kind of support, seem to play a crucial role in finding ways to live well despite the diagnosis. However, the collection also bears out that diversity in dementia calls for greater diversity of approaches. More needs to be done, for instance, to raise awareness and educate certain minority communities about dementia, to develop culturally appropriate services, and to eliminate the 'postcode lottery' of dementia care (June Hennell in Whitman 2016: 155).

Rukiya Mukadam's account 'Time to break the taboo,' in Whitman's collection, for example, describes how dementia is considered shameful in South Asian communities. Mukadam, an Indian doctor who practised in Malawi for thirty years, recounts how family members with dementia are kept away from social encounters to avoid embarrassment. Dementia and other conditions remain taboo, since illness is considered as having been caused by the individual's or a family member's sinful behaviour (Mukadam in Whitman 2016: 239–41). While it is risky to generalise from one account, Mukadam's testimony supports social science research which points to the fact that South Asian communities are less likely to access dementia services due to pronounced stigma, stemming from 'religious and cultural beliefs about mental health' (Innes 2009: 74). In her survey of research on dementia in different cultural contexts, Innes shows that 'face-saving' (85) and 'courtesy stigma' (74)—that is the stigma attached to family members of a person with dementia—also seem at issue in Chinese and Korean families, in which dementia is 'hidden in the family' (Innes 2009: 75). While notions about filial duty to care in certain communities might limit access to services (77), research on minority populations in the US and the UK also highlights that other key factors contribute to whether a diagnosis is sought and given, and whether dementia services are subsequently accessed: these include, amongst others, the lack of culturally sensitive tests (77), the lack of age-appropriate (78) or culturally appropriate services (respecting religious or dietary requirements) (87), and the lack of care providers who are able to communicate with the person with dementia and their family members in their own language (90).

While Innes' survey highlights that there is a need for dementia services to ensure that cultural and religious backgrounds are taken into account when designing dementia services, it also underlines that there are great similarities in the experience of dementia irrespective of cultural background. If dementia research, and also the dissemination and study of dementia narratives, needs to address differences across diverse socio-economic and sociocultural backgrounds, the differences that emerge across different groupings should not obscure either individual differences *within* groups or commonalities *across* diverse cultural groups.

Memory

Memory loss is frequently perceived to be *the* defining characteristic of dementia, especially of the Alzheimer's type. However, memory is not just one thing—a single faculty of the mind—but a variety of processes, ranging from semantic, episodic, and procedural to short-term or working memory (Gallagher and Zahavi 2008: 70). And yet, dementia is often equated with semantic (word loss) or episodic memory loss (the loss of autobiographical memories). Understanding Alzheimer's as 'merely' the loss of semantic memory, however, underestimates the profound changes that the disease effects. Christine Bryden succinctly describes this more existential shift in being-in-the-world in her memoir *Dancing with Dementia* (2005):

> You see, it is far more than simply memory loss. We are confused, we have problems with our sight, with our balance, with numbers and with direction. ... We have no sense of time passing, so we live in the present reality, with no past and no future. We put all our energy into the *now*, not then, or later. Sometimes this causes a lot of anxiety because we worry about the past or the future because we cannot 'feel' that it exists.
> (Bryden 2005: 99)

Since memory loss is such a defining characteristic of the condition, autobiographical accounts unsurprisingly often focus on the challenges of living with progressively impaired memory. While these challenges relate to all kinds of everyday activities, one aspect that is thematised in all accounts is the impact that memory loss has on *communicating* one's experience—both generally and in life writing specifically.

In producing his autobiographical journal *Partial View: An Alzheimer's Journal* (1998), Cary Henderson used a tape recorder to impart his thoughts about what it is like to be living with Alzheimer's. The use of the tape recorder is instrumental in his project of contributing to an 'understanding from the patient's point of view' (4) as it provides a 'memory device ... to keep your ideas long enough so somebody else can hear them' (7). For Henderson, then, the tape recorder extends his ability to tell his story beyond the stage where he is able to write or type. At the same time, Henderson's difficulty in learning to handle the tape-recorder highlights the extent to which dementia impedes the acquisition of new skills: 'I still haven't mastered this, apparently very simple thing of—uh—pushing down the two sides to get the machine to work. Pushing down two buttons ought to be the easiest thing in the world' (7). His account underscores then the extent to which memory loss includes procedural memory.

In his journal, Henderson also describes the disorientating effects of the loss of short-term memory. In doing so he challenges common perceptions about what the behaviour of people with dementia *means*—that is, he suggests that it is meaningful rather than meaningless. As Karen Lyman (1989: 602) notes, one of the adverse effects of the biomedicalisation of dementia is that all behaviour is henceforth interpreted as symptom of the disease pathology, and thereby robbed of its meaning. In particular, Lyman criticises health professionals for misinterpreting wandering as 'deviant' or 'problem' behaviour needing to be restrained (1989: 600). Henderson's account highlights how, rather than being an aimless activity, wandering represents an attempt to reconnect with the world and recover meaning: 'Once the idea is lost, everything is lost and I have nothing to do but to wander around trying to figure out what was it that was so important earlier' (24). 'When I'm wandering around, I'm trying to touch base with—anything, actually' (24), Henderson comments.

While challenging the view that all behaviour by people with dementia is meaningless, Henderson's wandering highlights the extent to which memory and cognition can be understood as 'embodied, embedded cognition'[11] or, in other words, as 'extended' (Clark and Chalmers 1998) beyond the physical mind or brain to include the social and physical environment. Our environment can be considered part of our memory system since not only notes and calendars act as memory devices but simple, everyday objects orient us in time and remind us of the task at hand. Beyond using technical devices as memory aids, Wendy Mitchell (2018), for instance, describes how she leaves things in sight to help her remember. These objects might be folders with instructions on how to get to a conference, but they may also include everyday objects and kitchen equipment. Once her possessions are in boxes or inside closets, they cease to exist—leading her in one case to buy ever new cheese graters. Laughing at the amount of cheese graters, ten in all, that she has accumulated, she comments to her daughter, 'The strangest thing is, I don't even like cheese that much … Let alone grated cheese' (189). To circumvent the problem that she cannot remember what is behind closed doors of any kind, Mitchell later places photos on her kitchen drawers and closets to remind herself of what is behind them (209)—one of many adaptations to her condition that help her function despite her progressing symptoms.

34 *Storytelling, experience, and empathy*

Both Henderson's *Partial View* and Mitchell's *Somebody I Used to Know* also highlight the unsettling effects of the loss of procedural memory. 'A simple task like stepping into the shower becomes fraught with uncertainty. Two taps become literally a burning question: which one is cold?' Mitchell writes (232). She further imparts how dispiriting it is to try and have a shower and discover she has forgotten to wet her hair before applying the shampoo, or how it has become impossible to figure out how to switch on an unfamiliar shower, let alone change the temperature (248). Henderson similarly describes his problems with simple, everyday activities, such as opening a can of dog food. His anxiety is exacerbated by the fact that he has lost his sense of time and therefore does not know how long his wife has been absent:

> This was a real, first-rate panic. I opened up the can with a—let's see, what did I use for that—uh, well, whatever came at the moment. I had to find some way to give the doggie some food. But this was one of those things you're—must get into if you're going to have a life with Alzheimer's. I'm too clumsy, because of the damned Alzheimer's, my feet and legs, oh well, my hands, to do their job, and the best I can is kind of wiggle them and try to get mad and other silly things. But after tearing up the can, and tearing up a can is a real experience, but maybe my wife, one of these hours, will be feeling better and she can really open the can. Right now, the doggie seems to be in fairly good shape—I am not sure I am.
>
> (31)

While this passage evokes the emotional impact of his deteriorating abilities, it also highlights the particular affordances of using a tape recorder to produce his journal. Contrary to other memoirs, Henderson's narrative arguably 'enacts'[12] moments of memory loss. In most other memoirs smooth, coherent, and rhetorically powerful prose starkly clashes with the language difficulties that the authors describe. In fact, the subsequent editing and polishing of the writing usually eliminates the 'diseased' or 'disabled self' from the text itself (Burke 2007a). Symptoms are described retrospectively rather than enacted. This is the case not only for language difficulties but for confusion, hallucination, paranoia, and moments of forgetfulness. In using a tape-recorder coupled with sensitive editing, Henderson's journal provides insight into his confusion. His musings reflect his word-finding difficulties, the loss of a train of thought, as well as expressions of anger, anxiety, and paranoia. The effect of this closeness between experience and expression is a heightened sense of awareness of 'what it is like' or, at least, what it *may* be like to be struggling with cognitive decline. The more polished accounts, by contrast, may at times make it difficult to imaginatively enter into the troubling experiences of the author as the reader is presented with such a reassuringly competent counterpart. And yet, as a number of authors of dementia memoirs have commented, writing often does come more easily than speaking, and the 'coherent' self presented in writing must therefore not necessarily be seen as less 'authentic.'

These comments address complex issues of representation in autobiographical writing by people with dementia. While I deal more thoroughly with issues of self-presentation and narrative identity in Chapter 3, this issue necessitates a short aside here. For one, when authors such as McGowin, or more recently Rohra (2011) and Mitchell (2018), express themselves in coherent language, their authenticity is questioned. Indeed, the very diagnosis of Alzheimer's is called into question by members of the general public, as well as clinicians, who often have only stereotypical images of late stage Alzheimer's in mind and cannot conceptualise that a person with dementia may be able to be so articulate. Wendy Mitchell discusses this issue on her blog, while explaining how much easier she finds it to express herself in writing, and in her own time, than in immediate interactions with others. She thereby defends the authenticity of her account.

Nonetheless, her printed memoir was written in collaboration with a professional writer, and contrary to Zimmermann's view (2017) that dementia autopathographies have moved to a post-modern aesthetic of representation, which incorporates fragmentation and confusion, Mitchell's memoir, in fact, represents the most eloquent first-person account to date: employing, for instance, the literary device of a you-narrative in which her present self, affected by Alzheimer's, addresses her 'then self,' before the onset of disease, in brief vignettes about her past life. These vignettes are situated within an otherwise coherent and linear account of her present experience of living with and raising awareness of young-onset dementia.

Mitchell's memoir raises the question of how we read autobiographical narratives by people with dementia. Do we read them as straightforward representations of reality? How do we assess the verisimilitude and 'truth-value' of these texts, an issue in all life writing, and what role does our assessment play for the political force these narratives develop? Since my aim in this chapter is to introduce readers to the experience of living with dementia by giving the words of people with dementia centre stage, exploring these issues here would go beyond the scope of this chapter. Instead, I hope to correct the tendency of ignoring the voices of people with dementia when talking about this condition. In Chapter 3 I return to more theoretical questions that attend to life writing in dementia and ask what is at stake, when the authors of dementia autopathographies use their stories to reclaim social identity and write back against nefarious stereotypes of dementia. I ask how the choice of genre, medium, and metaphors affects the narratives. In particular, I explore the complex problem of counter-narratives in dementia life writing and their relation to the contested notion of narrative identity.

Language

> Words slice through my mind so fast I cannot catch them and marry them to the eternity of the page.
>
> (DeBaggio 2002: 27)

As the quotation from DeBaggio's memoir *Losing My Mind: An Intimate Look at Life with Alzheimer's* (2002) so powerfully evokes, language production and reception become increasingly fraught areas in dementia. And yet, as equally demonstrated by DeBaggio's use of surprising metaphors to describe how hard it has become for him to find, and retain, the right word, language use in dementia can also become more creative, as the brain finds ways to circumvent problems of retrieval. Since language provides the primary tool to communicate with others, the impairment of language also has serious repercussions in the social sphere. Henderson, for instance, describes the effects of word-finding difficulties and slowed cognition on his ability to take part in conversations:

> I really can't converse very well at all. So that's very limiting. I can't think of things to say before somebody's already said it and they've superseded what I have to say. The words get tangled very easily and I get frustrated when I can't think of a word.
>
> (18)

However, as Henderson points out, there is also another reason why conversations with others are limited: 'when you have Alzheimer's', he notes, 'nobody really wants to talk to you any longer' (Henderson 1998: 18). Henderson further points out that people with dementia often experience a kind of 'social death' (Lyman 1989: 601), as others no longer engage with them, and instead either address the caregiver or spouse, or shun interaction altogether (see also Aquilina and Hughes 2006, Kitwood 1997).

Like Mitchell, DeBaggio and Henderson highlight the advantages of language production at the pace of the person with dementia. They advocate for forms of slowed interaction. Writing or tape recording can be done as the thoughts occur, and the person with dementia experiences a more cognitively alert moment. Furthermore, the process is less likely to be disturbed by time constraints, 'nervous tension,' or distractions that occur during face-to-face interaction (see DeBaggio 2002: 180, McGowin 1994, Ryan, Bannister, and Anas 2009: 145).[13] Indeed, DeBaggio describes the impact of Alzheimer's on one's expressive capacity as the experience of living in 'two worlds':

> In one I am afflicted with Alzheimer's, gasping as words slip through my lips with effort and suffering imprecision. This is the world in which I have to tell my companion I can't remember the word to make the sentence. In the other, slower world where I write on paper or directly on

the computer, vocabulary is more fluid and I often surprise myself when the perfect word finds its way into the sentence without effort. This has puzzled me from the first sentence I wrote for this book. It is only now eight months later, I begin to see more clearly how necessary it is to slow the pace to achieve a former normality.

(2002: 180)

However, not only language production, but language reception becomes progressively impaired in dementia. Henderson evocatively describes how his capacity to read is affected:

Reading's almost impossible, for one thing—things don't stand still. Words don't stand still. It appears to me that it's wavering. I can't pin it down—the words—they can be over yonder and over yonder and I can't catch them.

(Henderson 1998: 23)

The link between perception and the ascription of meaning has broken down: 'I can see the words, I can pronounce the words, but they don't seem to mean a whole lot' (23). And yet, Henderson is clearly *aware* that he has problems in understanding what people tell him:

'A lot of things that I don't understand, even after somebody tells me. If I could signal in some way and tell them, oh sure, I heard it, but the ramifications of whatever the heck it was that I heard, I kind of missed.

(35)

Henderson's account elucidates how this lack of understanding frequently contributes to a sense of feeling left out and even a sense of paranoia (81).

Language reception can be particularly challenging when the person with dementia has no visual cues to go by. Many authors describe how they stopped using the telephone as they no longer recognised who was calling or felt under pressure to fill gaps in the conversation. However, as Mitchell points out, contemporary forms of communication, such as video calls, or chat apps such as WhatsApp, by providing visual cues or slowing interaction, may allow people with dementia to communicate more easily and fluidly with friends and family. Embracing these new forms of communication is one of the ways that Mitchell continuously adapts to her changing abilities.

The effects of dementia on verbal communication, then, challenge us to explore the potential of nonverbal communication (Killick and Allan 2001). Exploring the potential of nonverbal communication is not only relevant for the caregiver, but also for the person with dementia who may use nonverbal cues to interpret the meaning of an utterance and draw on nonverbal means to express herself.

Perception, movement, and the senses

> I do believe Alzheimer's does include what your feet do and what your hands do, as well as what your brain does.
>
> (Henderson 1998: 8)

As will have become clear by now, 'memory' is instrumental to engage with the world, including movement and perception. *Apraxia*—that is, problems in planning the coordination of movements to accomplish a learned, purposeful task, 'what your feet and what your hands do,' as Henderson puts it, is among the symptoms of dementia. Often these losses go hand in hand with *agnosia*, the loss of the ability to recognise visual, auditory, or other sensual stimuli due to problems in processing information. As Bea, a woman interviewed by Snyder, explains: 'Sometimes what I'm looking for will be lying right in front of me and I won't see it. I don't always misplace things; they're right there, but I just don't recognize them' (Snyder 1999: 21). Examples of apraxia have already been discussed above as examples of the impact dementia has on procedural memory. Here, however, I explore the far-reaching implications that problems with movement and perception can have on people with dementia with regard to their ability to engage with and make sense of their world.

In her phenomenological account of illness, Carel (2008) draws attention to the fact that illness changes the geographical landscape one inhabits. She provides the example of how using a wheelchair changes the experience and navigability of a space. As the epigraph by Henderson underlines, the possibilities of bodily movement are curtailed in dementia. This limitation arises not necessarily because it is no longer possible to move hands or legs, but because as Wendy Mitchell puts it, the 'brain and legs aren't talking to each other; the communication is lost' (8). Further, Mitchell describes how her interaction with the world becomes more and more riddled with uncertainty: 'getting into a lift now is a tentative thing. I'm never sure where the edge is, placing my feet carefully on the floor, unsure whether I might fall off a ledge' (211). Henderson's journal equally attempts to capture and communicate something of this experience. Henderson's words 'I used to be able to talk to people and walk *without wondering if the pavement is actually there*' (8; emphasis added), for example, are accompanied by a heavily unfocused photo of his feet walking across a dizzying space of gravel. Here photographic style is used to evoke a sense of 'parallel experience' (Toker 1993) in the reader. That is, the lack of focus and perspective as if from Henderson's point of view captures for the reader something of the sensory experience of the dizzying effect of losing control over one's footage.

Nancy Andrews' photography does not merely accompany the text, nor does it objectify Henderson—although there are some instances of 'uncomfortable' representation. Rather, it provides a parallel, interpretative account of Henderson's words and life. So, for instance, a bird's-eye view shot from the top of a long, public staircase, with Henderson posed at the bottom, gripping the handrail, seemingly hesitant to ascend, communicates something of the emotional tone of Henderson's fear of stairs: 'I'm scared to death of climbing stairs ... I've got to hold on pretty tightly, then I'll go screaming meemies, the uncertainty of one's footage. ... You can't live at the bottom all the time, though' (11). Photographic style here is used to heighten the reader's awareness of how the subjective experience of space and motion changes in dementia.

Various autobiographical accounts draw attention to the fact that environments with too many stimuli—several people talking at once, background music, noisy restaurants—are impossible for a person with dementia to process (Bryden 1998: 67, Henderson 1998: 68). The difficulties presented by these environments are captured in Henderson's journal by the photographer Nancy Andrews: during a family gathering Henderson sits at the table, eyes averted, hands clasped, seemingly withdrawn. He is surrounded by several people talking and children who are playing (noisily, one presumes) on the floor (Henderson 1998: 68–9). While this outside perspective risks enforcing the stereotype of the person with dementia as withdrawn or an 'empty shell,' Henderson's words lucidly describe the difficulty for people with dementia to process stimuli in such situations—underscoring that the person and mind are anything but 'empty':

> Whenever there's a gathering of people, it seems, at least in my mind, to be a lot of confusion. I just feel the need for quiet. ... if there's not much going on ... I can think better. If there's anybody else in the room, it seems like—more than just one person—I do sort of lose my grip.
> (Henderson 1998: 68)

Accounts of living with dementia vividly communicate how the experience of objects, spaces, taste, sound, and movement changes in dementia. Mitchell describes how the world seems to have 'turned up its volume overnight' and moving through a busy intercity space becomes impossible without ear plugs (184). Colour contrasts become more important in order to distinguish objects. And dark objects (a rug or a TV screen) might simply be processed as a hole—a deeply unsettling experience. Such shifts in sensory experience may radically alter the author's sense of being-in-the-world (see also Ratcliffe 2008) and destabilise her very sense of self. Bryden, for instance, when describing the overwhelming confusion of a night out with friends, emphasises how her difficulties in processing disparate information impact directly on her sense of self: 'I felt *I was fading*, the sounds were getting distant, faces were difficult to focus on, and I found it harder and harder to concentrate on what people were saying' (Bryden 1998: 67; emphasis added). As the world fades, or the previously stable relationship to the world fades, the previous experience of self seems to fade with it.[14] And yet, use of the dominant metaphor of fading away is in stark contrast with the way the authors, in these journals, continue to be the centre of perception. As Bryden or others share their experience of dealing with hallucinations or multiple stimuli, they remain the subjects of experience. Therefore, these accounts highlight that while there is a *shift* in self-experience, it does not make sense to speak of a *loss* of self per se.

Apart from having increasing problems processing visual and auditory information, autopathographers also describe visual, auditory and olfactory hallucinations. Mitchell describes being shocked by hearing gun shots (133) or seeing her deceased parents—and then having to try and work out whether what she sees is real or not (192). McGowin provides a vivid account of having olfactory hallucinations: the unpleasant sensation, for instance, of smelling cat pee while others cannot smell anything (McGowin 1994: 125). However, McGowin's account also highlights that there are at times unexpected pleasures in her symptoms: 'I can sometimes enjoy the sweet fragrance of night-blooming jasmine, when no one else can. It is my own private sensation' (125). Equally, Mitchell sees the vision of her parents as 'gift ... a much loved glimpse of the past' (193). Based on her own experience of hallucinations, Mitchell asks readers to validate the experience of people with dementia, rather than try and 'pull [them] back into the present day,' by reminding them 'over and over' that loved ones have died (193).

What is remarkable about these memoirs is that their authors find ever new ways of adapting to the symptoms of dementia. By taking a disability approach to dementia, they underscore the extent to which symptoms can also be managed. Reading first-person accounts for the strategies their authors develop to counter increasing disabilities might be one way in which these narratives can contribute to developing support for people with dementia, to help them to live as well as possible, rather than seeing the diagnosis as a death sentence.

Overall, however, the disruption of habitual encounters with the world has profoundly pernicious effects on the authors' sense of self. DeBaggio, for instance, describes how after having been baffled and shamed by the failed attempt to use a photocopier, his return home presented a turning point in his (self-)experience:

> On the way home I had a peculiar feeling that the sidewalk wavered every once in a while. At intersections I was careful to look in all directions. It was a walk in which I lost something I may never get back.
> (2002: 116–7)

Autopathographies by people with dementia, then, attest to the way in which seemingly effortless processes of sense perception are fundamental in our experience of feeling at home in the world. Such narratives express the loss of this 'at-home-ness' and attempt to convey a sense of this experience to the reader.

Emotions and cognition

Memoirs by people with dementia abound with examples of deeply felt expressions of emotions: from frustration and anger to guilt, worry, appreciation, and love. While highlighting the persistence of emotions, these narratives also reflect on the subtle and less subtle ways in which emotions and cognition are changed in dementia—leading to substantial changes in how the authors experience themselves. DeBaggio, for instance, evokes the sense of his mind 'becoming one-dimensional' of having 'almost lost [the] ability to hold two thoughts simultaneously' (2002: 142). Bryden (1998) similarly describes how her inner thought processes are becoming unfamiliar as they become more 'stretched out, ... more linear, more step by step' (48–9). This loss of 'vibrancy,' 'buzz,' and 'interconnectedness' (1998) is paralleled on an emotional level:

> My emotions seem a little awry. Sometimes I am a bit more teary than before, for no apparent reason. But more often I seem to have what feels like a sort of emotional blank, which to my daughters looks like a lack of sparkle, of charisma. I don't get as excited as I used to, and I just feel a little 'flat'. It takes too much energy to react with emotion: where once it seemed automatic, now it takes actual mental effort to consider a situation, and then how to react to it.
>
> (92)

Bryden's description highlights the sense in which emotional responses are a cognitive activity (Damasio 2000) and the extent to which this cognitive life is constitutive of her sense of selfhood: 'I'm like a slow motion version of my old self,' she writes (Bryden 1998: 49). And yet, Bryden sees some benefits to this change: 'It's not all bad, as I have more inner space in this linear mode to listen, to see, to appreciate clouds, leaves, flowers ... I am less driven and less impatient' (1998: 48–9). Like other authors, then, Bryden suggests that one can live well with dementia, and despite the fact that the disease is usually described in terms of a 'living death,' it may also entail positive changes in the life of the person with dementia.

In one of his essays, Taylor (2007) puts yet another spin on these emotional changes. He describes how he is beginning to care less about his forgetfulness and the lack of correspondence between his world and his caregivers' reality. The feeling of no longer caring is experienced as both threatening and a relief. It prompts him to ask whether he is 'turning into an android that really doesn't care where it is, what is happening around it, what is happening to it' (57)—drawing on a dehumanising metaphor to conceptualise people with dementia. However, he also depicts his growing lack of concern as positive:

> In the past, behaviour like that would upset me. In the recent past, it would frustrate me. In the present, it just doesn't seem to bother me that much. Why are others around me so concerned? I forgot – so what?
>
> (58)

Read alongside his deep expression of fear about the future, this flippant remark does not ring entirely true, but it does speak to the fluctuation in his emotional responses to the lived experience of his disease. It is one of the strengths of the seriality of both essay and blog formats that they allow for varying responses, attitudes, and emotions to be registered over time, rather than providing a fixed teleological outlook—as in most retrospective memoirs.

If emotional changes can lead to an increased appreciation of the here and now, Henderson also highlights the negative impact the disease has on his emotional landscape: 'There's so many things about Alzheimer's that are rather bewildering,' he writes. 'Sometimes you can have mood swings that are really awful I think. Sometimes I feel on top of the world, a couple of days ago I did and today I just feel absolutely devastated' (Henderson 1998: 32). As DeBaggio recounts, dementia can also have an impact on the (seemingly unmotivated) strength of an emotional reaction:

> Strange things are happening. I blew up this morning with surprising force and frustration. The cause? The newspaper hadn't arrived. ... Little things wear down my emotional equilibrium. First vocabulary fractures; then my emotions explode like snowflakes in an angry blizzard.
> (DeBaggio 2002: 168)

The writers of dementia autopathographies sometimes experience their emotions as alien, out of control, or unmotivated. At the same time, they reflect on the potential benefits of some of the changes wrought by the disease. Importantly, by putting their emotions in the context of their life experiences, their narratives help to underline the continuity and validity of emotional reactions in people with dementia. Like other behaviour, emotions expressed by people with dementia are often seen through the lens of pathology, rather than being seen as legitimate reactions to a frustrating or undignified experience. In particular, the expression of negative emotions, such as anger, is classified as 'challenging behaviour' (Killick and Allan 2001). The social context of the situation in which this anger arose is frequently overlooked. A closer look at the experience of living with dementia highlights how these expressions of emotions, while affected by disease processes, remain meaningful. This recognition, in turn, may help attune caregivers to acknowledging and in turn validating what these emotions express.

Importantly, too, dementia autopathographies draw attention to the fact that intense negative emotions, such as grief, represent a natural reaction to the experience of living with dementia and dealing with losses, as well as the fear of future losses. Kate Swaffer (2016), in particular, highlights how grief counselling should constitute an integral part of post-diagnosis support for people with dementia. She argues that many of the symptoms of dementia might be exacerbated by depression that could be alleviated and improved if people with dementia were given adequate support and counselling.

Time

> The scariest thing is, I guess, the fact that I have no sense of time. I have not the slightest idea—my brain doesn't—what's ten hours away or two hours away.
> (Henderson 1998: 47)

It is hard to imagine what it may be like to live in the state that Henderson describes here. And yet, as Rita Charon notes,

> 'Because the experience of time might be one of the most telling aspects of the divide between the sick and the well, health professionals have an urgent need to examine and make at least imaginative sense of how patients might experience time.
> (Charon 2006: 121)

In dementia, the experience of time is transformed in numerous ways. The person affected by the disease arguably becomes 'lost in time,' due to the progressive inability to remember the current date, month, season, or year she is living through. DeBaggio describes this state of affairs while highlighting that certain temporal markers are of less importance to the person with dementia than they are to others (see also Henderson 1998: 44):

> *I awake in the dark morning without awareness of what day of the week it is. I wait for the newspaper or the radio to locate me in time. The day of the week, the hour of the day has little meaning for me even when I remember. I float in my own chaotic world, grateful to know I am still alive.*
> (DeBaggio 2002: 148; italics in original)

A person with dementia may also be lost in time in the sense that she may seem to be 'living in the past.' In such instances past autobiographical memories are being experienced *as* the present, or they colour the present to such a degree that the person is no longer aware of significant aspects of current reality. Such shifts are unlikely to be represented in autobiographical writing, since the writing project in itself relies on a certain amount of present-day information being available to the author. DeBaggio's graphic description of a night of delusion, during which he calls out in distress to his wife as his 'Mommy,' provides a rare exception to this rule:

> I was lost and had begun to regress to another time. I called her 'Mommy' and I asked where Daddy was in mantra-like singsong. I saw my mother where Joyce had been. I sat up in the bed and reached out to touch her in the dark air of the room but my tingling fingertips met nothing. My mother had been dead for decades, *but time melted away.*
> (DeBaggio 2002: 203; emphasis added)[15]

There is, however, a third way, frequently overlooked, in which people with dementia may become 'lost in time.' Temporal units are experienced differently as memory loss significantly loosens the sense of being moored to a particular time and place. Even small units of time can no longer be made sense of as they cannot be linked to a coherent whole, a narrative 'before' and 'after.' Life writing by people with dementia is rich in phenomenological descriptions of such experiences of being lost in time, such as Henderson's unsettling experience of not knowing how long his wife has been absent and therefore becoming concerned about the well-being of his dog. Henderson draws attention to the pervasiveness of this temporal unravelling:

> No two days and no two moments are the same. You can't build on experience. You can maybe guess what's going to happen a little while from now—minutes from now, hours from now—we don't know what to expect.
>
> (Henderson 1998: 47)

It is hard to imagine the disorientating effect such a transformed experience of temporal sequences must have and what the world may look like for a person experiencing these symptoms of dementia. In her memoir, Bryden quotes an email communication from a friend living with dementia, who evocatively describes the effect:

> Most of the time I live in the space I can see and the time called 'now' ... it is almost a 'virtual world' ... I move ... and a new space opens to view ... even my rooted-ness to my place in space feels tenuous ... as if I might be torn loose, uprooted, blown away.
>
> (Bryden 2005: 99)

As this extract suggests, living in the 'now' is not a comfortable experience. While a number of memoirs advocate a *carpe diem* approach to life and express their authors' willingness to live each day to the full and make the most of their remaining capacities, Taylor draws attention to the fact that the symptoms of dementia that create this continuous present may in fact undermine the ability to enjoy the present. 'Living in and for the moment assumes the ability to know what is going on, what [one is] doing in a given moment,' he writes (Taylor 2007: 131). This ability, however, is slowly eroded as the temporal unity of experience is disrupted.

Like in other progressive illnesses, time is also experienced as a valuable commodity. Writers of first-person accounts wonder how much time they have left, particularly, how much time they have left at a certain level of functioning. The dominant cultural narrative of dementia as progressive loss can make the future seem uncertain and simultaneously petrifying. And yet, the underlying uncertainty also contributes to the authors' sense of urgency. The authors are pushed to seize the day, to make use of every opportunity. Whether seizing the opportunity for a ride on the biggest rollercoaster in Blackpool or a flight in a glider: 'Life doesn't have to be dull and risk-free just because you have dementia,' Mitchell writes (266). For many of these authors, seizing every opportunity also involves going out and advocating for people with young-onset dementia for as long as possible.

The social world: intimate relationships and strangers

> I'd like a larger world than I have right now.
> (Henderson 1998: 24)

In many ways, this quotation from Henderson's journal speaks to all the aspects of experience discussed so far that are changed in dementia. In selecting these words as an epigraph for this section on changes in the social world, I aim to underline how this particular aspect of being-in-the-world in dementia is determined less by changes on a neurological level than by changes in other people's reactions. Therefore, it is one of the few aspects of dementia that could be reversed or at least alleviated (see Kitwood 1990, 1997). Many of the memoirs highlight the extent to which interactions with others—strangers, health-care professionals, friends, and family members—are changed after the diagnosis of dementia. The person with the disease may lose the ability to behave according to social norms (Carel 2008, Goffman 1963) or may become more dependent on others, thereby upsetting the nature of previous relationships. Importantly, research has shown that social relationships are severely undermined, not only by the disease itself but also by the process of disease labelling (Lyman 1989). The labelling of the behaviour of people with dementia as pathological results in limited opportunities for them to assert agency and control over their lives and to interact socially (Lyman 1989: 600–1). One of the most devastating effects of the stigma attached to dementia is that it often leads to social isolation and loneliness, a form of 'social death' (Lyman 1998). Indeed, people with dementia describe the stigma attached to dementia as a fear of contagion:

> We've never tried to hide that I have Alzheimer's. But everyone acts like they don't want to get near because they might catch it. They don't know how to deal with it.
> (Snyder 1999: 22)

The authors of dementia memoirs describe the harrowing experience of being ostracised by strangers and friends alike who may be alarmed by their behaviour, verbal mishaps, or slowness to respond (see also Snyder 1999: 60). They also express their guilt about how their social isolation impacts on their spouses' or children's lives.

However, diagnosis need not necessarily lead to isolation and abandonment. DeBaggio describes the support and encouragement he received from friends and readers of his botanical newsletter after sharing his diagnosis. Although too often Alzheimer's may curtail the formation of new relationships, the memoirs provide evidence that this is not a necessary consequence of the disease. Henderson describes forming new bonds with health-care professionals through being involved in their research project. While appreciating their kindness and personal qualities, his involvement in research also provides him with a new role that boosts his self-esteem. As he writes, 'when I get to Durham and I have something I like to do, I'm kind of on a high. It's something that I can do that not everybody can do, and it makes me feel good about this' (Henderson 1998: 63). Furthermore, many memoirs highlight the importance of forming new relationships through support groups and long-distance communication with other people with dementia. They underline the value of friendships based on a shared understanding of each other's experiences. While the memoirs often criticise health-care professionals for callous behaviour, they also describe instances of supportive and lasting relationships with understanding neurologists, family doctors, or psychiatrists (Bryden 1998: 4, 6, Lee 2003: 20–1). Indeed, Bryden's autobiographies underscore the potential for forming significant new relationships despite dementia. Bryden meets and falls in love with her husband after having struggled with the symptoms of dementia for a number of years (Bryden 2005). Her experience underscores that people with dementia can form new bonds and maintain personal relationships, if given the chance.

Nonetheless, intimate relationships with partners, children, or other family members are bound to be affected by the condition's progression. In some instances, formerly estranged relations between family members may in fact improve due to the way dementia affects both the caregiver and care-receiver. It is a common trope in filial caregivers' memoirs that parent-child roles become inverted by dementia. Autobiographers living with dementia explore their own reactions to this often-unwanted inversion of relationships in their writing. Across the board, people with dementia fear becoming a 'burden' to their families and will often state that they do not want their children to become their caregivers. Their growing dependence on others is frequently coupled with fear, anger, and frustration:

> Sometimes I give Erika a hard time just to be nasty. I guess it's because I'd like to be doing things myself instead of having someone telling me to do this or do that. I'm a little boy now. I have a mommy to take care of me. It's not a very good feeling. I'd much rather be out there doing something else.
>
> (Snyder 1999: 85)

However, the authors of dementia memoirs also express their deep thankfulness and appreciation for the roles their children or partners have taken on: 'My wife is trying extra hard to make things tolerable for me—to give me things to do and make me feel good. I really, really do appreciate that' (Henderson 1998: 28). While occasionally feeling left out in social interactions, Henderson also acknowledges the love and support he has received from his family: 'I think love is the key to all this stuff and love is something that my wife certainly has given to me and the family too and there's nothing that I can see to complain about' (65). Furthermore, he underscores the pivotal role his wife plays in anchoring him in life: 'I'm afraid of losing contact. She's the only one who understands me and I'm hard to understand' (28). Henderson's account, among others, draws attention to the fact that relationships are never one-sided. The authors with dementia frequently voice concern for *their* 'loved ones' and show an empathetic insight into what their family members may be experiencing. As Henderson notes, 'I think probably all of our caregivers, bless their souls and hearts, they do go through a little bit of hell themselves—a lot of it—and a lot of it because of us' (37). Dementia then changes not only the internal landscape of persons with dementia but their social world—and with it the worlds of their companions and family members.

And yet, those authors writing about dementia without a significant other at their side, such as Helga Rohra and Wendy Mitchell, often also see an advantage in their unattached state—for one because they do not suffer to the same degree a sense of guilt towards their partners as they see etched on the faces of others with dementia. Living alone also has practical advantages, though. Not only does living alone mean that nobody will move things around, Rohra and Mitchell both describe how it trains their cognitive capacity. Without a 'back-up-brain,' as Swaffer jokingly describes her husband, Mitchell and Rohra need to use their own resources to continue to deal with life. They often see family caregivers take over tasks from people with dementia and thereby inadvertently contribute to the faster loss of faculties (Mitchell 2018: 247–8). 'Use it or lose it' is their motto. Their narratives then represent powerful calls not to further disable people with dementia by being overprotective or too impatient to let them accomplish tasks on their own.

The experience of flow in dementia

> I appreciate and sometimes immerse myself in the process rather than only or mostly on the outcome. I like doing things. I like and appreciate the doing. Doing is how I know I am alive, and how I appreciate being alive.
>
> (Taylor 2007: 105)

What Richard Taylor describes here is clearly akin to the notion of 'flow' that the clinical psychologist Kate Allan has been exploring in the context of dementia. Allan describes the experience of flow as being

> characterised by a total and intrinsically enjoyable focus on an activity that balances skills with challenges, and provides clear and immediate feedback. It results in a merging of action and awareness, loss of sense of self-consciousness, and altered experience of time.[16]

While the discussion so far has focused largely on the negative ways in which dementia changes the person's sense of being-in-the-world, life writing by people with dementia also provides many positive examples or instances that can be understood in terms of flow.

For instance, DeBaggio considers writing not only a therapeutic means of distancing himself from the disease, allowing him 'to leave thoughts of the disease locked up in the computer' (DeBaggio 2002: 7), but also a means of actually being-at-one-with-the-world. *'The only time I feel alive now is when I am writing, under the spell of work and memories'* (DeBaggio 2002: 121; original emphasis). This sense of 'feeling alive ... under the spell of work' can be understood in terms of flow experience—of being completely immersed in an (enjoyable) activity. DeBaggio is bound up with his keyboard in this activity of writing rather than constituting separate subject and object in the world. At this stage, typing still comes automatically and seems to enable his thinking rather than disrupt his relationship to the world around him by interposing a baffling instrument he can no longer use.[17] This sense of being at ease in his body and his environment contributes to the satisfying sense of feeling alive. Similar instances of flow, of being-at-one-with-the-world, are also highlighted in other dementia memoirs.[18]

Arguably, writing is an unlikely candidate for a sustained experience of flow as the symptoms of dementia progress, and many memoirs—DeBaggio's included—comment on how the ability to write becomes increasingly impaired. Henderson's account, by contrast, highlights less cognitively demanding activities that can provide a sense of enjoyable immersion. Music, his 'only constant companion,' offers such an opportunity:

> I've whiled away many many hours listening to music. I can just listen to music and feel that I'm doing something that I just love to do. I can't make music anymore, but I can certainly use it for my own intentions—which are just to be beautiful.
> (Henderson 1998: 42)

His words are accompanied by an uplifting image of him physically expressing his enjoyment of music (43). Overall, Henderson's account underlines the importance of the appreciation of aesthetic objects, whether man-made or natural. Henderson takes pleasure in the changing colours of autumnal leaves and watching birds in his bird sanctuary. He writes, 'Things are a lot more precious than they were' (77). In other words, although dementia disrupts his experience of the world it also leads him to a deeper appreciation of all things, great and small.

While there are numerous further examples of what Bryden describes as 'dancing with dementia,' one final example shall suffice: many authors comment on the value of being in contact with animals. Henderson describes his relationship to his dog as one of care and mutuality.[19] The dog provides him with an excuse to leave the house and walk when he is feeling 'antsy' (48), but, more importantly, the dog provides a non-judgmental loyal companion, someone to play with, talk to, and simply watch. As Henderson puts it, his dog is 'somebody ... you know is not going to talk back. And you can't make a mistake that way' (13). For Bryden stroking a purring cat is an activity that provides her with the kind of 'brain time-out' that she finds necessary after being overstimulated (1998: 82). Mitchell, from a previous fear of animals, comes to enjoy cat-sitting her daughter's pet and feels a deep sense of calm when with the cat (2018: 167). As with music, there is a certain flow to being with and caressing an animal that is directional but non-instrumental and that does not necessitate the same kind of purposeful planning as other activities. As such, it can provide a reassuring sense of being-at-one-with-the-world, counter to the many examples of shifting self- and world experience in dementia.

Thus, life writing by people with dementia offers rich experiential detail on how both self-experience and world experience are prone to change in dementia. At times, the difficulties of engaging with the world are experienced as attacks on the person's very sense of self. The memoirs underscore how this sense of 'losing oneself' refers not only to the loss of characteristics or abilities that are considered central to one's sense of identity, but also to habitual and background ways of being-in-the-world. At the same time, these memoirs underline the fact that there continues to be a certain perspective on the world. *Somebody* experiences these changes, perceives an altered world, and feels disorientated or diminished. This person, with all the constantly shifting abilities, continues to be a unique centre of perception on the world. Research suggests that this first-personal givenness of experience continues in the late stages of dementia, beyond the possibility of communicating it in words (Kontos 2003, 2004, 2005).

Attending to the ways people with dementia describe their shifting experience in the earlier stages may provide crucial means of interpreting nonverbal expressions of attitudes, preferences, and emotions in 'behavioral or symbolic gestures' (Snyder 1999: 10) in later stages of the disease. Even in these stages, numerous channels of communication remain open, and we are called upon to acknowledge and try to interpret these *embodied* ways of communicating (Snyder 1999: 32–3). Arguably, such embodied ways of communicating are rarely translatable into written accounts of the disease. Although the use of photography in Henderson's collaborative journal partially explores the potential of embodied expressions of feelings—such as when Henderson strokes his grandchild's head, laughs with his wife, and sits slumped at the table—written memoirs are limited in the ways they can communicate through the body and communicate embodied selfhood per se. In the next section I therefore turn to a different medium, documentary film that draws on the potential of visual and auditory modes in exploring these aspects of the phenomenology of dementia. David Sieveking's documentary *Vergiss Mein Nicht* (Forget-Me-Not) provides medium-specific affordances when it comes to representing the embodied nature of the symptoms of dementia, embodied aspects of selfhood, and embodied means of communication in dementia.

From the caregiver's perspective: intersubjectivity in David Sieveking's documentary *Vergiss Mein Nicht*

The German documentary *Vergiss Mein Nicht* (Forget-Me-Not) (Sieveking 2012) explores the way Alzheimer's changes not only the person with dementia but the entire family. David Sieveking is narrator, protagonist, and film-maker alike. The documentary was filmed—with the help of a cameraman and sound technician—during several extended periods Sieveking spent living with his parents—during which he at times took over the role of primary caregiver for his mother Gretel. The documentary, of course, represents an edited version of Gretel's life, based on decisions of how (using what camera angle, type of camera, etc.) and when to film (what stage in her life and illness, or during which activities). Further the narrative representation of events is shaped at a later stage in the editing process by the decisions of what to cut and how to frame the narrative through words and music. Nonetheless, due to its mimetic potential, the documentary provides abundant material for an investigation of the ways that dementia changes the experience of the physical and social world. I examine the portrayal of the symptoms of dementia as entry point into the documentary itself and into the broader question of how viewing a person living with the symptoms of dementia on film may be different from reading about that person in print.

In particular, the documentary opens up the possibility of representing instances of embodied communication; at issue are various forms of nonverbal communication, such as touch, gesture, facial expressions, and posture as well as the role of body movement and tone of voice in nonverbal and verbal humour. What I am calling embodied communication also includes aspects of the voice of the person, such as modulation, tone, and intonation, i.e., what linguists call paralinguistic features of communicative acts—features that help constitute the meaning of an utterance in ways that go beyond its semantic content. Documentary film provides the perhaps unique possibility, within dementia life writing, of exploring how people with dementia continue to express themselves through vocal modulations and bodily movements. As the forms of embodied communication just mentioned provide an important means of gaining access to Gretel's state of mind, a large part of this analysis will be devoted to the way the documentary represents and reflects on these means of communication.

My guiding questions here include the following: What opportunities does documentary film provide for contemplating aspects of embodied selfhood in dementia? And how do the affordances of film differ from written memoirs by people with dementia? What is left out of my analysis here is a consideration of the ethics and politics of documentary film-making since Chapters 4 and 5 deal explicitly with the problems of representing 'vulnerable subjects' (Couser 2004) in dementia life-writing. These include such issues as gaining consent or violating the person's privacy. Given the mimetic potential of the medium, all of these issues may be considered particularly salient in documentary film-making.

Viewing symptoms of dementia

As hinted at previously, the mimetic quality of filmography allows for a rich representation of the symptoms of dementia. The documentary highlights the ways that the loss of memory impacts on many areas of human functioning and experience. It is therefore even more difficult than in written memoirs to discuss distinct areas of self-experience affected by the disease. I will nevertheless attempt to draw out some of the relevant areas that the medium of film speaks to in a particular way.

For example, the documentary provides valuable insight into the complex ways that language is affected by dementia. In presenting the viewer with Gretel's speech, rather than an indirect representation of her speech—as in written caregivers' memoirs—the viewer witnesses the repetitions, non-sequiturs, and word-finding difficulties that form the symptoms of Alzheimer's disease. In the first scenes of the documentary Gretel's linguistic impairment seems to 'mark' her as a person with dementia. There is a moment of vicarious shock or empathy with the narrator figure David who is confronted with a decided change in his mother since his childhood—having just established the opening narrative opposition between 'now' and 'then' that is so typical of many caregivers' memoirs. However, as the narrative progresses, the viewer gets used to the idiosyncrasies of Gretel's speech. So rather than undermining her expressive capacity and marking her as 'demented,' the documentary illuminates the way that language is not simply lost but retains much of its communicative function throughout the course of the disease. The film shows language in context: the setting of the conversational discourse renders intelligible even language that presents syntactical or semantic errors, or lapses in coherence or cohesion.

A scene depicting Gretel undergoing neurolinguistic tests—a standard procedure in the diagnosis and tracking of the progression of dementia—highlights the extent of Gretel's semantic difficulties. More importantly, however, it underscores the degree to which such testing undermines the patient's sense of self-worth. Gretel is clearly baffled by the test procedures. She has difficulties naming the images presented to her and attempts to withdraw from the situation by closing her eyes. The scene presents one of many instances in which Gretel's body language and facial expression clearly express her feelings or attitude, here her emotional discomfort.

The documentary also reveals the many ways that bodily engagements with the world are changed in dementia—for instance, by tracking the changes in Gretel's gait. In line with Henderson's description of his attempts to 'touch base,' it seems that touching objects in her environment helps

Gretel to situate herself. So, for instance, the viewer witnesses her sliding her hand along the counter at a doctor's office as she walks along. Much later in the film, she and her husband return to Hamburg, the setting of their love story. In a shop, Gretel touches all the sweets on display. Touching seems to allow her to establish a link to the world.[20] With an understanding of how dementia impacts on habitual ways of being-in-the-world, self-referential tactile behaviour, such as grasping one's own hands or stroking one's legs, can take on a new meaning. Contrary to seeing such repetitive actions as meaningless, they suggest that the person with dementia is attempting to establish a link with the world and familiarise herself with her own body and her environment. Touch, however, as indicated by the image of Henderson stroking his grandchild, and as I suggest below in my analysis of its communicative potential, also has a relational function.

The documentary brings to the fore how sense perceptions such as taste and smell may change with Alzheimer's. In additional information on the DVD, the viewer learns that Gretel developed a culinary preference for butter in the course of her disease. In Sieveking's discussion of this preference with a gerontologist, it emerges that Gretel's 'butter-addiction' may be in line with recent scientific insights into how early memories may gain importance later in life. It has been shown that for Holocaust or Gulag survivors the motives, wants, and exigencies of this episode of their lives came to be constitutive for the way that motives and needs were structured later in life. The fact that Gretel lived through the war, during which fatty foods such as butter were a scarcity, may therefore account for her growing obsession with butter. This aspect of her conduct also attests to the subtle ways that memories may structure experience and surface in behavioural patterns. This tendency has been highlighted by people working on so-called 'challenging' behaviour in dementia, such as the clinical psychologist Graham Stokes. Stokes (2010) provides numerous narrativised case studies of how behaviour that was treated as merely pathological—and seen as 'outlandish and bizarre' (8)—could actually be attributed to individual traits or past experiences and thereby interpreted as understandable reactions to the current situation.

In filming Gretel's daily life, the documentary registers many moments of confusion. Gretel is confused about how to handle objects (such as clearing the table or dealing with dirty dishes), about the identity of the person she is with, and about recent events in her life. So, for instance, after a long car journey to Switzerland to join her husband, she seems to retain no memory of the hours just spent in the car. Further, she has trouble recognising her husband and distinguishing between her husband and son—presumably because her son had recently taken over the role of primary caregiver. Although she seems happy to be reunited with her husband, her confusion is palpable in her facial expression, tone of voice, and bodily movements.

Yet the documentary also registers moments of being-at-one-with-the-world. As in the autopathographies discussed above, such moments may involve a bodily sense of well-being or a satisfying sense of being-with another person. Gretel shows a surprising grace, joy, and fluidity when she plays ball with her adult children. Further, as I discuss below, she also shares moments of 'communion' with others, relying on embodied modes of communication.

In sum, due to its mimetic quality, documentary film can provide insight into a wide array of symptoms associated with dementia. The outside view of the camera may, however, limit an understanding of how these symptoms are experienced by the person with dementia. Insight into Gretel's state of mind can, at times, be gleaned not only from her comments but from her facial expressions, gestures, and postures. Since paralinguistic information of this sort provides such a crucial form of communication in dementia (Killick and Allan 2001)—and since the documentary captures such paralinguistic cues in a medium-specific way—I turn now to the film's treatment of nonverbal or more generally embodied communication.

The communicating body in film

In contrast to life writing by people with dementia, which is necessarily confined to the stage when the person can still tell a more or less coherent verbal narrative, documentary film-making provides the possibility of representing nonverbal means of expression at later stages in the disease. Although Sieveking's documentary is of course edited and narratively arranged, it nevertheless provides a mediated space for the presence of the person with dementia. Gretel, the film-maker's mother, is continuously on screen. Her words, gestures, expressions, and movements are thus available to the viewer—albeit at one step removed from face-to-face encounter. Given Ratcliffe's observations on how we understand other people's state of mind directly through body language and gesture (2007), documentary provides fascinating possibilities to represent the phenomenology of illness nonverbally within a narrative genre.[21]

Sieveking describes how, before the onset of his mother's illness, the family thrived on intellectual discussions. He notes how in his family, 'the word' was 'everything.'[22] This remark echoes Killick and Allan's observation that 'Sometimes it seems as if we were all living according to the slogan "Words come first!"' (44). This way of being and doing things in the world has significant impact on the perceived potential of people with dementia to express themselves, to build relationships, and to shape their environment, as the disease syndrome is linked to various forms of language impairment and the eventual loss of language itself.

One of the commonplaces in popular understandings of dementia has been that since people with dementia lose the ability to communicate, we have no way of accessing their states of mind and no way of knowing *what it is like* to be living with dementia. No doubt, language plays a crucial role in the way our species engages with and acts in the world. However, in overstating the role of language, or rather in underestimating the contribution of nonverbal behaviour to interaction, we risk missing the continuing expressive potential of people with dementia. Shaun Gallagher and Dan Zahavi, point out that 'we can perceive the joy, sadness, puzzlement, eagerness of others ... in their movements, gestures, facial expressions and actions' (Gallagher and Zahavi 2008: 182). Contrary to mentalizing accounts of intersubjectivity, they hold that we gain access to other people's minds through perceiving their bodies in a situation or meaningful context (183). Accordingly, 'we experience the other directly as a person, an intentional being whose *bodily gestures and actions* are *expressive* of his or her *experiences or states of mind*' (183; emphasis added).

Sieveking's documentary highlights the expressive potential of people with dementia in two ways. First, by portraying how Gretel communicates through and with her body, the film draws the viewer's attention to the potential of embodied communication in people with dementia. Second, the narrative also traces how the experience of living and communicating with somebody who has dementia brings about a sea-change in the way family members relate to each other. As Sieveking describes it, they learn to relish the potential of touch and physical intimacy, not only in relation to Gretel but also to each other. Sieveking appreciates that through her new way of being-in-the-world his mother was able to teach him a valuable life lesson. Sieveking's father similarly highlights a positive side to his wife's illness since, as he puts it, it allowed him to rediscover his love for her.[23] The Sievekings are not alone in seeing dementia as a context for growth and learning, as the words of Michael Ignatieff, author of the novel *Scar Tissue*, confirm:

> I learned as much from my mother when she couldn't speak to me, when she couldn't communicate, when she simply stared and received our kisses on the cheek, as I learned when she was joking and laughing.
> (Ignatieff 1994, qtd. in Killick and Allan 2001: 52)

Yet contrary to Ignatieff's view that not speaking equals not communicating, Sieveking's documentary draws out many ways that communication is nonverbal. This is not to say that verbal and nonverbal communication are in opposition to each other: 'Although there are forms of nonverbal communication which do not involve words at all, in the majority of instances the two dimensions are intimately intertwined,' Killick and Allan write. 'Facial expression, qualities of voice, and gestures help the listener to decode and interpret words' (Killick and Allan 2001: 45). In language use generally, as in dementia, verbal and nonverbal cues act together to convey the full meaning of an utterance or gesture.

Killick and Allan speculate whether language impairment leads people with dementia to develop a keener sense for engaging in and interpreting nonverbal modes of communication. This hypothesis is corroborated by people with dementia who describe how they have to rely on nonverbal cues to make sense of what others say. Gretel's keen attunement to nonverbal cues and the emotional gist of a conversation comes out in a scene where her husband Malte recounts a quarrel with his wife's professional caregiver, Valentina. Although Gretel may not be able to follow the details of the narrative, she is clearly aware of its unpleasant nature and that it relates to her. Furthermore, her partial understanding seems to make her feel responsible for the situation. Her worried look and her query 'What did I do?'[24] indicate her concern. The scene provides a poignant reminder to caregivers not to assume that people with dementia are oblivious to what is going on around them and that they no longer closely monitor what is said in their presence. As this example highlights, the remaining capacity for understanding can lead to unnecessary negative emotions, a sense of misplaced responsibility, shame, or anxiety.

Through her bodily movements, postures, and gestures, Gretel clearly expresses feelings of distress, fear, or hurt—such as her sense of abandonment when her husband leaves her at the train station, leading her to turn away and avoid his goodbye kiss [22: 48]. However, her bodily movements also express her joy—as when she throws up her hands in greeting her older sister Ise. She reaches out to others, appreciates physical intimacy, wants to hold hands, and happily links arms with her caregiver Valentina. As Killick and Allan (2001) note,

> the potential of touch in enhancing well-being and promoting communication with people with dementia has yet to be explored properly. Most of us feel comforted and affirmed by touch which is employed in a respectful way, and for those with the condition it could make all the difference between being able to remain in meaningful contact with others, and losing a sense of connectedness.
>
> (63)

Touch, the documentary suggests, plays an ever-growing role in dementia: as a form of communication and therefore as a means to maintain relationships.

As many memoirs about dementia indicate, humour remains a crucial means of communicating in the context of dementia. Seeing the funny side of certain situations can help alleviate the stress of dealing with the symptoms of dementia, both for caregiver and care-receiver. Humorous exchanges, as John Bayley (1999) recounts in the memoir of his wife Iris Murdoch's dementia, remain possible when intellectual discussion no longer is. The sharing of laughter, then, is both a means of communication and of maintaining relationships. Gretel signals the humorous intent of her words through facial expressions, such as playfully lifting her eyebrows, as well as through her intonation and the modulations of her voice. On their drive through Switzerland, Gretel and her son David pass 'Die Jungfrau,' a famous mountain named 'the virgin.' After the name has been pointed out to her, Gretel quips: 'And who was that? Well it wasn't me, not *me*, for sure.'[25] She places unnatural stress on the 'me' ('ich' in the original) to highlight that by no means could she have been called a virgin. Tone of voice, intonation, bodily language, and facial expression all work together to communicate her humorous intent. Most instances of Gretel's humorous engagements with others do have a strong verbal content. Yet Killick and Allan, in their work on communicating with people with dementia, also point to the importance of humour based on bodily movements. They highlight that 'much of what occasions smiling, and even outright laughter, appears to come out of relationship' and they argue that by paying attention to the comical exchanges between people with dementia 'we can learn to encourage our own moments of sharing in the sheer fun of existence, often without a word being spoken' (Killick and Allan 2001: 57). Humour, like touch, can provide an important means of being-with and building a relationship with people with dementia. Both remain, also, ways in which people with dementia can reach out to others and express their subjectivity.

Embodied selves and relational selves

In its mimetic portrayal of living bodies, *Vergiss Mein Nicht* provides particularly rich examples of forms of embodied selfhood. In one sense, the continuing presence of Gretel on the screen as a living body, a unit of identity, strongly discourages viewing her as a non-person, as someone who has 'lost her self.' The documentary allows the viewer to get to know Gretel as a person; she is a person undergoing dramatic changes, but all her potential as human being and her unique subjectivity remain intact. The film also reaffirms the common-sense notion of identity that we operate with in everyday life, which is based on the identity of a living body over time. No philosophical concept of identity has ever been able to resolve the paradox between identity and change that living beings present. Gretel's body persists and so does Gretel. While aspects of her social identity—her roles or *personae*—change, at no point in the course of her illness does she cease to be herself.

A key aspect of her embodied identity, as represented in the documentary, is her unique voice. While autobiographies by people with dementia focus on the political notion of voice, in the sense of giving voice to a disadvantaged or stigmatised group, here 'voice' represents Gretel's unique personality in its embodied, literal sense. Her tone of voice, the use of intonation and modulation to convey humour or distress, as well as dialectal influences on her speech all attest to her unique personality. So, for instance, dialectal influences resurface when she returns to her hometown, Stuttgart, and talks to her sister, a strong dialect speaker. The shift to the phonetic variations of the Swabian dialect can be seen as a form of embodied autobiographical memory, that is, a procedural memory from a former period in her life. However, this shift is also, significantly, a marker of relationship. Dialect speakers will often revert to their dialect when speaking to close family or old friends, even if they otherwise predominantly speak a standard variant of the language. Gretel's shift marks her sense of belonging in relation to her sister. Indeed, Gretel's appreciation of relationships, in her nonverbal gestures, touch, and verbal expressions, may be seen as a pervasive and important aspect of her continuing selfhood.

The documentary also highlights Gretel's appreciation of physical pleasures, such as eating butter, enjoying a waffle, or smacking her lips when drinking a glass of wine. Furthermore, playing ball, going for walks, or listening to music provide moments of engagement with the world through her body and her senses. Some of these may be new developments, some draw on long-term procedural memories or previous habits and preferences, and some may not persist into the later stages of the disease. Nevertheless, these actions on Gretel's part highlight the bodily and social resources of positive experiences of being-in-the-world that do not rely on higher-order cognitive functioning. As Murna Downs, caregiver and professor in dementia studies, puts it,

> I am not so sure that I would hope for a world without dementia, for in a world without dementia we would be without the ones we love who have taught us that remembering and planning and naming and knowing are not the key human activities, but rather that feeling and being and touching and singing have enormous riches and depths that we are often too busy to relish in our race to rationality.
> (Downs 2000, qtd. in Killick and Allan 2001: 62)

Human activity, as Downs highlights, is embodied, sensual, and vocal. People with dementia, against popular perception, retain numerous means of engaging in human activities with others.

The documentary also suggests that we understand embodied selfhood not merely as residual body memories that represent core characteristics of the person's previous identity (such as Kontos's examples of someone still being able to read the Torah or of making knitting movements). The film highlights how important it is to recognise the embodied nature of selfhood in terms of the continuing presence of an inner life world which relies on a continuing first-personal givenness of the world. Gretel's inner life world is continuously revealed through her verbal expressions, facial expressions, gesture, and posture. Furthermore, by drawing on Millett's adaptation of the notion of ecological niche value, one can argue that the film represents a woman who, despite language difficulties and the growing inability to navigate the world, retains the potential for mutual relationships with other people. Her cognitive disabilities challenge her family to develop new, and at times more intimate, ways of being together.

The film also underscores that Sieveking's changing relationship with Gretel is not one-sided, based purely on catering to her disabilities, but reciprocal. Too often, a person with dementia is no longer seen for themselves but becomes 'a bundle of needs'—representing a 'burden' for the caregiver. The film underscores Gretel's potential to 'give back' in a relationship. So, for instance, in a scene where David has clearly reached the end of his tether in terms of trying to get her to co-operate in necessary activities of daily living (such as going shopping), Gretel's refusal and withdrawal suddenly turn to concern for her son. She opens her eyes to ask him how *he* is doing. When he replies that he is not doing too great, she asks why and then immediately goes on to try and cheer him up and enlist *him* in a joint activity—in this case a trip to her home town, Stuttgart. The scene underscores that people with dementia may often 'develop an especially sensitive facility for reading information which comes through nonverbal channels' (Killick and Allan 2001: 63), given that Gretel's concern is a reaction to David's tone of voice and posture. It also underscores that people with dementia remain relational agents and are able to show concern and love for others, not just the passive recipients of care. Even in the last scenes of the film that were shot close to her death, this dynamic persists. The film movingly closes with Gretel's radiant smile as her husband and son join her at her bedside. Her joyful reaction highlights her continuing recognition of these people as all important to her.

In short, the documentary provides unique ways of conceptualising embodied selfhood in dementia, for representing the embodied experience of living with dementia, and for exploring the many forms of embodied communication that remain available to people with dementia across the course of the disease syndrome. In showing how relationships remains reciprocal and how dementia can stimulate positive change and growth within familial caregiving relationships, this documentary, as Zimmermann also notes, 'challenges the general public as well as the medico-clinical researcher to reconsider their conceptualisation of the condition as one of decline and loss alone' (Zimmermann 2017: 127).

Conclusion

Non-fictional dementia narratives, in the form of autobiographical writing and documentary film, are a powerful means of evoking the changing life world of the person with dementia. The authors of first-person accounts illuminate how dementia influences their emotions and cognition, and with it, their very sense of self. Furthermore, they describe how symptoms of dementia impact on their ability to interact with the world, while also highlighting the many ways that they continue to take pleasure in their life and experience moments of feeling at one with the social and natural world. The narratives attest to the fact that we do not *have* a body but *are* a body (Carel 2008); the changes illness works in our bodies significantly alter our way of being-in-the-world, and ultimately our sense of self. Life narratives by people with dementia record these changes and the complex ways that body, self, and environment interact. Due to the nature of their production and the specific constraints of the genre they adhere to, the narratives cannot, however, address the phenomenology of dementia in the later stages of the disease. While some of the authors cling to a narrative self and fear that there will be nothing left once the ability to speak and remember has left them, others take a more optimistic view of the continuing ability to flourish and live a meaningful live. They challenge their readers to support people with dementia rather than succumb to the notion that nothing can be done to improve the lives of people with progressive neurological conditions.

Caregivers' memoirs may be considered to provide equally rich accounts of the changes brought about by dementia. However, due to their outside view, they may not provide the same kind of access to the phenomenology of dementia that life writing by those affected can. They are also more likely to focus on narratives of loss and the burden of caregiving than first-person accounts by people with dementia. Nevertheless, despite taking on an outside perspective, the emergence of caregivers' life writing that draws on visual media, such as graphic memoir[26] and film, speaks in illuminating ways to questions of embodiment. Here Sieveking's documentary serves as a counterpoint to the written autopathographies. The audiovisual representation allows for detailed accounts of the embodied nature of the disease. More importantly, perhaps, the documentary underscores the potential for embodied communication and the persistence of forms of embodied selfhood in dementia. While I am not suggesting that these are entirely outside the reach of written memoirs, documentary film provides medium-specific ways of conceptualising selfhood in dementia: (1) the body functions as indicator of remaining selfhood that is recognised by others; (2) bodily expressions suggest an inner life world and the persistence of a first-personal perspective in dementia—as expressed through embodied communication; and (3) this form of communication also highlights the persisting capacity for mutual relationships in dementia.

Life writing about dementia also raises theoretical and ethical questions, however. How do people with Alzheimer's, for instance, engage cultural scripts in their autopathographies to counter dominant notions of people with dementia as 'living dead?' And what textual, technical, or relational strategies can these authors use to extend their capacity to voice their experience (beyond the stage in their disease in which they can remember their life in detail, type, handwrite, or otherwise create coherent narratives)? How can people from less advantaged backgrounds—whether socioeconomic, educational, or in relation to their disease progression—tell about their experience of dementia? What risks are inherent in collaborative storytelling, in terms of patronising, exposing, over-editing, or otherwise misrepresenting the person with dementia?

Caregivers' memoirs and documentaries raise similar concerns with regard to the power relation between the person with dementia and the person in charge of shaping the narrative: what ethical issues are at stake, for instance, in representing persons who can no longer challenge the way they are represented, or provide meaningful consent to being involved as primary 'object' in a documentary film? Part II of this study addresses these issues with regard to autopathographies and collaborative life writing in Chapter 3 and caregivers' life writing in Chapter 4, respectively. That is, part II turns more squarely to the aesthetic, ethical, and philosophical implications of dementia life writing.

The present chapter, instead, pursued an agenda typical of first-wave medical humanities research: that is, of demonstrating that life writing both by people with dementia and by their caregivers provides a rich resource to consider the question of what it's like to be living with dementia. Grounded in first-hand experience, these texts speak from a position of experiential authority. Importantly, first-person accounts by people with dementia position their authors as 'experts from experience' (Whitman 2016) that may challenge the at times erroneous 'expert' knowledge propounded by health-care professionals. However, autopathographies in particular are also limited by their mode of production in relying on written discourse. Due to the nature of the disease syndrome and the limits it places on communicating complex thoughts and emotions, the forms of life writing discussed here may not be able to evoke a sense of what it's like for the person to experience more severe symptoms of dementia.

It has been commonplace in first-wave medical humanities to consider *fictional* illness narratives rich resources for care professionals to engage with the life world of illness and to expand their (necessarily) limited biomedical view of a given disease. Indeed, reading fictional narratives is considered a means to improve the quality of care and promote more empathetic healthcare professionals (Charon 2006). In the next chapter, accordingly, I turn from life writing to fiction, in order to explore how fictional narratives may simulate the experience of dementia. In the process, I investigate the question of how literary representations of dementia shape our understanding of the condition, what textual strategies are employed to simulate an inside view of dementia and evoke narrative empathy, and what role empathy may play in developing dementia-friendly care. In the process, I challenge the view that reading fictional dementia narratives can lead in any direct way to pro-social action and that literature necessarily acts as a 'tool for the good,' whether in the context of the medical humanities or in society more generally.

Notes

1 The term 'phenomenology' is frequently used to describe first-person accounts of 'what it is like' to have a certain experience. This usage differs from the technical usage which describes a philosophical discipline that aims to discover the underlying structures that make it possible to experience the world (Gallagher and Zahavi 2008: 10, 20, 26). I use phenomenology both in the non-technical sense, when referring to the description of *qualia* or 'what it is like' (Nagel 1974), and in the narrower, philosophical sense, when focusing on structures of

experience that are relevant to understanding dementia but that may be masked by approaches that rely on dualistic views of mind-body and self-world.
2 For further documentaries on dementia that present a range of different styles see *Complaints of A Dutiful Daughter* (Hoffmann 1994), *First Cousin Once Removed* (Berliner 2012), and *Glen Campbell: I'll Be Me* (Albert and Keach 2014).
3 Davis (2004) emphasises loss of self to legitimate family caregivers' grief.
4 These terms represent different points on what could be considered a continuum on notions of 'selfhood,' ranging from (social) identity to (perspectival) self. While I discuss notions of selfhood and identity across this range of meanings, I make no hard and fast distinctions among the terms.
5 Recent neuroscientific studies reveal the extent to which emotions are a function of the brain and therefore also prone to be affected by brain damage or disease (Damasio 1994, 2000, 2010).
6 I understand this term to refer to the fact that humans are relational beings—constituted by their relations but also endowed with the capacity for relationships. This notion has gained currency in a range of disciplines and under a number of guises. Relational models of identity have also figured importantly in life writing studies (Eakin 1998, Friedman 1988, Henry 2006, Mason 1980, Miller 1994, Smith and Watson 2010).
7 Apart from Alzheimer's disease, some of the authors were diagnosed with multi-infarct dementia, Lewy body dementia, frontotemporal dementia, or a combination of these. What unites these authors is that the condition manifested itself early in life (before the age of 65).
8 The number of dementia blogs is too vast to list. Morris Friedell's blog had a significant impact on patient advocacy in the 1990s and early 2000s and can still be found at http://morrisfriedell.com/struggle1.html. Similarly, Taylor's collection of essays was first published as blog at www.richardtaylorphd.com/blog.html. An example of a blog by a person with Lewy body dementia can be found at http://parkblog-silverfox.blogspot.co.uk/. Wendy Mitchell's blog continues after her memoir was published in 2018: https://whichmeamitoday.wordpress.com. Kate Swaffer's blog https://kateswaffer.com/daily-blog/ provides a forum for the Australian and global dementia advocacy movement.
9 These include Bryden (1998, 2005, 2015, 2018), Couturier (2004), Davis (1989), DeBaggio (2002, 2003), Donohue (2009), Graboys and Zheutlin (2008), Henderson (1998), Lee (2003), Mobley (2007), McGowin (1994), Mitchell (2018), Rohra (2011), Rose (1996, 2003), Schneider (2006), Swaffer (2016), and Taylor (2007).
10 Although Lucy Whitman's collection of personal stories by people with dementia *People with Dementia Speak Out* (2016) is more diverse in terms of age and ethnicity, she regrets not having been able to include authors from the LGBT (Lesbian, Gay, Bisexual, Transgender) community. In an appendix, she highlights the particular stigma and recurring experiences of discrimination—including in care settings—that people from the LGBT community face and she stresses the need to address the specific care requirements of this group (2016: 289–90).
11 See the discussion in Ratcliffe (2007: 107).
12 The term 'enacts' is not strictly speaking correct since these are still instances of mimetic verbal representations. In using this term, I mean to highlight the immediacy of the account and the lack of retrospective summary in representing symptoms. Basting (2001) similarly uses the term 'performance' to call attention to this effect.
13 The recent dementia diaries project—audio diaries that are shared on the website https://dementiadiaries.org/—offers another means to allow self-expression and communication in dementia without placing storytellers under the constraints of mainstream publishing.

14 See Ratcliffe (2008) on shifts in 'existential feelings' in psychiatric illness.
15 The discrepancy between narrative voice and narrative experience is noticeable here. It is not clear to what extent this episode is something DeBaggio remembers, from an inside perspective, or presents a reconstructed account of events, based on information provided by his wife.
16 www.st-andrews.ac.uk/psychology/people/pgprofiles/kma2/. Last accessed 31.03.2015.
17 Compare Heidegger's distinction (1962) between objects being 'present-at-hand' (*Vorhanden*) versus 'ready-to-hand' (*Zuhanden*). Objects usually present themselves to us as 'ready-to-hand.' Standard examples include the use of a keyboard or of a tool: we do not 'encounter' them as objects distinct from our activity, but instead they are bound up in our activity and typically they come to our conscious awareness as 'present-at-hand' objects only when they fail to function and therefore become conspicuous (Ratcliffe 2008: 44, 45).
18 Truscott (2004a) elaborates ways to achieve such flow in her autobiographical journal article.
19 Compare, in this connection, research into animal-assisted therapy in dementia (see Marx et al. 2010).
20 It is not incidental that the verb 'to grasp'—to understand the meaning of something—is a metaphorical extension of our haptic potential for holding an object. See also Lakoff and Johnson (2003) on the bodily substrates for metaphors that form the basis of everyday language.
21 Fiction films provide similar affordances. See Chapter 2.
22 Sieveking states 'Alles ging über's Wort' in an interview contained in the additional material on the DVD (see 'Potsdamer Filmgespräch mit Andreas Dresen'). All translations are my own.
23 'Ich bin der Demenz eigentlich dankbar dass ich die Liebe zu meiner Frau noch einmal neu entdecken konnte', as quoted by David Sieveking (see 'Potsdamer Filmgespräch mit Andreas Dresen').
24 'Was hab ich gemacht?' [1:20:28].
25 'Oh, und wer war das zum Beispiel? Ich war's nicht. *Ich* war's nicht' [42:08].
26 See Chapters 4 and 5.

2 From the outside in? Experience and empathy in fictional dementia narratives

Dementia is often positioned as a disease that 'we,' people not affected by the disease, can know nothing about. The previous chapter has demonstrated that despite increasing cognitive and linguistic challenges a growing number of people with dementia have been able to share their experience of living with the syndrome through blogs, published memoirs, and other forms of autobiographical writing. The chapter also foregrounded the potential of certain forms of life writing, such as documentary film, to highlight that even in later stages of the disease people with dementia remain intentional beings able to communicate their feelings through embodied communication—posture, gesture, facial expressions, and paralinguistics features such as pitch and tone of voice. Nonetheless, the progression of symptoms of dementia makes the communication of the disease experience through language and especially through conventional forms of life writing increasingly difficult. The present chapter asks what fictional narratives may contribute to an understanding of what it's like to be living with dementia (see also Bitenc 2012).

It is a commonplace of narrative theory that fiction provides the rare opportunity to inhabit another person's mind (see Cohn 1978, Herman 2011, Palmer 2004). Patricia Waugh suggests that fiction can convey 'what it feels like to be alive' (Waugh 2013: 24). Indeed, she suggests that 'to the extent that the novel creates a pre-reflective place which positions embodied minds in imaginary worlds and confers on them depth and thickness, we might think of it as the practical counterpart of theoretical phenomenology' (2013: 24). Rita Felski similarly speaks of novels as providing a form of 'social phenomenology' (2008: 89). She argues that through the technique of 'deep intersubjectivity'—a term borrowed from George Butte—readers 'come to know something of what it feels like to be inside a particular habitus, to experience a world as self-evident' (2008: 92). In evoking detailed storyworlds, both novels and films provide the possibility of exploring the experience of living with dementia within a particular physical environment and sociocultural context. Fictional films and novels may, I argue, be thought of as a form of *imaginative phenomenology*.

Furthermore, this chapter considers how, by simulating the experience of dementia, fictional narratives may elicit an empathetic engagement with the progressively impaired protagonist. Novels, it has been argued, elicit empathy for characters by promoting character identification and allowing readers to share a character's point of view. Martha Nussbaum defends the view that by evoking empathy for characters outside one's moral sphere, fictional narratives may promote global citizenship (Nussbaum 1997). In a similar vein, Rita Charon argues that novel reading plays a crucial role in expanding health-care professionals' ability to empathise with and acknowledge the pain of their patients (Charon 2006: 233).

However, Suzanne Keen, leading scholar on narrative empathy, challenges this so-called 'empathy-altruism hypothesis' (Keen 2007) according to which empathy with fictional characters leads to pro-social action towards real-life others. Keen also complicates the notion that narrative empathy is simply created by alignment of point of view. Empathic concern, instead, depends on a number of textual characteristics as well as the reader's personal traits and preferences. Keen's study nonetheless underlines that narrative empathy constitutes a robust element of the experience of novel reading. She explores the ways in which narrative empathy is evoked and how it is put to strategic use. Overall Keen's work exemplifies the value of exploring the formal means by which literary works arouse narrative empathy while remaining cautious about advancing overextended claims concerning narrative empathy's effects in the socio-ethical domain.

Based on my own corpus of fictional dementia narratives, I argue that further refinements in the theory of narrative empathy are called for if narrative empathy is to capture the full range of storytelling practices. What is needed is an even more nuanced understanding of the spectrum of empathic reading experiences. While I agree with Keen on the previously mentioned points, I demonstrate how a bottom-up approach, one that considers fictional accounts of the experience of dementia, may diversify the notion of narrative empathy. Further, a more fine-grained account of the working of narrative empathy has implications for debates about the value accorded to empathy in medical humanities research and education. Critically examining how empathy works and what work it does in the political and social domain seriously undermines the notion that empathy is necessarily a tool for the good (see also Whitehead 2017). On the contrary, as literary scholar Anne Whitehead argues, empathy is always already implicated in structures of power and privilege. Indeed, rather than acting as a sufficient condition for altruistic behaviour, it might equally act as mode of voyeurism or appropriation (Whitehead 2017: 60).

This chapter addresses how fictional dementia narratives, then, may simulate the experience of living with dementia and evoke narrative empathy. Further, it asks what role narrative empathy may play in developing dementia care. As a route into these questions I consider the dementia narrative *Still Alice*, comparing the novel by Lisa Genova (2007) with its film adaptation

(Glatzer and Westmoreland 2014).[1] I ask whether narrative empathy in films, as has been argued for novels, depends on seeing the world through the protagonist's eyes, and what distinct affordances for the arousal of empathy and for exploring the experience of dementia each medium provides.

After engaging with these questions, I investigate how experimentation with literary form may expand the limits of representing the symptoms of dementia in textual narratives. Recent criticism of the use of narrative to communicate illness experience often depends on a notion of narrative as linear, plot-driven, and tending towards closure (see Woods 2011). However, fictional dementia narratives range from linear and plot-driven to more experimental, less coherent and more lyrical modes of representation. I address how more experimental texts may contribute to the current theory of narrative empathy via the progressively impaired and partially unreliable narrator in J. Bernlef's *Out of Mind* (1988) as well as the configuration of multiple interior monologues in the stream of consciousness style used by B. S. Johnson in *House Mother Normal* ([1971] 2013). Then, in the concluding section of the chapter, I discuss the effect of narratives which do not explicitly thematise dementia but may nonetheless be read through the lens of neurodegenerative decline. To this end, I argue that Kazuo Ishiguro's novel *The Unconsoled* (1995), although not explicitly labelled and marketed as 'dementia narrative,' may be productively read as an exploration of the phenomenology of dementia. More specifically, I suggest that this novel's manifold textual ambiguities afford opportunities for empathetic engagement through 'parallel experience' (Toker 1993). I suggest too that the novel's resistance to being fully 'naturalised' as a dementia narrative in fact opens up the possibility for the reader to come close to the existential uncertainty that living with dementia entails. In a condition like dementia, where those affected may at some stage no longer be able to articulate what it is like to be living with this disease, works of fiction like Ishiguro's may afford special insights into what it's like to have or experience this illness.

Still Alice: from fiction to film

Still Alice tells the story of 50-year-old cognitive psychology professor Alice Howland who, in mid-career, is diagnosed with early-onset Alzheimer's disease. The narrative explores the link between neurons, memory, and identity. Further, the narrative hones in on how the social world of a person with early-onset Alzheimer's changes: how the disease alters and inverts both professional and personal relationships, and how the entire family is affected by the onset and progress of the disease. Yet contrary to many earlier dementia narratives, *Still Alice*—both in the novel and in the film version—does not focus on the experience of the people *surrounding* the person with dementia. Although the novel uses a third-person narrator,[2] events are largely focalised[3] through Alice. Hence, the symptoms—such as night-time wandering, confusion, or misinterpretations of reality—are viewed through her eyes and mind.

Due to the use of focalisation, Alice's symptoms enter into the composition of the narrative discourse. For instance, when Alice's thoughts begin to circle around, the narrative mirrors this symptom with almost verbatim repetitions of her thought processes. Yet the reader, briefed by the dust jacket and the prologue, has a better awareness of what is happening than the experiencing protagonist. This set-up frequently leads to instances of dramatic irony, where the reader knows things in excess of what the character knows. Such irony, however, limits the potential of the novel to portray an inside view of living with dementia. The evocation of 'parallel experience,' whereby readers are placed in an 'intellectual predicament analogous to that of the characters' (Toker 1993: 4), is restricted to only very brief moments of confusion, when there is a lack of information about some aspect of the storyworld. Such moments are usually resolved quickly. Generally, Genova uses detailed descriptions of contexts and characters to allow the reader to infer events or to identify characters, even when Alice no longer recognises them.

That said, parallel experience—or feeling 'as' the character does—may not be necessary in order for the reader to feel 'with' and 'for' Alice. Even though the novel does not elicit the *same* mental confusion in the reader as Alice experiences, it nonetheless presents a rich account of how the life world of the person with dementia changes. Seeing and experiencing these changes from Alice's point of view, and being privy to her thoughts and emotions, highlight the psychological impact these changes have on her sense of self and self-esteem. The use of internal focalisation raises the reader's awareness of some of the degrading and painful aspects of living with dementia: the hurt inflicted at being ostracised by her former colleagues and the emotional pain of witnessing her husband's growing estrangement from her, the deflating experience of neuropsychological testing or of being patronised by others, and the despair at losing control over her bladder and her words. Indeed, the double perspective of seeing with but also knowing more than the protagonist allows for readers to engage with the character with dementia while remaining aware of their own perspective. We are offered a certain degree of (imaginative) insight into what it feels like to have dementia, and yet we are the non-dementing other(s) ready to identify also with Alice's family, friends, and colleagues. Thus, we are offered an insight into how 'our' behaviour is perceived, critically at times, by the person with dementia (see Bitenc 2012: 315).

The theory of narrative empathy needs to address this double perspective. Rather than defining empathy strictly as the experience of sharing the *same* feelings as the character, the dual perspective that reading narrative fiction evokes may elicit feelings of sympathy, pity, or compassion on behalf of the character. Keen, in her study of narrative empathy, acknowledges that the term empathy is frequently used synonymously to sympathy; but she argues for a stricter definition of empathy as a 'vicarious, spontaneous sharing of affect' (Keen 2007: 4) in which 'we feel what we believe to be the emotion of others' (5). That is, she distinguishes between 'I feel your pain' as an example of empathy, and 'I feel pity for your pain' as an example of sympathy, or 'empathic concern' (4; 5). Despite this initial distinction, however, her account frequently conflates the stricter sense of empathy with a broader understanding of the term.

More generally, the current definition of narrative empathy lacks the necessary precision to disentangle the subject position of the empathiser from the 'object' of empathy. As hinted at in my formulation above, I suggest that the stricter notion of empathy may be better defined as feeling 'as' rather than feeling 'with' the character. Such experiences of 'feeling (exactly) as' another are very rare—if not impossible, since we always experience the world from our first-personal perspective on the world. As Meretoja argues, 'We always engage with other perspectives from within the horizon of our own life history, our own values, belief, commitments, and attachments' (2018: 130). If this aspect has been disregarded in discussing narrative immersion, so has it in the context of developing a theory of narrative empathy. While it is debatable, whether narrative fiction can create the possibility of feeling *as* another, feeling 'with' or 'for' a character—and here I would use the terms sympathy, pity, and compassion, despite their current unfashionableness—is certainly a pervasive element of reading fiction. These terms register how readers necessarily inhabit both their own subject position and that of the imagined other. Since empathy is the accepted term to discuss these types of reader emotions with regard to fictional characters, I retain it in my discussion. Nevertheless, I attempt to clarify when a textual strategy or filmic technique elicits empathy as synonymous with sympathy and when it is more likely to provoke an experience of 'feeling as' the character, roughly in line with Toker's notion of parallel experience— that is, where the narrative discourse is organised in such a way as to evoke a similar cognitive and emotional experience in the reader as that of the character. Toker's emphasis on cognitive experiences is crucial to considering the use of narrative empathy in narratives concerned with representing neurodegenerative decline. Are we made to feel (confusion, disorientation, and panic) as the character does, or are we, primarily made to feel pity for the character's situation? At the same time, Toker's concept highlights that the current theory of narrative empathy needs to address the wide spectrum of emotions and states of consciousness that literary narratives evoke.

Both the film and novel represent a wide array of experiences of living with dementia. In comparing the two versions, I focus on select examples that illustrate some of the parallels and the contrasts between the textual and the audiovisual medium. Overall, the 2014 film adaptation of *Still Alice* remains remarkably close to the original text. Some minor changes and a number of omissions—necessitated by turning a 300-page novel into a 90-minute film—do not significantly alter the text's main storyline or its key thematic concerns. What is more, as shown by additional material on the DVD, the producers and director seem to share Genova's concern with presenting the story from Alice's point of view. The novel allows insight into Alice's thoughts through frequent use of free indirect discourse and direct thought representation. Short of using either a narrative voice-over to communicate her thought processes or filming all scenes as if from Alice's eyeline, there is no obvious one-to-one method of transposing the novel's 'inside view' to film. Granted, the film does use a number of over-the-shoulder-shots, which roughly align the viewer with the protagonist's perspective; yet it largely employs medium-distance shots of Alice. We do not literally inhabit Alice's point of view, but instead read her mind and emotions through close scrutiny of her body language, facial expression, or tone of voice. This occurs much in the same way as we read other people's thoughts, intentions, or emotions in real life, according to contemporary phenomenologists. The use of close-ups or portrait position in moments of emotional intensity allows the viewer the close scrutiny of her facial expressions and gestures. So, for instance, during a visit to her neurologist, the camera rests on Alice throughout the entire dialogue. The neurologist's voice comes from off-screen, compelling the viewer to focus on the impact that his words have on Alice. We discern how the questions of the Mini-Mental State Examination (such as, 'Where are we?' 'What day is it?') seem laughable or demeaning to Alice. We also read in her face her embarrassment at being asked to bring someone with her to all subsequent appointments. In the novel, these thoughts and feelings are verbalised, but the visual representation is no less effective.

If we consider recent research on mirror neurons, and Keen's exploration of motor mimicry as a basic form of empathy, we can also see why film may evoke strong emotions in the viewer.[4] Witnessing Alice's struggle, as she has to inform her three children that early-onset Alzheimer's is genetic and that they have a 50 percent chance of inheriting the disease, is heart-rending. Similarly, her daughter Lydia's pained reaction, as she realises that her mother has just failed to recognise her for the first time, may evoke a strong emotional reaction in the viewer, resulting in empathy not only for Alice's plight but for the ways others are affected by her disease.

Nevertheless, while adept at evoking empathetic concern in the viewer, there are instances where the film seems less effective at portraying an inside experience of the disease than the novel. For example, when Alice loses her bearings while running a familiar route, the film employs a number of techniques to evoke a sense of this experience: the camera lens goes out of focus, the music soundtrack becomes eerie and discordant, and the sound of Alice's breathing comes to the foreground in order to communicate her panic (10:05). However, the sense of being lost—recognising individual buildings but not being able to place them in relation to a mental map—is not very effectively evoked by this representation. The lack of focus in the visual field of the camera is more evocative of vertigo than of the feeling of being lost.

And, compared to the novel, the lasting emotional impact of the experience, even after Alice has recovered her bearings, is glossed over.

The novel is also more effective in simulating how Alice becomes lost in time. As described in the previous chapter, one of the challenges of dementia is that, as recent memories become affected, people with dementia may come to live in multiple, competing time frames. Here the novel's use of thought representation is particularly salient. Thus, at one point the narrator reports Alice's thought that *'Anne's going to be so jealous'* (282; original emphasis) when, in fact, her sister Anne has been dead for thirty years, thereby signalling that Alice is experiencing life through her childhood time frame. In returning to her childhood, Alice cannot yet know that her mother and sister died in a car crash in her college years. When confronted with their death anew, she re-experiences her initial despair and sense of loss. Significantly, this confrontation with what to her is a new piece of information is also one of the instances that suggest that Alice's differing view of reality may lead to paranoia:

> John stood over them, drenched.
> "What happened?"
> "She was asking for Anne. She thinks they just died."
> He held her head in his hands. He was talking to her, trying to calm her down. *Why isn't he upset, too? He's known about this for a while; that's why, and he's been keeping it from me.* She couldn't trust him.
> (Genova 2007: 156; original emphasis)

While the novel does not explore the problem of paranoia further, it raises the issue of how to deal with situations when the perception of reality between the person with dementia and family caregivers diverges. The question arises as to whether to 'go along' with delusions, misconceptions, or confabulated memories or whether to confront the person with dementia with the caregiver's view of reality. Validation therapy, as developed by Naomi Feil (1989, 1992), argues we should acknowledge and validate the point of view and emotions of the person with dementia. However, this may not always be a straightforward possibility and may, when validating confabulated traumatic events, even be harmful, as Sue Miller suggests in her memoir of her father's dementia (2003). *Still Alice* validates the perspective of the person with dementia by foregrounding her point of view above all others. The novel thereby makes the emotional reactions of a person with dementia understandable. Genova's strategy here could be described in Keen's terms as either 'ambassadorial strategic empathy' or 'broadcast strategic empathy' in that its calls upon readers not affected by dementia 'to feel with members of a group [here: early-onset Alzheimer's patients], by emphasizing common vulnerabilities and hopes through universalizing representations' (Keen 2007: xiv). Most people, at some point in their life, lose a family member.

By highlighting how Alice experiences the concomitant feelings of despair afresh due to her memory disorder, readers may come to feel sympathy for her pain, rather than dismissing it as delusional. However, the novel also pinpoints the difficulties of finding common ground in such cases of diverging realities. In this example, for instance, it may be impossible for Alice's husband John to experience, or convincingly feign, sorrow at an event that happened three decades earlier. It remains an open question as to how to respond to the divergent perceptions of a person with dementia; what this novel does suggest is that people with dementia remain 'semiotic subjects' (Sabat and Harré 1994) and that their views and perceptions should be taken into account and met with respect.

At the same time, there are aspects of the filmic representation that, arguably, go beyond the limitations of novels. For example, the film portrays the extent to which the physical capabilities of a person with Alzheimer's are affected by the disease. We witness, for instance, how Alice eventually requires help getting dressed, since she is no longer capable of planning the order in which to put items on, nor the movements required to do so. At the same time, the way her husband John overrides her choice of clothes in this scene highlights how pervasive the loss of autonomy can be in dementia (1:16:38). Although Alice can still make a choice and expresses her preferences, her wishes are ignored. The film manages to capture how easily even apparently benign actions, such as helping a person to get dressed, can contribute to the infantilisation of people with dementia.

Further, while the novel glosses over Alice's growing inability to coordinate body movements, the film by contrast highlights the extent to which Alice struggles with routine tasks. Towards the end of the film we are shown how difficult it has become for Alice to tie her shoe laces. Her limber and confident movements from earlier in the film have slowed to a shuffling pace. Alice barely speaks and has difficulty getting words out. In the novel, the impact of Alzheimer's on physical abilities is hardly addressed. Alice seemingly moves without difficulty; at the end she can still carry and handle a small baby without problems. Arguably, the fluent third-person narrative, with but a few hints of Alice's word-finding difficulties incorporated into the discourse, masks the more global deterioration in Alice's abilities. This does, however, allow Genova to avoid stereotypical representations of people with late stage dementia. In this respect, it may be considered either a strength or a weakness of the novel that it ends before Alice enters the final stages of her disease.

The filmic representation, with Alice vacantly shuffling along beside her caregiver, may confirm common stereotypes of people with more advanced dementia as 'empty shells' or 'zombies.' However, the film also works against such assumptions by highlighting how Alice can still recognise and name emotions—significantly, love—in others and in herself. Nonetheless, it is somewhat disturbing that the closing scene in both film and novel suggests that in order for the subjectivity of the person with dementia to be recognised she must still be able to interpret and use words meaningfully. In the epilogue to the book and the final scene of the film, Alice's youngest daughter Lydia acts out a monologue from one of her plays in front of her mother. Lydia then asks her mother to tell her how it makes her feel, what it is about. In each case, Alice identifies the emotion as 'love.' The scene suggests that even a person with limited language capacities can still understand and express emotions. Yet it is problematic that Alice needs to be able to articulate her feelings and her understanding of other people's feelings in order for her to be recognised as a sentient human being.

Even though *Still Alice* emphasises the importance of linguistic expression, the narrative also asks us to consider more holistically how love and relationships play out in the context of dementia. Alice is still able to feel love and to respond emotionally to her family caregivers. As exemplified in this exchange, Alice's youngest daughter Lydia finds new ways of engaging with her mother and continues to recognise her mother's subjectivity. *Still Alice* suggests that our identities, though seemingly rooted in professional roles and our own memories, reside equally in our everyday encounters with others and our capacity for relationships. Relational identity here works in two ways. The daughters not only honour their historic relationship with their mother, but also validate a new form of relationship with her, which is not based on her role as mother or her ability to recognise her daughters. In the novel, Alice is represented as a capable advice giver, despite her otherwise limited capacities, and she provides comfort and love to her grandchildren. The film, perhaps more realistically and less sentimentally, underlines Alice's capacity to engage with others in the moment. Her relational identity and her humanity are enacted in such encounters with others.

Experiencing dementia/experimenting with the novel

In this section, I turn to the question of how certain authors have aimed to extend the limits of representing the experience of dementia, especially the later stages, in textual narrative. What techniques, within the limits of verbal narration, do these authors find to represent such symptoms as the loss of language, the loss of a coherent life narrative, and the loss of the feeling of groundedness in everyday life? What aesthetic and ethical challenges does the imaginative engagement with later stages of dementia pose? And what effect do these experiments with language have on the evocation of empathy in readers? Further, I ask how narrative fiction that engages in more experimental modes of representation may expand the current understanding of narrative empathy. Contrary to Keen's view, which suggests that avant-garde texts, in emphasising defamiliarisation and a shock aesthetic, undermine empathetic reading (or viewing) experiences, I show how literary experimentation may, on the contrary, lead to the kind of empathetic experience, or experience of 'feeling as,' that Toker describes as parallel experience; that is, the reader may be said to experience similar epistemological uncertainty as the character with dementia. Reconsidering the relationship between empathy and texts that consciously disrupt immersive reading experiences—through metafictional devices and drawing attention to their fictional status—allows me to highlight that empathy and understanding cannot simply be aligned with the notions of identification, immersion, and transportation but is intertwined, even evoked by cognitively active reading experiences.[5]

Out of Mind

J. Bernlef's novel *Out of Mind* (1988)[6] follows a few months in the life of Maarten, a 71-year-old Dutch retiree, who emigrated to the US during mid-adulthood. For a long time, it was the only fictional narrative to use a first-person narrator with dementia.[7] From the start, we are plunged into the immediate thought processes of the first-person narrator, who, even though he is in Genette's terms an autodiegetic narrator telling his own story, remains unsure and indeed wrong about a number of aspects of his situation, such as the time of day and day of the week. In using 'concurrent' present tense narration (see Margolin 1999), the narrative resembles a series of diary entries. The use of concurrent narration has significant effects on the narrative; it contributes, for instance, to a sense of immediacy. More importantly, perhaps, in contrast to retrospective first-person narration, there is no distance between the 'narrating-I' (who has a fuller understanding of events) and the 'experiencing-I.' Yet an organising consciousness can nonetheless be discerned behind the novel, one which makes the narrative intelligible to the reader.

An example from the text illustrates how the use of present tense narration and Maarten's lack of insight into the situation affect the narrative. While out for a walk with his dog, the retired Maarten comes to believe that he is on his way to a work meeting. Maarten seems simultaneously aware and unaware of the strangeness of the situation: 'I am the first to arrive, I can tell from the virgin snow all around. It is *perhaps a rather strange* and yet quite suitable place for an IMCO meeting, so close to the sea' (Bernlef 1988: 33; my emphasis); 'from time to time I glance briefly over my shoulder, because for the secretary to a meeting to be forcing a door open is not an everyday event, *I realize that*' (34; my emphasis). When he becomes fully aware of his situation—namely that he is retired and has broken into a holiday residence—he is overcome by nausea:

> I just manage to reach the porch. As I hang over the rail my stomach empties itself into the snow, a mucky brown, steaming pulp in which even Robert [his dog] shows no interest. I feel cold.
> What am I doing here? In the summer, people from Boston live here.
> (35–6)

The present tense here heightens the sense of immediacy and adds to the build-up of dramatic tension. It also allows the reader to follow the workings of Maarten's mind and emphasises the acute pang he experiences when he becomes aware of his delusion. However, it is important to note here that this is, of course, not the same as not knowing what is going on and therefore experiencing the situation *as Maarten does*. The reader remembers Maarten is a retiree and realises that Maarten's memory loss distorts his reality.

What happens, then, as Maarten's cognitive decline accelerates and his narrative becomes more and more fragmented, enigmatic and idiosyncratic—and therefore more difficult for the reader to decode? Bernlef's narrative techniques could be described as promoting parallel experience: at this stage in the narrative both the reader and the first-person narrator experience a sense of disorientation, the narrator-character with regard to his (fictional) reality and the reader in decoding the narrator's words. Nonetheless, the effect is not perfect since a number of techniques ensure that despite the narrator's decline the process of narrative transmission does not break down (Bitenc 2012: 308, 309).

Providing detailed descriptions of the storyworld is one such technique. Maarten minutely describes his perceptions and, in that sense, remains a 'reliable' narrator. Given that Bernlef's readers do not suffer from short-term memory loss, they will be able to identify characters by their clothes or other characteristics, or remember what happened previously in the storyworld, even when Maarten does not. To help the reader parse the time frame of actions, the author uses line breaks between paragraphs to signal that story time has passed. When Maarten experiences, a time shift that returns him to his kindergarten days, this, on the contrary, occurs seamlessly within the space of a short paragraph (Bernlef 1988: 5). Towards the end of the narrative Bernlef employs the use of brackets to indicate how Maarten retains dual awareness (as expressed, for instance, in second-order thoughts), even as his narrative disintegrates. The narrative voice here becomes split between a more confused version in the body of the text and a more lucid version in the brackets: 'The blonde girl from earlier (so I can remember her for a while at any rate) gets up and goes to the hall' (104); 'And a chair. (Was it already there or has it just been pushed forward?) I sit down. Notice that the rubbing has resumed. Not unpleasant actually' (100). Here Bernlef begins to drop the first-person pronoun and to employ short and sometimes fragmented sentences in order to mimic the decline in Maarten's linguistic abilities and the growing incoherence in his thought processes.

Towards the end of the narrative the voice in brackets—and the narrative as a whole—increasingly employs the imperative mode. Indeed, as the first-person pronoun is dropped in favour of 'he' or 'it,' the imperative mode seems to indicate the last vestiges of Maarten's first-person narrative voice. It seems as if Maarten is speaking to himself, trying to make his (uncompliant) body do what he wants it to do. The third-person pronoun indicates his growing sense of loss of self and self-control. Nevertheless, the perspective on the world or, as phenomenologists put it, the first-personal givenness of experience remains his own: 'Hands and feet it must have ... eyes open and shut: same place ... eyes open and shut again: same place' (122). Despite the technique of fragmentation and the emphasis on Maarten's dissociation from his body, the way Maarten remains the centre of consciousness and perception—the being that realises that he is in the 'same place'—paradoxically highlights his continuing identity, suggesting that lower-order cognitive functions might be sufficient to accord personhood or at least selfhood to a subject. In any case, the reader continues to see him as a character, a 'person' in whom we are interested and with whom we empathise (see Bitenc 2012: 312).[8]

As Maarten's symptoms of dementia progress, the narrative discourse fluctuates between the use of the first, second, and third person, highlighting the shifting and unstable nature of Maarten's sense of self. Through this back and forth between the first and third person the narrative does not follow a linear progression towards 'it-ness,' the vacant 'empty shells' of many contemporary representations of dementia, but highlights instead the narrator's persisting subjectivity.[9] In this part of the narrative, also, embodiment is foregrounded. For instance, Maarten begins to rely on physical sensations to feel himself, to feel at one with his body: by rubbing his hands on his legs or even pinching himself (see 124). Maarten attempts, even in the later stages of the disease, to make use of any opportunity to recapture his former sense of self, and the 'blissful feeling' of being-one-with-the-world:

> Get up, *you* ... go and inspect that piano from close by ... *he* walks to the little steps by the side of the stage ... toilingly clambers up ... keys that go up and down all by themselves [...] perhaps they can help *your* fingers ... teach them perhaps to play again ... to play from memory again ... that blissful feeling that *your* body is playing you ... that you yourself have become music.
>
> (128; my emphasis)[10]

The shift from the third-person pronoun 'he' to the second-person pronoun 'you' and possessive 'your' holds out the possibility that Maarten may overcome his sense of alienation from his own body. However, the pianola, with its own 'agency,' impedes Maarten's attempt to feel at one with the world: 'he sits down on the chair in front of the piano and feels the keys knocking against his fingers ... they push you away ... rebuff you' (128). Right after this passage, in fact, one of the most objectivising moments of the entire narrative takes place:

> They take it to a space where there are beds ... they make it sit on the edge of a bed ... they undress it ... they put pyjamas on it that look like

the pyjamas of those other men with their big, staring, half-bald heads on the tall, white pillows and all turned towards him ... they push a pill into his throat ... they pour water through it as if he were a funnel ... they lay him in the bed ... they walk past the row of beds together ... they are silent until they reach the door and call out together good night GOOD NIGHT they call and then it is dark.

(129)

The next paragraph begins with the eerie sentence, 'There is breathing everywhere.' Like Mrs Gradgrind in Dickens' *Hard Times* who on her deathbed pronounces that 'I think there's a pain somewhere in the room ... but I couldn't positively say that I have got it' (Dickens 1854: 191), Maarten seems to have lost the sense of himself and others as distinct persons. Nevertheless, the narrative itself upholds and communicates his subjectivity. The reader continues to read the words on the page as the perceptions, thoughts, and feelings of Maarten's consciousness. As Alan Palmer argues in *Fictional Minds* (2004) it takes very little (a personal pronoun, a name) for readers to project the extended consciousness of a character in fiction. Importantly, since readers are given insight into Maarten's thought processes, even as these become less coherent, they are likely to be able to decode the little language Maarten still uses when talking to his caregivers. In narratives focalised through the eyes of the caregiver, such as Michael Ignatieff's *Scar Tissue*, the reader, together with the caregiver, can only speculate on whether the utterances of the person with dementia make any sense. Narratives such as Bernlef's are thus ethically important in suggesting that the enigmatic utterances of people with dementia have meaning when we take into account the person's life history and their current perception of the world. Such narratives suggest that rather than automatically disregarding the seemingly incoherent utterances of people with dementia, it is imperative to try and make sense of them as best as possible.

The closing paragraphs of the novel highlight the important role that respectful and gentle physical contact plays in the care of people with more advanced dementia, while also emphasising the importance of relationships. During the night Maarten seeks the hand of an unnamed woman (possibly Vera or his mother), to find either the hand of another patient or more likely his own. In any case, Maarten experiences the physical contact as reassuring:

> ... she is among them somewhere ... seek her ... her hand we must seek ... this takes time [...] her hand will come to you ... here ... first take that hand that gropes aimlessly in the dark ... take it gently ... calm him ... now you no longer need to hold anything yourself ... she will do that from now on ... she carries you ... I carry you ... little boy of mine ... the whole long frightening night I will carry you until it is light again.

(129)

Again, the present tense highlights how Maarten experiences the past as the present. He seems to have returned to the scenes of early childhood where a loving female takes care of him. When on the following morning his wife Vera comes for a visit, it is clear that although Maarten does not recognise her voice, he takes comfort in her visit and in listening to her hopeful tale of renewal and repair:

> When it is already light and GOOD MORNING and someone says ... whispers ... the voice of a woman and you listen ... you listen with closed eyes ... listen only to her voice whispering ... that the window has been repaired ... that where first that old door had been nailed ... there is glass again ... glass you can see through ... outside ... into the woods and the spring that is almost beginning ... she says ... she whispers ... the spring which is about to begin ...
>
> (129)

It is notable that the novel ends with a section that is not only more coherent than those preceding it but also inherently hopeful. Despite the excruciating pain and confusion that have gone before, the nature imagery which closes the novel suggests a positive outlook on dementia. Arguably, Maarten's increasing loss of self-awareness and return to his childhood self allows for a more tranquil experience of his world. Maarten no longer perceives his environment through the traumatic experiences of World War II. (For a time, possibly because they are speaking American English, Maarten mistakes both doctors and nurses for his 'liberators' and is worried that they will treat him as a Nazi collaborator.) While the metaphorical spring in dementia that the narrative's ending projects may resemble the more tranquil period towards the end of the disease that caregivers at times describe, it also risks underestimating the continued potential for suffering in the person with dementia. Caregivers' memoirs, such as Sally Magnusson's *Where Memories Go* (2014), are powerful reminders that the last stages can be anything but painless. Yet, overall, *Out of Mind* questions the commonplace that the person with dementia loses all sense of awareness and the caregiver suffers more than the care-receiver. Fictional and non-fictional dementia narratives alike help expose such preconceptions as misrepresentations or misinterpretations of the experience of dementia.

House Mother Normal

If the publication of *Out of Mind* coincides with the rise of the Alzheimer's disease movement in the 1980s, then B. S. Johnson's experimental novel *House Mother Normal*, first published in 1971, predates, by a decade, the growing contemporary concern with dementia. Nonetheless, *House Mother Normal*, in its medicalised understanding of dementia and its concern over the running of care homes, resonates with contemporary explorations of dementia.

Johnson's novel consists of a frame narrative by the house mother of a care home and eight twenty-one-page-long interior monologues by the elderly patients in that home, presented in stream of consciousness style. Each of these narratives tells of the same sequence of events: dinner, 'work,' 'exercise,' and 'entertainments.' As we come to see these events through different characters' minds, we are able to piece together a sense of the actual events in the storyworld. The technique is similar to that found in modernist texts, such as William Faulkner's *The Sound and the Fury* (1929), where we come to make sense of the narrative of the mentally disabled character Benjy through subsequent retellings of the same events by other characters in the storyworld.[11] Here, compared to Faulkner's novel, the strategy of distributing *fabula* details is inverted, since we start out with the accounts of more verbally coherent characters and move towards those of the most severely cognitively impaired characters, George Hedbury and Rosetta Stanton. Importantly, Johnson exploits the overdetermined narrative structure in order to enhance the reader's mental map or situation model of the storyworld (Bernaerts 2014: 298). Not only do all narratives treat the same sequence of events, but the number of pages on which these events are evoked correlate with each other. So page 5 of each narrative relates to the moment in which the house mother gets her patients to sing the 'house hymn.' One of the effects of this '3-D reading experience,' as Lars Bernaerts calls it (2014: 298), is that we can complete the narrative 'puzzle' by referring back and forth between pages. This narrative reconstruction is particularly important vis-à-vis the most fragmented and incoherent narratives towards the end. Johnson's narrative structure also ensures that the reader continues to attribute consciousness to or project 'experientiality' (Fludernik 1996) onto word fragments, nonsense words, and even blank pages (see also Bernaerts 2014: 297; 305).

The text further differs in technique from *The Sound and the Fury* in that the patients' narratives are framed by the house mother's prologue and epilogue—the latter providing her version of the evening's events. '(you shall see into the minds of our/eight old friends, and you shall see into my/mind' (Johnson [1971] 2013: 5), the prologue reads. The instances of metalepsis in her narrative, i.e., the moments where different narrative levels and the ontological level occupied by the author get entangled with one another (Pier 2013), draw attention to the ways the supposedly mimetic 'insights' into each character's mind are mediated not only by the house mother but, in the final instance, also by the author: '(you always knew/there was a writer behind it all? Ah, there's/no fooling you readers!)' (204). Each of the patients' narratives is further framed by introductory remarks similar to case notes or patient charts; these notes include age, marital status, percentage of sight, hearing, touch, and movement, while also providing a list of the various diseases the patients suffer from. Importantly, a cognitive quotient (CQ) count—which could be compared to a score on a Mini-Mental State Examination—indicates the severity of the character's dementia.

While, according to Bernaerts these 'ironic' introductions set up 'a frame through which the fictional minds can be constructed and interpreted' (300) (since we know that we are moving from the least to the most severely cognitively and physically impaired narrator), this play with genre has the further effect of highlighting the insufficiency of reductionist medicalisations of human experience. The mimicry of contemporary patient charts, which supposedly contain all relevant information about the human subject, is contrasted directly with a rich phenomenological approach to embedded, embodied, and extended human minds.[12]

As is obvious even from this brief description of the text, the novel plays with many genres—most notably drama—and is at several removes from the conventions of the realist novel. Through the house mother's direct address to the reader the novel deliberately draws attention to its constructed nature. Furthermore, Johnson exploits fonts, formatting, and other material textual features to explore the 'qualia' of the subjective experience of dementia (see also Bernaerts 2014: 305). Line breaks, indents, different fonts, and the blank page indicate gaps, jumps, or slowness of processing in the character's consciousness. Indeed, Johnson uses a number of strategies and techniques, which Monika Fludernik would term 'typification,' to create 'a fiction of authenticity' (Fludernik 1993: 17, 19, qtd. in Herman and Vervaeck 2005: 95). Typical, clichéd turns of phrase and stylistic means that are supposedly inherent in oral language—such as swear words, exclamations, garbled syntax, hesitation, non-sequiturs, and so on—are employed in order to give the reader the sense that a representation is true to life (Herman and Vervaeck 2005: 96); in Johnson's case the technique is used to evoke a sense of how the mind of a person with dementia may work.

Given that people in the later stages of dementia struggle to verbalise their experiences, it is important to ask: by what standard do we measure the verisimilitude of these interior monologues or their hypothesised closeness to the phenomenology of dementia? Arguably, these interior monologues mimic actual speech acts of people with dementia, such as the fragmented speech and repetitive style of reminiscing, recorded in social science research (Hydén 2010, Hydén and Örulv 2009, Örulv and Hydén 2006, Usita et al. 1998) and collaborative life writing (Clegg 2010). However, the disadvantage of judging verisimilitude of consciousness representation on the basis of actual speech is that it presumes that thought is necessarily (or primarily) verbal. Also, Johnson's style of consciousness presentation—as mimicked to a certain extent in Naomi Krüger's recent novel *May* (2018)—must be considered a literary stereotype. In a condition such as Alzheimer's, questions of literary representation and their relationship to what is taken to be reality, though difficult to answer, remain ethically relevant. We must ask what is at stake when representing fictional inside views of people with dementia as either coherent or incoherent, embodied or disembodied, rational or emotional, like 'us' or unlike 'us,' to draw on just a few persistent binary oppositions.

In *House Mother Normal* the narratives represent a blend of immediate perceptions of the character's current environment—those relating to ongoing activities—with what might best be described as reminiscences or associative thought. Bernaerts (2014) notes that earlier readings of the novel may have overemphasised the element of 'memory narratives' or reminiscence in *House Mother Normal*. His own reading, drawing on cognitive models, instead emphasises the embodied nature of these fictional minds. He argues that by highlighting perception and emotion, Johnson underscores the characters' engagement with their environment and their 'action-oriented thought and plans or scenarios for the near future' (307). 'Memories (in particular memories of relationships and traumatic memories),' Bernaerts writes, 'are an important part of the minds evoked in *House Mother Normal*, but they alternate with thought induced by perception and oriented toward action, which brings the pensioners' minds back to the present' (307). Johnson employs this 'past-present-future' continuum (307), I argue, as exploratory modelling of the phenomenology of embodied minds affected by dementia.

The monologues, furthermore, include snippets of direct speech (marked by italics) and highlight the extent to which each fictional mind represents an 'embedded' and 'social' mind (Palmer 2004). Each character's consciousness is shaped by social norms and perceived wisdom and includes the perceptions of other characters' minds. The reader comes to see how characters respond to each other with either sympathy or dislike. Also, each character evaluates the same situation differently, based on their personal characteristics and values. As Bernaerts notes, fear and feelings of disgust towards the house mother are among the most pervasive and strongest emotions evoked and 'enhance the dynamics of the characters' mental action' (305). And yet, characters differ significantly in their evaluation both of the house mother and of her sardonic entertainments. These evaluations contribute to the complex individualised portrayal of each character's consciousness, while also shaping the reader's evaluation of the ethics of the narrative.

The novel's focus on a relatively brief space of time allows for detailed, seemingly real-time descriptions of thoughts and events. *House Mother Normal*, compared with other dementia narratives, is less concerned with maintaining a protracted narrative arc in which the character's progressive decline is portrayed. The text can thus explore the limits of language and coherence to a greater degree than other texts. If George Hedbury's narrative is, towards the end, marked by almost blank pages and only a few words, his fragmented language still makes sense insofar as readers have been 'briefed' about what is going on by other narrators. So, for instance, the following fragment refers to the house mother's vile game of 'pass the parcel':

                                              Package

   for me   pass, parc

              what?   (152)[13]

Similarly, the following passage may be seen to evoke George's sense of disorientation at suddenly finding that he is being pushed around in his wheelchair during the 'exercise' routine:

>   name   it
> moving   moving!
> everything's moving!
>
>   ?   (153)

Most notably, perhaps, George's internal cries of pain (155) during the cruel game of wheelchair tournament starkly emphasise his continuing capacity to suffer. The representation of his pain contrasts with the outside perspectives (both sympathetic and unsympathetic) offered to the reader in previous accounts. In other narrators' accounts, George is considered 'alright' (23) since he does not say anything that might dispute this interpretation. His internal monologue, however, draws attention to the fact that people with dementia continue to feel pain even when they may no longer be able to verbalise it.

As noted previously, the narrative progresses from the most mentally able to the most severely impaired character. Rosetta Stanton's 'medical chart' suggests a drastic stage of decline with her physical capacities ranked around five percent and her CQ count at zero. The first fourteen pages of her account contain only snippets of what to an Anglophone reader appear to be nonsense words, dispersed across an otherwise empty page.[14] However, on page fourteen, as she is addressed directly by Ivy Nicholls who is pushing her wheelchair during 'exercise,' Rosetta's 'narrative' suddenly becomes coherent: In response to Ivy's question *'How are you Mrs S?'*—which the reader will either have remembered or can return to on the corresponding page of Ivy's account—Rosetta's internal monologue reads:

>   I a m
> t e r r i b l e , I v y .   (175)

Indeed, this passage is in ironic contrast to Ivy's account. Following her questions to Rosetta, Ivy's monologue continues: 'No answer. I have never heard her speak since I came here CAN'T HEAR A THING CAN YOU, MRS STANTON?' (65). However, Rosetta's internal monologue proves Ivy wrong:

>   N o w I c a n   e v e r y
> w o r d y o u s a y.. I am a prisoner in my
>
> self. It is terrible. The movement agonises me.
> Let me out, or I shall die   (175–6)

Here Johnson is drawing on a common trope of dementia narratives. While some accounts argue that the person with dementia has lost her self and

Experience and empathy 81

resembles an 'empty shell,' other accounts insist that the self is 'locked into' the disintegrating body. Such accounts suggest that the person within persists, much as before, but loses the ability to communicate her subjective experience to others. Becoming a prisoner inside one's body is seen as an even greater 'horror' than the supposed state of selflessness. Johnson draws on this trope in Rosetta's monologue. In fact, he even seems to suggest that her loss of consciousness at the end of her narrative—represented by six uniformly blank pages—is a last act of agency, of willed oblivion. In response to Ivy's further conversational remark 'DON'T GET ANY LIGHTER, DO YOU, MRS STANTON?' (66), Rosetta responds in her thoughts:

```
              No, I  d o
n o t get      a n y
l i g h t e r,   I v y,
I    i n  –
     t e   n d
n o  t
t    o        g    e     t
  a    n      y –
t    h    i    n      g
   a         n         y
m         o        r         e


n    o
m              o         r              (176)
```

How does one read the six blank pages that follow? Do they represent her loss of self? Or do these blank pages, alternatively, constitute an attempt to represent the unfathomable experience of advanced dementia? Within the structure of the novel, with a set number of pages allocated to each character, the blank pages remain significant. They are not merely empty pages but a continued representation of Rosetta's consciousness. After first experiencing this consciousness through the eyes of others, the reader then communed with it and continues to engage with it, even in its 'blankness.' It is relevant, of course, that Rosetta's account does not consist of blank pages from the start. Readers try to parse the information they get as best they can, using the structural overlay provided by the text. The blank pages may then be read as a powerful representation of the loss of words, which is inexpressible by any other means than silence.

Of course, some readers may simply skip the blank pages; in which case they omit to 'read' the marked absence of thoughts or experiences that the author intended to convey. One could also argue that, here, Johnson confirms the trope of loss of self in dementia. Without actual text to represent the character's consciousness, the character may be considered 'as good as dead.' Rosetta may then be seen to inhabit the same space of the 'living dead,' on a textual level, that people with dementia are frequently understood to inhabit outside fiction. That said, in its theatricality and artistically overdetermined form, *House Mother Normal* repeatedly draws attention to its constructed nature. The aesthetics embody an ethical value in that the disruption of a 'naturalised' or immersive reading strategy repeatedly reminds readers that they are dealing with a *representation* of dementia as imagined by a specific author in a particular cultural and literary context.[15] The novel is designed to make its readers think about the problems of representing dementia and concomitantly the difficulties of accessing, inhabiting, or understanding the phenomenology of the condition. If, as I have argued in relation to *Out of Mind*, such disruptions of an immersive reading experience can have a distancing effect on the reader and may at times impede emotional engagement and empathy with the characters (Bitenc 2012), the foregrounding of the narrative as textual construct nevertheless fulfils an ethical function: by problematizing their own truth value these novels call the reader's attention to the risk of effacing the perspective of people with dementia in narratives written as if from their point of view.

At the same time, in providing a number of 'inside' perspectives, Johnson not only plays these narratives off against each other, but also orchestrates the novel such that each narrative comes to inform and enrich all subsequent (re-)tellings. Therefore, the configuration of parallel narratives allows readers to develop empathy, or some level of understanding of the inner life world of even the most severely impaired characters. As Andrew Motion suggests in his introduction to the novel,

> by the end of the book, when we are hearing from characters who are hardly able to speak, and whose states of mind are represented by blank pages, or pages on which only a few words or letters appear, we have acquired sufficient knowledge to sympathize with them despite their inarticulacy – or all the more because of it.
>
> (Johnson 2013: vii)

Given that even the least coherent narrative ends with a markedly coherent passage implies that even in this experimental mode, to recognise subjectivity, or to make it 'readable,' one must draw on coherent language. Nevertheless, in employing the associative style of stream of consciousness narratives, and emphasising the embodied, embedded, and extended nature of fictional minds, Johnson pushes against the limits of conveying an 'inside' experience of dementia that apply to realist novels.

In vividly portraying the characters' personal reactions to events, their likes and dislikes, their moments of pride, and their fond or painful memories, Johnson also manages to evoke a deep sense of the characters' humanity. Of course, the nature and extent of readers' engagement will depend, as suggested by Keen (2007), both on their personal characteristics and on their reading preferences. For some, an accessible and emotive work, such as *Still Alice*, which draws on the conventions of the realist novel, may be most effective in raising awareness for the experience of dementia. A reader who shares with Alice her professional background, as well as attributes of gender and age, may experience more empathic concern for the character than readers who differ from the protagonist in these respects. Similarly, reading preferences—such as disdain for anything smacking of the sentimental or, conversely, impatience with the modes of (post)modernist fiction—will influence the reader's manner of engagement with any given narrative. In my own reading experience, more experimental writing modes at times turn dementia into a kind of 'mind game';[16] these modes, while raising interest for the symptoms of dementia, are not always conducive to empathy or sympathy. However, these experimental modes afford innovative ways of representing certain aspects of what it might be like to live with dementia otherwise overlooked. Furthermore, they highlight the difficulties and ethical pitfalls attendant on representing people with advanced dementia who are no longer able to express their own experience or correct the way they are represented by others. If literature supposedly provides a means of experiencing dementia from the inside out, it also suggests how the phenomenological viewpoint of actual others with dementia may be erased. Fictional dementia narratives such as *House Mother Normal* both enact such an erasure (in Rosetta Stanton's case figured through the blank page) and draw attention to their own participation in this act. Ironically, while potentially effacing or 'overwriting' the subjectivity of people with dementia, these narratives also push against the effacement of these others in the cultural imaginary by fictionally giving voice to and imaginatively constructing the embodied consciousness of a subject with dementia.

The Unconsoled

I turn now to a novel that does not signal its status as dementia narrative but can be productively read through the lens of neurodegenerative decline. Indeed, I argue that not naming the condition opens up new avenues for exploring what it might feel like to live with the epistemological uncertainty that dementia frequently entails. In Kazuo Ishiguro's *The Unconsoled* (1995) the concert pianist Mr Ryder arrives in a central European city to participate in an event which seems of unprecedented importance to the future of this city. The first-person narrative is told by Mr Ryder himself. From the start, his telling is marked by uncertainty: by gaps in Ryder's knowledge about his situation, his recent past, his relation to others, and the nature of what is expected from him on his visit. While the narrative is presented through the limited viewpoint of a seemingly memory-impaired (autodiegetic) first-person narrator, Ishiguro at times extends the scope of his narrator's vision or knowledge to include an almost omniscient understanding of other characters' perceptions, thoughts, and memories. Ryder also narrates events at which he is not present, exhibiting the spatio-temporal freedom conventionally attributed to omniscient narrators. Even more strikingly, he is privy to other character's thoughts and memories that cannot be understood or explained within the conventions of a first-person narrator. And yet, in these instances (rather than shifting into a different narrative voice), Ishiguro insistently emphasises Ryder's perspective through the use of first-person pronouns. The narrative is marked, therefore by a clash between the narrator's disturbing lack of knowledge and deficient grasp of his situation and an excess of knowledge about other characters' perceptions, thoughts, and memories.[17] One of the effects of this technique is that the reader does not inhabit a stable perspective. Attempts to naturalise the many inconsistencies and sheer impossibilities of the narrative are undermined by the very instability of narrative voice and focalisation. The narrative resists being decoded via the conventions of 'realist' first-person narration, while nevertheless drawing on these conventions as dominant mode throughout. We come, therefore, to view the world through Mr Ryder's limited (and simultaneously incongruously expanded) viewpoint.

What allows a reading of this novel as a dementia narrative is that, on the story level, Ryder finds himself in situations that mirror what a person with dementia can be hypothesised to experience due to the symptoms of cognitive decline. At times, such situations take on a surreal or kafkaesque character. While Ryder does not seem to suffer from word-finding or other linguistic difficulties, he does, at one stage, entirely lose his ability to speak—and, in consequence, fails to speak up for his long-term friend. Ryder, straining to reveal his true identity to a committee of officious local women, can bizarrely emit only grunts. Flushed red by the strain to speak, he presents a disturbing spectacle. Shortly afterwards, he inexplicably regains his capacity to use language. While this sudden (and, as it turns out, reversible) language loss is not a realistic representation of dementia, the scene is evocative of how crucial language is in asserting our identity and in positioning ourselves positively in relation to others. Without language, the renowned pianist becomes a no one, unable to represent himself or intervene on behalf of others. Significantly, he also becomes an object of disgust to those around him.

Ryder also has a less than firm grasp on his recent autobiographical memories. And although the citizens expect him to play an inordinate role in upcoming events—a role which would appear to be in excess of what one might expect from a concert pianist—Ryder remains confused about 'the precise nature' (4) of the event as well as his role in it. Indeed, the narrative has, throughout, a nightmarish quality, in that Ryder is continually running late for appointments and never finds himself in the right place. He also frequently loses all sense of time, and since readers see events through his eyes they cannot unambiguously pinpoint the actual passage of time in the storyworld. The nightmarish quality of the narrative is enhanced by physical impossibilities within the storyworld.[18] Buildings frequently morph into each other as the protagonist navigates the confusing landscape of the city, and corridors and rooms change their shape as the narrator moves through them or returns to them. In a striking parallel with the experience of people with dementia in nursing homes, who often feel as if 'traces of ... their childhood home [were] pushing forward under the wallpaper of the care home' (Clegg 2010: 12), Ryder becomes convinced that his hotel room is one of his childhood rooms. I quote at length to give a sense of this experience:

> I was just starting to doze off when something suddenly made me open my eyes again and stare up at the ceiling. I went on scrutinising the ceiling for some time, then sat up on the bed and looked around, the sense of recognition growing stronger by the second. The room I was now in, I realised, was the very room that had served as my bedroom during the two years my parents and I had lived in my aunt's house on the borders of England and Wales. I looked again around the room, then, lowering myself back down, stared once more at the ceiling. It had been recently re-plastered and re-painted, its dimensions had been enlarged, the cornices had been removed, the decorations around the light fitting had been entirely altered. But it was unmistakably the same ceiling I had so often stared up at from my narrow creaking bed of those days.
>
> (16)

What is notable about this passage is its assured tone—as expressed through verb tense (simple past, past perfect) and the absence of modal verbs. Contrary to the use of concurrent narration in Bernlef's *Out of Mind*, Ishiguro uses conventional past tense narration throughout.[19] Nevertheless, there seems to be very little distance between the narrating-I and experiencing-I. Despite all evidence to the contrary (that he is on the continent and not in the UK and that all aspects of the room have been altered including the ceiling's dimensions) the narrator is entirely sure of his discovery: 'the sense of recognition growing stronger,' 'I realised,' 'unmistakably.' Indeed, further contemplation of the room triggers a detailed memory of a specific afternoon during his childhood. Arguably, in contrasting the vividness of Ryder's childhood memories with his recent memory lapses, and in allowing the narrator to experience no sense of contradiction at this superimposition of distinct geographical locations, Ishiguro at this point in the narrative (the conclusion of the first chapter) sets up the possibility of framing the rest of the narrative through the lens of progressive memory loss.

That said, reading this novel as dementia narrative does not provide the reader with an all-purpose interpretative tool which makes sense of the inconsistencies of the storyworld or the narrator's disorientating experiences. Instead, the narrative places readers in a situation where they will need to contend with a certain level of uncertainty, disorientation, and confusion which may be considered central to the experience of dementia. Similar to the dementia narratives I have discussed previously, Ryder's loss of the sense of time and his experience of getting physically lost are enacted in the narrative. Yet here the reader has no possibility of resolving these difficulties—e.g., by naturalising them either through reference to genre[20] or by reading them as indicators of the diseased narrator's mind. The mental map of the storyworld resists falling into place, and readers are left with a sense of confusion about the world they are inhabiting through Ryder's consciousness. This aspect of the narrative makes it an interesting case for considering the notion of parallel experience in relation to the phenomenology of dementia.

The Unconsoled also resonates with other dementia narratives in that the novel explores how cognitive decline may affect not only one's ability to navigate space and time but impact on one's social world. So, for instance, Ryder's eminent position as renowned pianist is slowly undermined as he struggles to meet the demands made on him and, finally, fails entirely to fulfil any of his responsibilities. This process is intimated from the start of the narrative in his very first interaction with the hotel's desk clerk. As the clerk begins to chat about the preparations for the elusive 'Thursday night' he mentions how a certain Mr Brodsky, clearly the conductor of the orchestra, has been 'doing splendidly' and is in the process of practising in the hotel's drawing room. Ryder's response indicates how little he seems to be in the know about events:

> 'Brodsky, you say.' I thought about the name, but it meant nothing to me. Then I caught the desk clerk watching me with a puzzled look and said quickly: 'Yes, yes. I'll look forward to meeting Mr Brodsky in good time.'
> (4)

Ryder, it seems, is astute at reading other people's reactions and quick to cover up idiosyncrasies in his behaviour due to his failing memory. This behaviour resonates with accounts of people with dementia, who report trying to hide their symptoms from others. In the later stages, set phrases, which are still accessible, are often used to keep social interactions going and to gloss over the inability to express oneself more precisely. Such set phrases then provide a means to continue functioning on a social level. In the novel, Ryder, like many people with dementia, retains the capacity to navigate social encounters relatively smoothly, despite an often substantial lack of knowledge.

Nonetheless, Ryder's relationships to significant others are severely disturbed by his memory loss. In the hotel, Ryder meets an elderly porter named Gustav. As they become more closely acquainted—incidentally, through Ryder's apparent ability to read the porter's mind—Gustav asks him to meet his daughter Sophie and find out what is troubling her. We then follow Ryder to a café where he meets Sophie and her son, Boris. Initially, seeing events unfold from Ryder's point of view, the reader expects this to be their first meeting.

> Turning, I saw a woman sitting with a young boy waving to me from a nearby table. The pair clearly matched the porter's description and

I couldn't understand how I had failed to notice them earlier. I was a little taken aback, moreover, that they should be expecting me ... Although the porter had referred to her as a 'young woman', Sophie was in early middle age, perhaps around forty or so. For all that, she was somewhat more attractive than I had expected. ... 'This is Mr Ryder, Boris,' Sophie said. 'He's a special friend. Of course he can sit with us if he wants.'

(32)

It soon becomes clear, however, that Ryder is well known to both Sophie and Boris, and indeed, it emerges that Ryder and Sophie have been in an intimate relationship for years. With this knowledge in mind it is difficult to make sense of why Ryder describes their initial meeting in the way he does, unless one posits that he has temporarily forgotten all about their joint history.

Ishiguro thus largely limits the reader's perspective on events to that of a partially unreliable, memory-impaired first-person narrator. Occasionally, the reader might, as in the passage just quoted, later suspect that Ryder is unreliable when the facts revealed contradict Ryder's reporting: 'Is this really what Sophie said?,' one might ask. Since, if Ryder has been acting as something of a father figure to Boris, then Sophie's introduction ('This is Mr Ryder, Boris') is incongruous. Indeed, Ryder's narrative later suggests that a previously harmonious (step)father-son relationship has only recently been disrupted by some unnamed event. In the meantime, Ryder remains fundamentally uncertain about his shared past with Sophie and Boris, and concomitantly about how to behave towards them. This is evident, for instance, when Ryder visits them in their home:

I followed the pair of them up two flights of stairs. As Sophie unlocked the front entrance the thought struck me that I was perhaps expected to behave as though familiar with the apartment. On the other hand, it was equally possible I was expected to behave like a guest. As we stepped inside, I decided to observe carefully Sophie's manner and take my cue from that.

(283)

This passage calls attention to the strategies that people with dementia may employ when they are uncertain about their relationship with others. Since the reader never gets the full story of their relationship and is therefore, like Ryder, left to speculate on events, the narrative technique brings readers closer to Ryder's experience of epistemological uncertainty. The parallel experience of uncertainty about the storyworld—about time, space, events, and relationships—may then intimate what it feels like to lose a firm grasp on one's life due to dementia. We become, like the narrator lost in time and lost in space, uncertain about our location within the storyworld and the (surreal or real) nature of the events taking place.

If Ishiguro's tale provides a resonant image of the phenomenology of dementia, it is also about other aspects of humans' lives as embodied, social agents. Ishiguro, of course, is a master at depicting regret—most notably, the missed opportunities in relationships—the word *not* spoken, rather than the word spoken hastily. This theme resonates in *The Unconsoled*, especially in the relationship between the aged porter and his daughter Sophie. However, the novel also puts a particular twist on the theme of dysfunctional relationships—one that may contribute to an understanding of how relationships may be impacted by progressive memory loss. Ryder seems to have had some kind of disagreement with Sophie but cannot remember any of the details. Nonetheless, he repeatedly experiences surges of anger towards her. There appear to be various sources for this anger. On the one hand, his anger seems to be motivated by the underlying reasons for the falling out, even when he cannot remember them. On the other hand, as events spiral out of control, Sophie becomes a convenient object for his anger at his own powerlessness. Ryder then begins to blame Sophie for everything that goes wrong. As is usual in Ishiguro, the characters never address these issues, never manage to reach an understanding of the other's point of view. In the end, the couple parts ways. Ishiguro's novel suggests how the capacity for misunderstanding is exacerbated when one of the partners suffers from memory loss and may lack insight into his own feelings. Although he does not engage in a direct exploration of dementia, Ishiguro here hints at some of the complexities inherent in interacting with intimate others when both the memory of recent interactions and even the history of one's relationship have been lost.

Concluding reflections on narrative empathy

In this chapter I pursued three questions: one, can imaginative fiction contribute to a better understanding of the experience of dementia? Two, how do narrative techniques which are used to simulate the phenomenology of dementia interact with the reader's experience of empathy? And three, what implications does this bottom-up analysis of narrative empathy have for current theories of narrative empathy and the role empathy plays in the medical humanities?

Much like life writing, fictional narratives evoke the varied life world of the character or person with dementia. They place the character in a specific social and cultural context, while exploring both the character's inner life, her relationship with others and with her physical world. Fictional narratives are therefore well placed to explore how, in Havi Carel's terms, the life world of a person changes due to serious illness (2008). Novels as well as films provide the kind of thick description that is necessary for a full understanding of sociocultural phenomena—including the experience of living with a neurodegenerative disease. Contrary to life writing, however, fictional narratives, and the novel in particular, may address the experience of the later stages of dementia by simulating an encounter with the progressively impaired character's mind. Nevertheless, it is important to stress that such representations draw on specific literary techniques and conventions and are based on culturally available conceptualisations of dementia—what dementia is taken to *be* and what it *means*. As part of this hermeneutic circle, narrative technique in turn influences the kind of understanding of the experience of dementia readers and viewers procure. Film, in particular, makes use of the embodied agency of both protagonist and viewer to further intersubjective understanding of the protagonist's motivations, feelings, or state of mind. In the novel, various experimental modes aim to expand the limits of representing serious cognitive impairment within language and narrative. Nevertheless, these narratives continue to act within the bounds of language and at least minimally coherent narrative acts.

Still Alice, *Out of Mind*, and *House Mother Normal* are all recognisable dementia narratives. These texts allow readers to enter the mind of the character(s) with dementia. They provide many possibilities for narrative empathy while also stimulating intellectual curiosity about the limits of seeing the world through the eyes of a person with dementia, since the reader necessarily retains a grasp on the narrative storyworld that exceeds that of the characters. Furthermore, instances of empathic feeling with, or rather feeling as the character, are evoked by creating processes of parallel experience in the reader. Nevertheless, since these narratives are explicitly marked as dementia narratives, and the authors use certain techniques to make their storyworld intelligible to the reader, we, as readers, experience a certain sense of dramatic irony—of knowing more and understanding more than the character with dementia does.

I suggested that the experience of narrative empathy—feeling *as* the character does, rather than feeling *with* (which is more akin to sympathy)—may be rather limited in coherent or 'conventional' dementia narratives, such as *Still Alice*. Contrary to Keen's view that certain literary avant-garde texts, in emphasising defamiliarisation and a shock aesthetic, undermine or actively eschew empathetic reading (or viewing) experiences, I showed how literary experimentation may create processes of parallel experience in the readers; that is, the reader may be said to experience an 'intellectual predicament analogous to that of the characters' (Toker 1993: 4). To explore the empathic possibilities of experimental fiction, I considered the use of a dementing and unreliable narrator, such as in J. Bernlef's *Out of Mind*, as well as the configuration of multiple extended stream of consciousness monologues, such as those employed in B. S. Johnson's novel *House Mother Normal*. Also, I suggested how a novel which does not announce itself as dementia narrative, such as Kazuo Ishiguro's *The Unconsoled*, provides means for evoking the parallel experience of certain symptoms of dementia in the reader.[21]

The potential of narratives which do not provide a clear disease pathology for their characters—that do not name the disease or label the character as a person with dementia—needs to be explored in more detail. Particularly in the context of the pathologisation of many aspects of human experience, such narratives may allow for an exploration of what it is to be human, without limiting our understanding to supposedly stable disease categories. I am aware that my reading of Ishiguro's novel as dementia narrative goes against the possibility of de-pathologising human experience. However, I maintain that the novel provides rich opportunities for exploratory modelling of the phenomenology of dementia, without necessarily having to be 'reduced' to merely being 'about' this condition. Importantly, while the novel opens up a promising means of coming close to the existential uncertainty that living with dementia entails, in the last instance, it resists being naturalised as a dementia narrative. Arguably, then, *The Unconsoled* employs what Hanna Meretoja (2018) considers a 'non-subsumptive narrative practice' with regard to exploring the phenomenology of dementia, since it does not 'reinforce cultural stereotypes by subsuming singular experiences under culturally dominant narrative scripts' (112).

This point brings me to the question where the dementia narratives discussed this far might fall on the continuum that Meretoja proposes as a tool to assess the ethical potential and dangers of storytelling. Meretoja (2018) suggests that narratives practices may be aligned along a continuum from 'non-subsumptive' to 'subsumptive narrative practices.' Subsumptive narrative practices are ethically suspect in that they might appropriate or erase the subjectivity of the other. Such practices, she argues,

> tend to hinder our ability to encounter other people in their uniqueness and perpetuate the tendency to see individuals as representatives of the groups to which they belong according to gender, sexual orientation, ethnicity, age, class and so on.
>
> (112)

We might add the category of disease condition or type of disability to this list. Importantly for my analysis, subsumptive narrative practices frequently use what Meretoja calls 'naturalizing strategies' (112) to 'mask their own nature as interpretations and manipulate the recipients by taking on an authoritative tone' (112). Like other scholars of narrative ethics, Meretoja values polyphony and self-reflexivity. By contrast, she considers 'monological narratives that invite immediate identification through naturalizing strategies ... more dangerous than ones that encourage awareness of multiple perspectives and of narrative construction' (131).

On this view, *Still Alice* might be considered the most ethically problematic narrative, since it represents the experience of the character through the dominant Alzheimer's script which focuses on cognitive deficits and decline. Further, it invites 'immediate identification,' by suggesting largely that Alice is like 'us,' the reader without dementia. The narrative ends before Alice progresses to a stage that is often considered beyond communication and beyond understanding. The risk is that by making the character with dementia like 'us,' Genova's narrative undermines the potential of truly understanding the experience of (later stage) dementia. As Andreea Ritivoi notes, 'it is important to resist positing similarity between ourselves and others if we are to maintain the possibility of understanding them' (Ritivoi 2016: 63 qtd. in Meretoja 2018: 121). And yet, as I discuss below, not engaging with the other's perspective, or positing them as radically 'other,' as the representation of consciousness in *House Mother Normal*, or particularly in *May* (2018) might suggest, is equally problematic.

Non-subsumptive narrative practices, on the other hand, challenge the process of appropriation and 'follow the logic of dialogue and exploration' (Meretoja 2018: 112). As inherently dialogic, polyphonic, and self-reflexive narrative, *House Mother Normal* might emerge as furthering the ethical potential of engaging non-subsumptively with others and challenging preconceptions about dementia by highlighting the degree to which people in the advanced stages of the condition still engage with the world as embodied and embedded subjects that retain their first-personal perspective on the world and capacity for emotions. By drawing attention to its own fictionality, the narrative also works against naturalising strategies. It alerts readers to the fact that the representation of dementia is a *representation*, with little or no claim to being an accurate representation of others experience. And yet, there are also moments of stereotyping in Johnson's account, as there are in other narratives. It remains debatable, then, to what extent 'narratives make possible an ethical relationship to the other' (Meretoja 2018: 89).

A number of open questions remain especially about how narrative technique and empathetic feelings interact. For one, the correlation between defamiliarising strategies and narrative empathy may be less straightforward than commonplace literary theorising suggests. It is questionable whether Brechtian shock aesthetics and techniques of defamiliarisation aimed at impeding 'the automatic transfer of the emotions to the spectator' (Brecht 1964: 94, qtd. in Keen 2007: 56) necessarily achieve such an effect. Felski (2008)—in discussing the phenomenon of 'enchantment' that Brecht notably worked against in his audiences (56)—makes the case that contrary to current doxa 'anti-absorptive devices are widely used for absorptive ends; artifice does not exclude immersion' (73). Of course, the link between immersive reading experiences and narrative empathy remains elusive as long as it is unclear what exactly is meant by immersive reading. Contrary to some definitions that suggest we become so emotionally absorbed in the storyworld that our reflective capacities are switched off until we emerge from this moment of enchantment, immersive reading may also include, at times even depend upon, significant cognitive (reflective and sense-making) activity in the reader.[22] I would moreover argue that certain modes of experimental fiction have an important contribution to make to the exploratory modelling of the phenomenology of dementia. These texts may be able to probe and extend the limits of engaging with the minds of the severely memory-impaired, or create instances of parallel experience in the reader. The parallel experience of trying to make sense of the narrative world may in itself be considered part of an immersive reading experience which nevertheless demands a high level of cognitive engagement. Furthermore, in its emphasis on deconstructing the illusion of reality, experimental fiction significantly contributes to an ethical probing of the risks of effacing the experience of real others by fictive imaginings.

The ethical problems attendant on representing dementia here become clear. Thus, while the narrative technique of broadcast strategic empathy in *Still Alice* is employed to further the 'recognition' of people with dementia and of their continued humanity—in the ethico-polical sense of recognition as 'acknowledgment' (Felski 2008: 29)—the question arises whether this narrative does not instead contribute to the 'othering' of people with more advanced dementia who can no longer use language coherently. As many critics would be quick to point out, the act of representing another's experience risks obliterating the radical alterity of that other and putting her actual point of view under erasure. Recognising oneself in the other—as when experiencing empathy—is considered a violation of the other's alterity (Lévinas 1961, 1979, Sartre 1943, Zahavi 2007). Indeed, the entire narrative approach to understanding others 'might be criticized for entailing what could be called a *domestication of otherness*. You reduce the other to that which can be captured in narratives' (Zahavi 2007: 199; original emphasis). Counter to a number of claims in first-wave medical humanities, literature, like philosophy, biomedicine, and neuroscience, may then equally be considered a totalising and reductionist enterprise.

Further, focusing on the other as an *object* of empathy may be seen to deny the other's subjectivity. Empathetic feelings in the context of literary reading may indeed be considered entirely self-centred or even selfish: Keen (2007) points out how feelings of recognition in the reader may lead to an 'erasure of suffering others in a self-regarding emotional response that affronts others' separate personhood' (xxiv). In this context,

> Empathy earns distrust for its apparent directional quality—an empathetic performance may appear condescending to its object or to an observer ... Feminists, postcolonial theorists, and critical race scholars in legal studies resist the universalizing of human emotions inherent in much of the commentary on empathy.
> (Keen 2007: xxiv)

Drawing on feminist and postcolonial theorists, Whitehead also highlights that empathy represents an affect that 'typically follows the paths already traced out by the circuits of economic and political privilege' (Whitehead 2017: 126). Most importantly, just like the scholars quoted above, Whitehead cautions that seemingly empathetic engagement with the experience of another might actually lead to acts of voyeurism or, as discussed above, appropriation of the other's experience.

Such a cautionary approach is warranted in the context of dementia narratives, due to the excess vulnerability of people living with the disease syndrome and their inability, generally, to write back again the way they and their experience are represented in contemporary dementia narratives. Nonetheless, a global dismissal of narrative empathy and of the attempt to understand others through narrative perspective-taking may be even more detrimental to people with dementia. Considering the use that narrative empathy has been put to in furthering social causes in the past, it may be premature to dismiss its effects in the current Alzheimer's advocacy movement. Not to engage with the question of what it may be like for people to live with the symptoms of dementia—and perhaps adapt attitudes and behaviours based on such imaginative exploration—might constitute an even greater ethical shortcoming in that the experience and needs of people with dementia may simply be overlooked or dismissed.

Considering that the link between empathy and pro-social behaviour in the real world is tenuous, the social relevance of empathetic reading experiences in relation to dementia care remains an open question. Nonetheless, anecdotal evidence suggests that fictional dementia narratives, such as the film *Still Alice*, affect the filmgoer's view of dementia—and even lead to a moral reassessment of the behaviour of various family members towards a relation with dementia. However, if fictional narratives have the potential to affect people's views—which I believe they do (see also Green 2004, Green and Brock 2000, Green, Garst, and Brock 2004)—they might equally lead to negative outcomes for certain groups within society. In Chapter 6, I therefore return to fictional dementia narratives to explore the possibility that rather than providing counter-narratives to either reductionist biomedical or dehumanising sociocultural conceptualisations, novels and films may in fact compound negative stereotypes of dementia. Furthermore, I explore in what way fiction intervenes in contemporary debates about dementia care in ways that go beyond questions of empathy and perspective-taking. Here I hope to have shown that whatever form of empathy novels and films evoke, and irrespective of whether this may lead to pro-social action on behalf of others, fictional narratives have the potential to raise awareness about certain aspects of the phenomenology of dementia—some of which may lie beyond the scope of non-fictional dementia life writing.

My overall aim in this chapter was to provide a solid case for literature's value as a 'practical counterpart of theoretical phenomenology' (Waugh 2013: 24) or, indeed, as a form of *imaginative phenomenology*. At the same time, by investigating the literary and filmic techniques that simulate an experiential reading or viewing experience, I not only hoped to underline the potential of imaginative narratives to explore the lived experience of others, but also to emphasise their necessarily constructed nature. In the context of representing people with progressive neurological decline, who at some stage lose the ability to communicate their experience and to challenge the way they are represented by others (see also Couser 2004), it is of no small ethical importance to pay attention to how stories about those persons shape what readers and viewers take to be their experiences of the condition. In Part II, I turn more squarely to these questions of identity, self-presentation, and representation in the context of dementia life writing.

Notes

1. Dementia films have seen a veritable 'boom' in recent years. See, among others, literary adaptations such as *Away from her* (Polley 2006), *The Notebook* (Cassavetes 2004), and *Small World* (Chiche 2010), science fiction comedy drama *Robot and Frank* (Schreier 2012) as well as biopics such as *Iris* (Eyre 2001) and *The Iron Lady* (Lloyd 2011). Furthermore, Alzheimer's features in a number of science fiction films and thrillers. These frequently follow the plotline of animal experiments for a new Alzheimer's drug that spiral fatally out of control, or involve the trope of either a monstrous carer or demoniacal/possessed person with dementia.
2. In Genette's terms (1980), this narrator would be categorised as heterodiegetic as well as extradiegetic—that is, as a narrator not involved in the events being reported and not a character in the storyworld who functions as an embedded teller. When discussing texts where the finer distinctions Genette's framework offers are not necessary, I mention the relevant narratological descriptors only in passing, or simply employ the traditional, but less precise, categorisation of narrators according to grammatical person (e.g., first-person or third-person narrator).
3. Focalisation was introduced by Genette (1980) to distinguish between 'who speaks' and 'who sees or perceives.' This distinction draws attention to how readers may experience the narrative world through a focal character's mind and perception at times distinct from the narrator's vision and voice.
4. For an introduction to mirror neurons see Iacoboni (2008).
5. Of course, all reading experience necessitates cognitive activity. What I mean to highlight are that texts which are challenging because they disrupt 'immersive' reading experiences, by experimenting with form or using gaps, can still further an understanding of the experience of dementia and thereby change readers' attitudes and beliefs—as has been argued for immersive reading experiences.
6. J. Bernlef is the pseudonym of Dutch author and poet Hendrik Jan Marsman. The novel was originally published in 1984 as *Hersenschimmen* by Em. Querido's Uitgeverij B.V., Amsterdam.
7. Recent years have seen the publication of a range of first-person fictional narratives. A number of texts pair the first-person narrative of the person with dementia with other first-person narrators: family members, and others who interact with the person with dementia, see Coleman (2014), Krüger (2018) and Rill (2015). Cavanagh (2015) uses a first-person narrator with early-onset Alzheimer's who insistently addresses his narrative to his teenaged son. For novels with a first-person narrator that employ a crime story plot, see Richler (1997), LaPlante (2011) and Healey (2014). In each case, the epistemological uncertainty that Alzheimer's entails in the first-person narrator is used to increase suspense. Roy (2009: 50) argues that Richler employs dementia as a narrative device to query, in postmodern fashion, whether there is ever a 'true' version of events. LaPlante and Healey, by contrast, engage more deeply with the question of what

it's like to suffer from dementia. Alzheimer's does not function merely as 'narrative prosthesis' (Mitchell and Snyder 2001: 47; qtd. in Roy 2009: 44), but instead the authors employ the murder mystery plot in order to explore the experience of living with dementia. For an earlier crime story with a third-person narrator that uses Alzheimer's as plot device, see Suter (1997).

8   Damasio's differentiation between 'core' and 'extended consciousness'—and the associated notions of 'core' and 'extended selfhood' (2000)—provide useful concepts to reconceptualise (self-)consciousness in dementia. However, since animals share core consciousness with humans, the concept of core consciousness risks feeding into dehumanising discourses about people with dementia. At issues is of course, whether the respect we accord, or should accord, humans shouldn't also be extended to other species with consciousness.

9   Krüger-Fürhoff similarly argues that the novel imagines 'a view from within that bears witness to the successive breakdown of perception and coherent language, but not of the protagonist's self' (2015: 105). Nevertheless, she asks whether Bernlef's aesthetics—drawing on modern and postmodern literary techniques such as 'stream of consciousness, semantic destruction, and alienation' are convincing 'on an ontological level' (104).

10 Since the ellipses here are part of the original, I use square brackets, here and elsewhere where this is the case, to indicate where I have omitted text.

11 Recent dementia novels, both with first-person narrators (Coleman 2014, Krüger 2018, Rill 2015) and with character focalisers (Downham 2015, Pritchett 2014), use a similar technique, although they vary in the degree of coherence they accord to the perspective of the person with dementia.

12 See Charon for the shortcomings of hospital charts in providing sufficient information about the patient as a basis for an empathic healing relationship (Charon 2006: 140–8). Charon develops the practice of 'Parallel Chart' writing to address the phenomenology of illness, and she demonstrates how this practice can yield clinical benefits (173–4).

13 While my quotations do not represent exact replicas of the original formatting, I follow the original text as closely as possible when doing so is relevant for my analysis.

14 In fact, the words are Welsh and a translation of the first few words ('galluoag'- *competent/able*; 'lwcus'- *lucky*; 'ynad'- *justice* or *to judge*) suggests that Johnson is adding another layer of meaning to his multilayered challenge to perceived norms. Johnson throughout the text inverts the sane-insane dichotomy; here by playing with the fact that English speakers without a knowledge of Welsh will read these words as nonsense when instead they make perfect sense.

15 Krüger-Fürhoff similarly draws attention to the culturally constructed nature of dementia narratives: 'we as readers, together with the literary authors of imaginary inner perspectives, are left with what we *think* dissolution of memory and break-down of language may feel and look like. These expectations are culture-bound' (2015: 104; original emphasis).

16 Bernaerts (2014) uses the term mind-game in his article on *House Mother Normal*. He comments on, but does not explore, how 'empathy and the attribution of pain are mitigated by irony' and the tragicomic tone of the novel (2014: 306).

17 Genette (1980) classified such 'infraction[s] of the dominant code of focalization in which a narrator provides more information than is licensed by this code' as 'paralepsis' (Dawson 2013: 23). Dawson argues that first-person omniscience constitutes 'another category of narrative voice' (2013: 196). Scholars of 'unnatural narratology' propose to classify such cases as instances of an 'unnatural mind' (Iversen 2013), as 'telepathic first-person narrators' (Alber 2014), or as explained by the concept of 'impersonal voice' (Nielsen 2004).

18 See Alber (2013) on impossible spaces in narrative worlds.
19 The end of the narrative represents an exception as it employs the auxiliary modal 'would' to indicate the counterfactual, hypothetical future scenario playing out in the narrator's mind.
20 The novel, despite many fantastic elements, emphasises the otherwise 'naturalist' setting of events rather than invoking the conventions of science fiction or fantasy—conventions which would allow readers to explain incongruous aspects of the storyworld through the possibilities of fantastic storyworlds.
21 There are of course limits to the notion of parallel experience, since the reader retains her capacity to remember what has gone before in the narrative.
22 Green and collaborators (Green 2004, Green and Brock 2000, Green, Garst, and Brock 2004) by contrast suggest that cognitive scrutiny correlates negatively with the degree of immersion, or what they call 'transportation into a narrative world,' following Gerrig (1993). While their research on how fictional narratives change attitudes and 'real-world beliefs' still leaves many questions unanswered, it strongly suggests that there is a correlation between transportation and the extent to which reader' attitudes shift after reading a narrative. Their evidence suggests that fictional narratives influence readers' beliefs, which, in turn, has implications for considering the role of narrative and narrative ethics in bioethical decision-making, see Chapter 6.

Part II
Life writing, self-writing, and creating identities

3 Life writing at the limits
Narrative identity and counter-narratives in dementia

The question of how serious illness disrupts a person's sense of self or identity has been a central concern in the medical humanities from its inception (see amongst others, Frank 1995, Kokanović and Flore 2017). In response, illness narratives have emerged as a means to grapple with the changes in identity that illness brings in its wake. While any serious health condition affects the capacity to tell an illness narrative and concomitantly to reconstruct identity through life writing, neurodegenerative diseases such as Alzheimer's pose particular challenges to the process of autobiographical writing. And yet, in few other conditions is the issue of how identity is produced, communicated, and recognised more at stake than in the context of dementia—since the persistence of selfhood or identity continues to be sweepingly denied in people with this condition. Shying away from the ontological question of what selfhood or identity is, I want to explore the potential and limitations of one of the most widespread tools for claiming identities—narrative. Further, I suggest ways in which the categories of narrative coherence and counter-narratives need to be rethought in the context of identity narratives in dementia. The use of identity narratives as counter-narratives in dementia is both politically relevant—considering how personhood in Western societies is tied to debates about human rights and euthanasia—and pragmatically fraught.

In this chapter, I consider first-person accounts by people with dementia, so-called autopathographies as well as collaborative life story work with people with dementia (Clegg 2010) in order to shed light on the possibilities and limitations of the notion of narrative identity in the context of progressive neurodegenerative diseases. I probe the limits of narrative coherence in constructing identity, while also stressing the ethical imperative of attending to identity narratives in the context of dementia life story work and life writing. I suggest that in the context of collaborative dementia life narratives, as compared with other sorts of life writing, a relatively greater proportion of the task of co-creating coherence and co-constituting the interlocutor's identity may shift to the editor, listener, or reader.

Further, I investigate how narrative identity links with the concept of counter-narratives which has gained currency across a range of disciplines

(Bamberg and Andrews 2004) and which is particularly pertinent in the context of narratives of illness and disability (Couser 1997, Frank 1995). I ask to what extent dementia life narratives may function as counter-narratives to the dominant cultural construction of dementia as 'loss of self' and 'death before death,' and how genre influences the construction of counter-narratives in dementia life writing.

To contextualise my discussion, I briefly outline the debates surrounding narrative identity and counter-narratives—while suggesting the implications of these debates for life writing by people with dementia. I then consider two types of case studies—first-person accounts by people with early-onset dementia and collaborative life story projects in nursing homes, in particular the collection *Tell Mrs Mill Her Husband Is Still Dead* (Clegg 2010)—to elucidate how the notions of narrative identity and counter-narrative come into play in these particular life writing environments.

Narrative identity in dementia: friend or foe?

Life is narrative. It is through narrative that we create selfhood. If we fail to produce an acceptable narrative, our normalcy is questioned. These are some of the tenets and implications of the narrative identity thesis—widely accepted today across a range of disciplines (Bruner 1991, 2003, 2004, Dennett 1993, Eakin 1999, 2008, Ricœur 1991a, b, Schechtman 1996, 2007). Since dementia causes memory loss and severely affects cognitive functioning, the disease eventually erodes the ability to tell a coherent life narrative. If selfhood is tethered to the ability to tell one's life story, people with dementia will be seen to have lost their selves. Consider Jerome Bruner's claim that 'there is now evidence that if we lacked the capacity to make stories about ourselves, there would be no such thing as selfhood' (2003: 86). Galen Strawson (2004), by contrast, vehemently challenges the view that selfhood is constituted through narrative. He attacks both the 'psychological Narrativity thesis'—according to which 'human beings typically see or live or experience their lives as a narrative' (Strawson 2004: 428)—and the 'ethical Narrativity thesis'—a normative view that 'experiencing or conceiving one's life as a narrative' is 'essential to a well-lived life' and crucial 'to true and full personhood' (428). Although Strawson's argument has its problems (see Battersby 2006, Eakin 2006), his work has stimulated a timely debate, relevant to people with dementia, about the ethical implications of the view that identity or selfhood is constituted through narrative.

In the following, I address the implications of narrativist accounts of selfhood for people with dementia. I outline both the strengths and limits of the narrative account when it comes to capturing the processes by which identity is expressed, constituted, or negotiated in the context of dementia. In doing so, I adopt a position within the debate that can be characterised as a 'moderate' or 'qualified' narrativist approach.

One of the central problems that has emerged from the debate about the narrative constitution of selfhood is that the terms 'self,' 'life,' and 'identity' are frequently used interchangeably.[1] Critics of the narrativist approach to selfhood have pointed out that not all kinds or levels of selfhood can be adequately accounted for narratively and that to require selfhood to be articulated in narrative can be problematic. Expecting life to conform to the genre of a quest narrative (Frank 1995, MacIntyre 1981), and basing an evaluation of this life purely on the success or failure of this quest, places too large a strain on any ordinary human being—if such a being exists. It also places inordinate strain on the lives and narratives of those affected by illness and disability, failing to take into account the natural course of decline towards the end of life—and disqualifying people with dementia from leading any kind of meaningful or valuable existence.[2]

Scholars such as James L. Battersby (2006) recognise the plurality of possible selves and doubt that the notion of self can ever be exhaustively captured in a narrative, or even numerous narratives (37). Nonetheless, they continue to accord narrative a central function in human sense-making. Battersby argues that it is important to scrutinise the uses to which narrative is put in the social domain. Paul J. Eakin, similarly, rejects strong narrativist formulations of identity.[3] He nonetheless pays tribute to the 'power of narrative not only as a form of self-representation but as an instrument of self-understanding' (Eakin 2006: 184). At the same time, Eakin underscores 'the very real imperialism of narrative requirements that structure our social encounters and define us as persons' (186). Eakin concludes that 'it's all very well to attack "narrativity," but it's much harder to escape it in self-presentation. We're part of a narrative identity system whether we like it or not' (186). Instead of worrying about the 'lofty norm of the examined life,' as Strawson does, Eakin argues that we need to attend to the 'deep-seated social conventions that govern narrative self-presentation in everyday life' (181–2). Eakin points out that in contemporary Western culture we are expected to be able to produce a self-narrative and that failing to do so leads others to deny in us the very existence of selfhood. Such social conventions are immensely relevant to people with memory loss. There is a difference, however, between posing narrative as essential to selfhood (strong narrativist claim) and recognising its social function in contributing to the formation or articulation of a particular kind of identity (moderate narrativist claim). In the context of personhood debates, strong narrativist claims—such as Bruner's claim that the inability to tell a self-narrative leads to the 'death' or 'loss' of self—can be detrimental to people with dementia and should be considered ethically suspect.

A further objection that can be levelled at the strong narrativist approach is its lack of attention to the nature of embodiment. Dementia affects all areas of cognition and not just the capacity to tell a life story. Phenomenologist Dan Zahavi therefore argues that *if* selfhood is lost in dementia, the capacity to tell a self-narrative cannot reasonably be considered its sole cause (Zahavi 2007: 192). More importantly, Zahavi queries whether it is accurate to speak of lost selfhood in people with dementia at all. Zahavi conceptualises selfhood as the 'first-personal givenness' of experiential life (2007: 188). Selfhood, on this view, is bound up with experience itself and is not constituted through narrative. Thus, Zahavi cautions that 'when speaking of a first-person perspective one should consequently distinguish between *having* such a perspective and *being able to articulate* it linguistically' (191; my emphasis). He concludes:

> It is by no means obvious that Alzheimer's disease brings about a destruction of the first-person perspective, a complete annihilation of the dimension of mineness and that any experience that remains is merely an anonymous and unowned experiential episode, so that the 'subject' no longer feels pain or discomfort as his or her own.
>
> (192)

Indeed, the embodied first-person perspective on lived experience persists even into the last stages of dementia. In other words, it is erroneous to assume that dementia entails a loss of self.

In my analysis I take into account the argument that whatever the ontological criteria for *selfhood*, we are part of an *identity* system in which 'identity narratives, delivered piecemeal every day, function as the signature for others of the individual's possession of a normal identity' (Eakin 2006: 182). As Eakin highlights, 'The verdict of those for whom we perform [identity narratives] is virtually axiomatic: no satisfactory narrative, no self' (Eakin 2001: 120). In the world we inhabit, narrative plays a crucial role in claiming rights, assigning responsibility, and having one's selfhood or identity recognised (see also Ritivoi 2009). People with dementia may struggle to tell their life stories, and their stories may consequently be classified as 'broken narratives'; that is 'problematic, precarious, and damaged narratives told by people who in one way or another have trouble telling their stories' (Hydén and Brockmeier 2008: 10). The problem with the notion of 'broken narrative' is that it suggests that the life or identity narratives people with dementia tell in ongoing interaction previously existed in some idealised, 'whole,' and coherent form that has been damaged by the onset of illness.[4] Instead, just like in other acts of conversational storytelling, the fragmentary nature of these stories involves the listener in a process of co-construction. Since people with dementia continue to use narrative to position themselves both in social interaction and through collaborative life writing, we need to investigate how these narratives are used and how coherence is created intersubjectively.

It makes sense to take on Strawson's criticism that a diachronic or narrative self-experience is not necessarily the only or the best way to experience one's being in time. But it equally makes sense to acknowledge the practical importance that the narrative organisation of memory (Fernyhough 2012) and the narrative performance and constitution of identity have both intrapersonally and socially. Not all life experience can or must be narrativised to constitute part of one's life or one's sense of self. However, lacking the means to narrativise one's life experience can put one on shaky terrain when it comes to positioning oneself in relation to others, this process being integral to what it means to be a person.

When considering the question of narrative identity, I am therefore inclined to argue that it is less a question of whether identity *is* narrative or *has to be* but whether we *negotiate* or *perform* identity through narrative. The narrative self is not an ontological given but a social practice and a potential means of self-understanding and understanding others—including the possibility of misunderstanding. The notion of embodied, experiential selfhood as proposed by Zahavi and others usefully adds to our understanding of different aspects of selfhood in dementia. The fact that a body-self or experiential self persists in dementia seems out of the question. It also seems clear that the person with dementia can at some point no longer communicate her perspective through narrative or constitute herself narratively in social encounters. Nevertheless, both social science research (Hydén 2018) and collaborative life writing projects show that people with dementia continue to attempt to negotiate identity through narrative—and do so further into the disease than may have seemed possible. Such attempts demand our attention and participation in terms of providing 'narrative scaffolding' (Hydén 2018). At issue is an ethical claim in which the task of performing or constituting narrative identity shifts from the teller to the listener (or reader), to a comparatively greater degree than in other storytelling situations.

Reconsidering master and counter-narratives

Life writing studies, the medical humanities, and disability studies converge exactly around the issue addressed by Eakin: that is, the question of how people perform identity narratives that serve their tellers. Performing identity narratives may be used to counter disempowering ways in which one has been socially and culturally positioned. Generally speaking, counter-narratives arise in response to a given culture's masterplots (Abbott 2008: 236)—alternatively described as 'dominant discourses,' 'discursive configurations,' or 'master narratives.' Counter-narratives are thus linked to identity politics, in that members of a marginalised group may challenge the way their identities are constructed in the mainstream. In the medical or health humanities, illness narratives are frequently considered paradigmatic examples of counter-narratives since they challenge the dominant discourse of biomedicine and the negative cultural constructions of illness and disability. I want to explore whether life writing in dementia functions in a similar manner. To address this question, I first develop some of the general issues relating to the concept of counter-narrative, and consider these issues in the context of more traditional (i.e. not always explicitly collaborative) autobiographical writing by people with dementia, before moving on to collaborative life writing in the collection *Tell Mrs Mill Her Husband Is Still Dead*.

A first look suggests that the process of countering might be more complex and fraught than the word 'counter-narrative' suggests. For one, scholars working in fields related to gender, ethnicity, or race underscore the extent to which counter-narratives are inextricably entangled in the master narratives they set out to subvert (Bamberg and Andrews 2004). Arguably, by invoking the very master narratives they aim to counter, these narratives contribute to upholding the dominant discursive configurations. Master narratives may also be so ingrained in the ways we think that it becomes impossible to communicate without them. As Bamberg points out, one is forced to enlist masterplots in order to make identity claims that are intelligible (or acceptable) to others (Bamberg 2004: 361). This need to employ master narratives in one's self-presentation is also evident in dementia autopathographies; and yet by enlisting models of competent and coherent narrative selfhood the authors of these narratives may unwittingly undermine their aim to present a counter-narrative to the dominant discourse on dementia.

Further, both the concepts of 'master' and 'counter-narrative' are difficult to define. However, they provide useful heuristic tools for understanding the functions of narratives in negotiating issues of identity in dementia. According to Carlos Kölbl, a master narrative represents 'a narrative version (or rather discourse) that is most commonly spread within a particular population' (Kölbl 2004: 28)—in this case, high-income Western democracies. As regards the content of this discourse, I argue that the master narrative of dementia can in shorthand form be described as 'loss of self' and 'death before death' (Behuniak 2011, Herskovits 1995). Dementia is seen to equal a tragic progression of losses, in the course of which the person with dementia becomes 'emptied out' and her life and person become of little, if any, value. This view of dementia finds expression in a cluster of pernicious metaphors. Since the dominant construction of dementia is perpetuated and transmitted through 'cultural artefacts such as books, films, [and] newspaper articles' (Kölbl 2004: 28), literary and cultural criticism present productive means for investigating this discursive configuration.

Cultural representations of dementia do not operate on their own, of course, but are underpinned by larger ideologies bound up with Western philosophy and contemporary biomedicine. The dominant cultural construction of dementia in the West is informed by cognitivist notions of personhood as well as a reductionist materialist understanding of how body and mind—in this case the brain and the mind—interact. In short, if the mind is nothing but the brain, severe neuropathological breakdown entails 'loss of self.' By defining personhood on the grounds of rationality and cognitive capacity alone, people with dementia become non-persons. The dominant discourse on dementia therefore has far-reaching implications for how societies think about and behave towards those who bear this disease label.

I define as counter-narrative any narrative—or in the context of collaborative storytelling, any conversational *move* (Goffman 1981, qtd. in Hydén 2010: 40)—that resists the dominant discourse on dementia or challenges its effects (such as infantilisation, neglect or abuse based on dehumanising or disabling views of people with dementia).

Despite the problems attendant on theorising master narratives and counter-narratives, I argue that these concepts represent valid and important ways to address the question of how dementia is understood in contemporary Western societies. As a neurodegenerative disease that affects language and memory—capacities that are supposedly 'what makes us human'—dementia raises complex ethical and political issues. In light of recent care scandals in the UK, continuing discussions about the allocation of scarce economic funds, the privatisation and commodification of 'care' itself, and ongoing debates about the practice of euthanasia, how we understand dementia and how we define the rights of people with dementia are questions that will only become more pressing in the future. By referring to people with dementia as 'vegetables,' 'shells,' or 'living dead' we risk stripping these people of their personhood and their human rights (Burke 2007b, Herskovits 1995). By contrast, the stories told by people with dementia show how they may productively use autobiographical and confabulated stories in order to claim identities for themselves, to counter the negative cultural construction of dementia, and to critique the care environments in which they live.

The problem of counter-narratives in dementia: reading first-person accounts

To explore how autobiographical writing by people with dementia may function as counter-narrative, I ask what specific strategies (such as genre, metaphor, plot, or theme) first-person accounts employ to counter the stigma of dementia. Other relevant questions are as follows: Can these accounts be considered 'successful' instantiations of counter-narratives? How might one assess the success or failure of counter-narratives? Is it even feasible or possible to disentangle masterplots and counter-narratives from each other—or are they always enmeshed with one another? And finally, do the conventions of autobiography—in that they rely on the narrator's ability to tell a coherent story and thereby confirm agentive, autonomous, and cognitivist notions of personhood—undermine any potential the texts might have for countering the dominant discourse on dementia as 'loss of self' (see also Burke 2007a)?

An important first question to consider is how the conventions of autobiography shape the narratives. Autobiography generally demands a 'comic plot,' one where the narrator is better off at the end than at the beginning of the story (see Couser 1997). The expectation of a happy outcome and the predominance of 'triumph narratives' in contemporary representations of illness (Conway 2007) prescribe certain forms of closure. Genre may then curtail the possibilities of representing neurodegenerative diseases—here, by demanding that the authors put a positive spin on their illness experience. This is in stark contrast to the progressive decline that the disease syndrome entails. Of course, one may also argue for a converse relation. Authors of dementia autopathographies may be purposefully enlisting the 'comic plot' of autobiography in order to paint a more positive picture of dementia and thereby counter the notion that dementia entails a 'death before death.' Martina Zimmermann notes that Thomas Graboys's account of living with Parkinson's and Lewy body dementia employs a 'triumphalist storyline while offering an exploration of the author-narrator's limits' (2017: 91). She argues that this use of storyline may help address a larger audience and 'purposefully further necessary sociopolitical discussion' (91–2). In modelling their life narrative on the *bildungsroman*, shaping their narratives as conversion tale (see Bryden 1998, 2005), triumph, or quest narrative (see, amongst others, Lee 2003), these authors draw on generic conventions to help them fashion their stories as counter-narratives.

As might be expected in a story about degenerative illness, however, the fit between the genre model and autopathography will by necessity only be partial. With regard to the quest narrative, in which spiritual enlightenment and personal growth constitute the 'holy grail,' many authors argue that dementia has taught them to live in the moment and appreciate the here and now. In his autobiographical essay, dementia activist Richard Taylor complicates the view that this is always possible. He notes how 'living in and for the moment assumes the ability to know what is going on, what [one is] doing in a given moment' (Taylor 2007: 131). Yet this ability is slowly eroded in dementia as the temporal unity of experience becomes fragmented and disjointed—casting doubt on the potentially facile moment of 'closure' or 'redemption' suggested by either the recurring *carpe diem* motif or the comic plot of many of these autobiographies.

In general, Taylor's essays provide a complex response to the widely employed strategy of countering stigma through a positive reinterpretation of life with dementia. Taylor's reply to the rhetorical question 'What's the Upside to Having Alzheimer's Disease?' is initially 'Nothing that I can think of, right off the bat' (77). And yet he subsequently lists a number of positive changes in his life due to the disease. Among them are an increased closeness to his family, gratitude for all he has, and the 'deeper appreciation of what [he] should and should not respond to emotionally' (78). However, he self-consciously reflects that while these responses to his disease 'feel good' he wonders whether rather than being the 'upside' of Alzheimer's this is, in fact, how he should have lived his life in the first place (78). He concludes, 'Still, I couldn't say, as some others with Alzheimer's do, that I am glad I know that I have Alzheimer's, glad that I got the diagnosis early' (78). Taylor, thus, does not participate in the practice of finding 'redeeming significance even in terminal illness' (Couser 1997: 16).

Furthermore, as compared with linear narration, Taylor's collection of essays allows for a more nuanced understanding of how dementia affects experience and especially the author's sense of self. Thus, later essays in the collection frequently undermine the claims or conclusions of previous essays. Rather than presenting the reader with closure and a stable viewpoint, Taylor's shifting life experience and attitude towards dementia are documented as his life unfolds. Personal essays, as Couser notes about diaries and journals,[5] may present an advantage over retrospective autobiographies, precisely in that they 'do not await the resolution—whether in recovery from or accommodation to dysfunction—that seems to license most retrospective autobiographical accounts of illness and disability' (Couser 1997: 6). Or as Zimmerman puts it 'a collection of essays skilfully circumvents the lack of happy closure' (2017: 100). Nevertheless, Taylor's voice and particular style provide coherence to the essays and allow for them to be read as one person's act of reclaiming his identity from the dominant cultural construction of Alzheimer's as 'living death.' Pace Zimmermann, then, who argues that due to the collaborative nature of first-person accounts we should merely focus on the *content* of these narratives, I would argue that even if these narratives rely on some (more or less explicit) form of collaboration, the style and tone of these narratives cannot be entirely disregarded.

Writing about dementia, further, has both a personal and a political dimension. Most autopathographers stress the therapeutic quality of writing about their experience, thereby suggesting that narrative self-making can have psychological benefits.[6] They also consider their blogs and writing as memory bank, a way to capture and remind themselves of what they have done. While some authors stress the importance of writing as a personal and private process of coping with their experience, many also see their writing as an important contribution to the dementia advocacy movement. In criticising the callous, unfeeling behaviour of health-care professionals and the lack of understanding of friends or strangers, the authors of these memoirs challenge the notion that people with dementia lack insight into their own experience and may therefore be considered unaffected by inhumane or undignified treatment. They write back against the 'epistemic injustice' perpetrated against people with dementia, who are no longer considered experts on their own experience (Fricker 2007 quoted in Capstick, Chatwin, and Ludwin 2015). They also challenge, what Kate Swaffer (2016) terms 'prescribed disengagement,' that is, health professionals' advice that there is nothing to be done and that the newly diagnosed should go home and get their end-of-life affairs in order. Instead, these authors show how they still have a role to play and how they can make significant contribution to society, in particular through their advocating for the rights and needs of people with early-onset dementia.

In speaking out against discriminatory behaviour and helping to create a better understanding of the disease, dementia autopathographers therefore aim to alleviate the stigma attached to dementia. Their writing also constitutes a means of reclaiming agency. As Lucy Burke notes, 'to write is to align a person with a narrative voice, and to make a claim for social recognition and personhood' (Burke 2007a). This view is also taken by Ryan and her collaborators. They describe how writing provides the authors of dementia autopathographies with the socially recognised roles of writer, storyteller, teacher, advocate, and wisdom figure (Ryan, Bannister, and Anas 2009: 151). These new roles may go some way towards making amends for the loss of other social roles. Indeed, autobiographical writing can be seen as a means of 'reclaiming social identity' per se. Here the notion of 'positioning' comes into play, since the experience of being negatively positioned may, indeed, be detrimental to one's sense of identity. These autopathographies attest how certain roles and identities become unavailable to people with dementia due to the progression of their disease, as well as the disabling reactions of others. For instance, the authors of dementia autopathographies are often forced into early retirement due to their illness. They struggle with the sense of feeling useless, no longer a 'fully functioning' member of society. As Cary Henderson highlights in his memoir, the loss of social roles—the ability to work, be a parent, and have hobbies—has a deep-seated impact on his sense of feeling fully human (1998: 35). Writing, then, can provide a means of self-assertion and self-creation that is immensely important to people with dementia who are being deprived of former social roles (Basting 2003a). Indeed, some authors find that dementia gives them a new purpose in life, and dementia advocacy (writing, speaking at conferences, participating in research, and sitting on Alzheimer's boards) takes the place of former paid employment.

And yet, these narratives also illustrate the degree to which the dominant cultural narrative of dementia negatively impacts on the author's sense of self and well-being after diagnosis. In her collection of essays, Kate Swaffer (2016) describes how hard it was to develop a sense that life beyond a diagnosis was possible and worth living. She further highlights how negative conceptions of dementia make it difficult to mobilise public and health resources to support those living with the condition. Thomas DeBaggio's two memoirs *Losing My Mind* (2002) and *When it Gets Dark* (2003) equally provide illustrative examples of how the cultural construction of dementia informs the author's self-conception. Contrary to Zimmermann's view that first-person accounts are 'more utilitarian than autobiographical in nature' (2017: 22), DeBaggio's illness narratives come close to being fully fledged autobiographies. *Losing My Mind* includes three narrative strands: the first concerns his past life experiences from birth to the early 1970s; the second describes the progression of current symptoms, the 'stories of humiliation and loss' containing 'the rough details of [his] tangle with Alzheimer's' (2002: ix); and the third is constituted by scientific reports on recent Alzheimer's research. While the first strand is rich in autobiographical details, the second strand outlines the effects of a disintegrating memory on DeBaggio's sense of self: 'This narrative represents a mind-clogged, uncertain present. It is filled with memory lapses and language difficulties and the sudden barks of disappointment and loss' (ix). DeBaggio highlights the importance of memory and of language in his sense of self. In fact, DeBaggio sees the moment of losing language and the ability to communicate as the end of selfhood per se, thereby colluding with the dominant conceptualisation of Alzheimer's as 'death before death':

> Although my body may still be sputtering along, the day will come when I can no longer write a clear sentence and tell a coherent story. That day will be the actual time of death. The person in me who lives on until natural death occurs is only a show left by the deadly laugh of Alzheimer's.
> (117)

DeBaggio evidently has a strongly narrativist and diachronic outlook on his life and identity. He describes how the stories he encountered through radio plays, television, and journalism shaped his own identity; how literature provided him with a model for living; and how it continues to provide comfort in his present situation. In Strawson's terms, DeBaggio is living according to the 'psychological Narrativity thesis' in that he seems to 'see or live or experience' his life 'as a narrative or story of some sort, or at least as a collection of stories' (Strawson 2004: 428). Nonetheless, DeBaggio is clearly aware that the imagination and the act of storytelling reshape memory—and thereby the identity narrative one constructs. For instance, DeBaggio ironically comments on the way his parents reconstructed their past as benign, despite the fact that they lived during an era of enslavement, lynching, two world wars, an influenza epidemic, and the Great Depression. Similarly, DeBaggio reflects on the unreliability of his own memories in shaping his sense of personal identity. In this way his memoir not only produces a narrative version of selfhood but reflects critically on the relation between narrative, memory, and self in that production.

Further, despite propounding a narrativist view of identity, DeBaggio also hints at other forms of selfhood. Reflecting on a piece of rock he has been given by a friend, DeBaggio writes:

> This coldly solid piece of the explosive past reminded me of the earth's longevity and the firmness of the past in contrast with our ephemeral present. Like many old objects it is without verbal account but nevertheless it is *full of meaning* and a reminder of the permanence of time. Unlike our own wispy recollections, this rock is a survivor of memories beyond our knowledge, a mute reminder that *the past lives silently in the present*.
> (108; my emphasis)

This passage suggests that memory may be embodied, or that the physical body may provide a base for selfhood. However, the 'meaning' of the object 'without verbal account' depends on a reflexive human other who can recognise the stone as 'survivor of memories beyond [the perceiver's] knowledge.' Likewise, the person with advanced dementia who is mute and unable to project her sense of self requires another to recognise her past life and the continuing meaning of her life that continues 'silently in the present.'

This passage in DeBaggio echoes Richard Taylor's conviction that despite biological and psychological changes, at the end of the disease process, he will still be himself:

> I have no idea who I will be when I am wheeled out for the final act on the Alzheimer's stage. But I do know I will *be* ... I will still be me ... perhaps a *me* different from what I have ever been before.
> (Taylor 2007: 118, original emphasis)

However, as noted previously, Taylor's conclusions are never simple. Throughout his essays, Taylor struggles to define the degree to which his brain and his self are one, the extent to which he exists separately from his disease pathology (89). Taylor also stresses the impossibility of 'knowing the truth about people with late-stage Alzheimer's.' To claim insight into the later stages, he argues, is like

> claiming to know the form and content of the fourth or fifth dimension. We are limited by our own thinking and language to imagining something we cannot see, hear, feel, touch, or taste. We can take what we know and project it, but we are still within the confines of our own minds.
> (24)

Among other things, Taylor reminds us that due to its progressive nature, dementia is not 'one thing.' Accounts by people with early stage dementia may thus have only limited purchase on what the later stages look or feel like. Indeed, those who speak out about their experience are generally not representative of the wider population of people with dementia in terms of ethnicity, race, age, or class, and their experience may therefore not necessarily reflect those of others with dementia (Innes 2009: 64). Furthermore, dementia autopathographies are clearly constrained by the modes and conventions of their production. Indeed, these texts may be seen to compound the stigma attached to dementia, by relegating stigma to the later stages.[7] The authors claim that although they have been diagnosed with dementia, they are not (yet) to be equated with 'vegetables,' 'zombies,' or 'shells.' However, by using these negative tropes themselves for their prospective selves (see in particular Davis 1989, DeBaggio 2002) and also by using life writing to assert agency, these authors potentially confirm the master narrative of dementia as 'loss of self' and 'death before death'—suggesting that only when you can tell a (more or less) coherent life story, are you still a valuable human being.

The form of autobiography, as dictated by genre conventions, constitutes an ethical problem if we tie narrative form—'how the subject is realised through writing'—to social recognition in personhood debates (Burke 2007a: n.p.). 'For it is precisely these fictions of autonomy [perpetuated through the conventions of life writing],' Lucy Burke writes, 'that render the vulnerable and disabled beyond the pale of social, political and often legal recognition' (n.p.). In this context, McGowin's memoir *Living in the Labyrinth* (1994) has been singled out as an example of how narrative form, and its reception, may be ethically problematic. Basting notes that in McGowin's account the symptoms of dementia are described rather than 'performed': The language of her memoir is 'cleansed of the disease ... spelling, grammar and memory of dialogue and events are pristinely intact' (Basting 2003a: 89). The memoir also includes a number of rhetorically powerful arguments. Basting notes, quoting McGowin at length, how well McGowin is able to articulate 'the contradiction between her own feelings of self-worth and the depletion of her cultural value as a victim of Alzheimer's' (90):

> If I am no longer a woman, why do I still feel I'm one? If no longer worth holding, why do I crave it? If no longer sensual, why do I still enjoy the soft texture of satin and silk, against my skin? My every molecule seems to scream out that I do, indeed, exist, and that existence must be valued by someone!
> (McGowin 114, qtd. in Basting 2003a: 90)

While Basting suggests this passage captures the frustration she has seen in the behaviour of people with more advanced dementia, she nevertheless states that she finds McGowin's eloquence 'almost disturbing' (90)—presumably due to its lack of 'authenticity' as the voice of a person with Alzheimer's.

However, criticising dementia autopathographies for being too coherent represents a double-edged sword. Zimmermann, in her history of Alzheimer's disease life writing, is concerned with whether what she calls 'patient narratives' are 'credible in narrative terms' (2017: 96). In her analysis of Taylor's essays, Zimmermann, for instance, seems to concur with common stereotypes about people with dementia when she suggests that Taylor's 'highly accomplished tone' must be reliant on 'editorial support' (2017: 101). Despite the growing number of dementia autopathographies—in blog, essay, or book form—these authors still face the problem that in terms of 'speaking out' about their experience they are 'damned if they do, and damned if they don't.' If they are able to coherently tell about their experience, then their diagnosis of dementia is frequently challenged—a situation that many describe as deeply upsetting. Anyone who can still talk or write, cannot have dementia, the logic goes. 'People have looked at my blog and questioned how I can possibly have dementia,' Wendy Mitchell writes.

> It's sad when the things you continue to do make people question whether you have dementia. They're not inside my brain to hear or see the hallucinations. Would it make them feel better to see me on a foggy day, the type where I curl up under my duvet and hide away from the world? Would that make the disease fit better into the pigeonhole they've allocated it?
>
> (Mitchell 2018: 259)

Accordingly, authors of dementia memoirs use strategies of legitimization in their writing and in their presentations to counter any challenges to their status as authentic person with dementia.[8]

If, on the other hand, their writing is not sufficiently coherent to appeal to mainstream presses or satisfy the expectations of readers, then their views and experiences are once again likely to be disregarded. However, dementia affects the cognitive capacities of individuals differently, and for some writing might come more easily than speech, and for others it may be the other way round—in which case they may rely more on interviews and collaboration with a writing assistant to get their story told. In any case, determining the cognitive capacity of people with dementia based on their writing proves both impossible and represents a misguided approach. People's abilities exist and come into play in interaction with their environment: both through tools and through the help of other people. Since even in cases where the writing assistance was substantial, the authors describe how they edited each chapter painstakingly to ensure it represented their views and experience, it seems somewhat hasty to question whether the tone, style, or instances of humour stem from and represent the named author.

More recent memoirs often explicitly acknowledge the writing assistance involved in providing a smooth, coherent, and accomplished narrative (see, for instance, Rohra 2011). Wendy Mitchell's highly literary memoir that uses you-narrative to address her pre-diagnosis self in brief vignettes does not explicitly describe the process of collaboration with writer Anna Wharton, but Wharton is named as co-author on the book's title page. However, not all contemporary forms of dementia life writing provide coherent narratives promoting fictions of autonomous selves. Cary Henderson's collaborative life writing project *Partial View* (1998) acknowledges not only the collaborative nature of dementia testimony but also the interdependent and relational nature of identity (see also Burke 2007a). Furthermore, Henderson's account, through its repetitive and syntactically flawed style, 'enacts' or 'performs' the symptoms of dementia. Thereby, the text fully acknowledges the difficulties Henderson experiences. While Burke is aware that collaborative texts 'raise their own ethical difficulties,' she lauds them for raising the problems explicitly, 'rather than subsuming them behind what has always been a fiction—that of the autonomous, independent subject' (Burke 2007a: n.p.). Burke's discussion of Alzheimer's testimony resonates strongly with Angela Woods's recent challenge to the uses—and potential abuses—of 'narrative' in the medical humanities, in that Woods questions the current promotion of one model of selfhood within medical humanities research—that is, of the self as an 'agentic, authentic, autonomous storyteller' (Woods 2011: 2)— to the exclusion of more shifting, interdependent, relational, or embodied models of selfhood.

By providing a collaborative account and highlighting the process of its production, Henderson's memoir challenges the agentic, authentic, and autonomous notion of selfhood. However, it also provokes the reader to reconsider the extent to which narrative 'coherence' in a life narrative is necessary for it to count as a claim to personhood. Henderson's memoir is illuminating, since it lacks any kind of overarching narrative frame and it includes hardly any references to the author's past. It lacks the usual plot device of pitting 'then' against 'now,' or of providing a chronological narratives from first symptoms, the difficult path to diagnosis, through personal struggle and grief to acceptance and a renewed purpose in life that many first-person accounts chart. And yet Henderson's insights into his current situation, his appreciation of nature and music, his paranoia, anger, and fear, as well as his deep compassion for his family care partners provide a powerful sense of self. The inscription of his 'now-self' through the use of brief musings is no less powerful than, for instance, DeBaggio's narrative that is more heavily focused on his 'past-self.' Despite minimal coherence between and sometimes within sections, Burke notes how 'Henderson's personhood is asserted in the very act of narration' (Burke 2007a: n.p.). Unlike other dementia life writers, Basting comments, 'Henderson does not rely heavily on memory to define who he was and, simultaneously, who he is. His narrative voice lives in the present moment, rather than describing the disease with the distance for reflection that more traditional narratives provide'—and, I would add, *require* (2003: 94). In short, small stories (Bamberg 1997) and not just life stories with a protracted narrative arc or in the form of a quest can function as a means for reclaiming identity and countering stigma.

Nonetheless, in relying on the performance of 'neurotypical' selves able to tell coherent life narratives, most of these memoirs ultimately reclaim selfhood only for people in the early stages of dementia. They may therefore, as Burke points out, 'collude with precisely those norms that underpin the stigmatisation of dementia in the first place' (Burke 2007a: n.p.). Disability scholars question whether autopathographies can ultimately 'counter' the dominant construction of dementia as loss of self (Basting 2003a, Burke 2007a). Burke worries that in tying life writing to social and political recognition we are 'still working within a paradigm that potentially robs those unable to produce their own narratives of their personhood' (Burke 2007a: n.p.). She raises the question whether to tell 'a good enough story' about Alzheimer's may not 'require a different genre—a new set of conventions—fully to speak to the damage wrought by the condition and to the significance of relationships and intersubjectivity to the illness experience' (n.p.). I argue that collaborative life story work represents just such a 'new' genre of dementia life writing.

Coherence in 'broken' counter-narratives: 'Mrs Mill' and other stories

In this section I argue that collaborative life history work with people with dementia not only extends the possibilities of representing the experience of cognitive decline, but also pays tribute to the intersubjective, interactive, and relational nature of identity (see also Basting 2001: 79). I investigate what happens when we shift our attention from the published autobiographies of individuals to seemingly incoherent or 'broken'[9] narratives told in the context of a collaborative life writing project such as the Trebus Project.[10] These narratives challenge the extent and the nature of 'coherence' expected conventionally of life stories. They alert readers to different *forms* of coherence in collaborative dementia narratives and appeal to readers to actively participate in the creation of coherence.

The artist David Clegg has been producing collaborative life stories with people with dementia since 2001. *Tell Mrs Mill Her Husband Is Still Dead*[11] is one of the publications to emerge from these collaborations. Clegg's Trebus Project shares certain goals with both life history work and dementia advocacy. In collecting the (life) stories of his participants, Clegg operates somewhere between the practices of ethnography, collaborative life writing, and creative writing; with the result that the narratives cannot be clearly assigned to any of these genres or disciplines. Despite its parallels with life history work and patient advocacy, Clegg nevertheless regards his work as artistic practice—describing the words he collects as 'the building blocks' of his 'sculpture' (11). Clegg's procedure raises complex questions about who these stories belong to and how they are to be received. Do we read these narratives as social history, testimony, and/or identity narratives? Or do we assess them as collaborative art work? In which case, do we ascribe artistic intentionality to the storytellers or to Clegg (and the numerous other editors)? Due to the nature of the collaboration process these questions cannot finally be resolved. The very nature of these narratives therefore demands an interdisciplinary approach. In developing such an approach, I map out a framework that leverages the ideas of identity narrative, narrative coherence, and counter-narratives to generate new hermeneutic tools for understanding these collaboratively told (life) stories. I propose an integrative approach that draws on life writing studies, literary criticism, conversational storytelling analysis and small story research to yield productive strategies for engaging with these accounts—strategies that will need to be further extended and diversified in future work.

Before I provide examples of how counter-narratives are constructed in collaborative storytelling, a few preliminary notes on the collection as a whole are in order. *Tell Mrs Mill* contains nearly 50 stories by people with dementia. Sometimes these narratives consist of conversations between participants, but usually each chapter is devoted to a single storyteller. Pseudonyms are used in all but one case. Clegg's practice differs here from the usual conventions of life writing. Despite having acquired consent for his work, he shields the narrators' identities—by changing names, addresses, and occupations. This practice shows that Clegg is sensitive to the difficult ethical issues attendant on representing 'vulnerable subjects' in life writing (Couser 2004). Nonetheless, it is somewhat surprising that Clegg chooses to obscure the storytellers' identity since, according to his introduction to the collection, many of the participants 'told their stories because they would be published not despite it' (Clegg 2010: 13). Indeed, Clegg adamantly criticises care homes for isolating 'the people it is supposed to be protecting' and for cutting off 'avenues of real communication' (13)—under the pretext of adhering to patient confidentiality. In contrast to the 'institutional need to censor' or to 'sanitise' life stories, Clegg underlines how most of his participants 'insisted that their story be told "warts and all"' (13). By allowing the storytellers' unique voices to shine through, Clegg exposes their disability. By shielding their privacy in order to mitigate the effects of this exposure, however, he undermines the storytellers' authority. Collaborative life writing in dementia clearly raises complex ethical issues not easily resolved by any one set of rules or conventions.

Conversational storytelling research yields many productive tools and concepts for reading the stories in *Tell Mrs Mill*. However, there are limits to this method of inquiry due to the very nature of the stories themselves. The narratives in *Tell Mrs Mill* are, for the most part, a far cry from the detailed transcriptions that appear in conversation analysis. Since Clegg's part in the conversation has been edited out, it is unclear how his contribution shaped the stories. Many stories were, furthermore, elicited over the course of numerous visits. The process of editing may then have rendered the final product either more or less coherent. I have no way of reconstructing the editorial process. However, this reconstruction is not necessary in order to get a sense of how the storytellers use narrative to position themselves both in the ongoing interaction and in the context of the publication of their life story (when they retained the sense of this second level of engagement). That said, the editorial process, as I outline below, does play a prominent role in the way we read these narratives as counter-narratives.

Let us turn now to the stories themselves. The collection is striking for the sheer variety of selves it represents. One is drawn into the storytellers' life histories while also gaining insight into their current situation in the nursing home. Many narrators are openly critical of the care environment and the rigid structure of the institutions they live in. They criticise care staff for curtailing their freedom, denying them their individuality, and invading their privacy. On this account alone, these stories can productively be read as counter-narratives to the potentially dehumanising, or at the very least infantilising,[12] treatment of people with dementia in nursing homes.

The narrators use autobiographical stories to make identity claims. Sometimes these narratives may lack coherence—when the temporal order becomes disjointed, referents are unclear, or multiple versions of events contradict each other. Hydén and Örulv (2009) show how we can understand even such seemingly incoherent narratives by paying attention to how the narrators use the evaluative sections of their narratives to make identity claims. According to Hydén and Örulv, evaluation 'tells the audience something about the teller or the narrator'—significantly about 'his or her moral standing in relation to what transpired in the story' (210). Evaluative sections of a story are used to present a continuous identity, to present oneself as the 'same person' as previous to the onset of dementia with the 'same moral qualities' (212).

Many of the stories in *Tell Mrs Mill* function in this identity-building way. For instance, Aidan stresses how he has always been a 'loner' and how his independent nature has kept him from becoming an alcoholic embroiled in bar fights—unlike many others from his socio-economic background. By telling stories about his past and aligning his present self with them, Aidan emphasises continuous traits of his identity. For Isabella, engaging in the Trebus Project represents a continuation of her lifelong involvement in political advocacy. Remembering her experience of visiting an abattoir, Isabella notes, 'But now I've seen people with dementia treated just as badly ... people in care... people with dementia... drugged and sedated with a cup of tea and a digestive biscuit' (Clegg 2010: 111).[13] The story content (inhumanity towards animals) is made pertinent to her current situation and employed as a searing critique of current dementia care practice.

More generally, Isabella calls attention to the vulnerable position of people with memory loss:

> Dementia care in this country doesn't exist ... the problem is ... a great many people who are supposed to be carers ... have contempt ... for the loss of memory and the mental problems that that leads to ... and take advantage of it. They behave in the most diabolical way and think they can get away with it ... because ... no one would believe the poor woman with dementia.
>
> (112)

In her lively stories about her previous political battles as well as her damning evaluation of the current state of care, Isabella maintains her identity as political activist. Isabella's counter-narrative therefore functions on a number of levels. It undermines the notion that people with dementia undergo a loss of self since her narrative allows Isabella to present a continuous identity.

Life writing at the limits 117

She performs this identity in interaction with Clegg but also through the wider dissemination of her narrative on publication. Furthermore, she criticises the stigma attached to dementia and challenges the way people with dementia are treated.

As the story of a former Hitler Youth suggests, the teller of autobiographical stories can also make identity claims by distancing herself from past actions and highlighting changes over a life time. Here the storyteller, Eva, dissociates herself from her youthful enthusiasm for Hitler by describing herself retrospectively as 'silly' and 'weak' (23). While her anecdote of offering a bunch of flowers to Hermann Göring may or may not be confabulatory, it vividly evokes her sense of having been swept up in a wave of mass enthusiasm. When it comes to making identity claims in her present situation, though, it is central that Eva retrospectively evaluates her girlhood self, specifically in relation to this incident, as 'proud and stupid' (23). She thereby claims a different moral stance towards her youthful attitudes, resolving the conflict that subsequent knowledge of the Holocaust caused in her sense of herself as moral being. She performs this new identity and highlights her distance from her previous self by integrating self-quotation into her story. As Hydén (2010) notes,

> Telling autobiographical stories is a way to expand the present reality and thus expand one's own identity. By introducing new versions of the self, the teller is able to relate to these figures, by identifying with them, by rejecting them, or by claiming that a change or development has taken place, a development that may be continuous or discontinuous.
>
> (39)

This 'narrative expansion of identities' through which the teller can introduce new aspects of herself into an ongoing interaction provides the means by which a speaker, as in Eva's case, negotiates her identity with the present audience (Hydén 2010: 39).

Eva's collaboration with Clegg also represents another instance of countering the dominant discourse on dementia. Validating her life experience as part of a life history project, the collaboration underlines that her life is anything but valueless. People with dementia witnessed a time which is slowly passing out of living memory. They have something important to tell us about how things were for them. The stories not only provide counter-narratives to the dominant construction of dementia, but, for instance, by describing what it was like to live in wartime London, as a number of stories do, they also challenge the retrospective glorification, or sentimentalisation, of the past.

Although a referential relationship to 'life' is central to autobiography studies (Eakin 1992, Lejeune 1988), the criterion of referentiality may recede into the background in collaborative dementia life writing—without, however, dropping out of the picture entirely. Recent work on confabulation in dementia illuminates how even confabulatory stories are used to make identity claims. To recognise these claims, however, we need to expand the notion of narrative coherence. Maria Medved and Jens Brockmeier's view of narrative as 'primarily a communicative activity' (Medved and Brockmeier 2010: 25) opens the door for recuperating relevance in fragmented and possibly confabulatory autobiographical narratives. They underscore how the narratives told by a brain-injured person may be psychologically coherent, by highlighting a central pre-morbid personality trait. Other authors have stressed the relevance of 'emotional,' 'metaphorical,' or 'thematic' coherence in confabulatory stories by people with dementia (Crisp 1995, McLean 2006). Jane Crisp (1995) proposes a framework in which the relevant criteria for evaluating stories by people in advanced stages of dementia 'would no longer be the literal truth or falsity of the details,' but among other things, 'the overall point of the story—the underlying message or thematic and metaphoric meaning it suggests' (135). Crisp underscores that it is important to note 'the qualities to which the storyteller [of confabulatory stories] is laying claim':

> Sometimes these are fantasized qualities of strength, activity, resourcefulness and power, which serve to compensate for an actual position of weakness and dependency. ... Less positive stories may present the teller as ill-treated, trapped, confused and miserable; qualities that make a direct claim on the listener's sympathy, reassurance and aid.
>
> (139)

In her case study of the story told by Mrs Fine, a woman with dementia, Athena McLean (2006), shows how the tragic plot of 'wronged wife' allows Mrs Fine to make an empathy-eliciting identity claim. The plot segment also helps Mrs Fine make sense of her current living situation—in that the notion of having been disinherited explains why she finds herself in the seemingly reduced circumstances of a nursing home. While details of her story cannot be considered 'true' to real-life events, McLean highlights the 'emotional truth' value of the story (171) and the extent to which it helps Mrs Fine make sense of her situation.

Nonetheless, neither Crisp nor McLean lose sight entirely of the criterion of referentiality in making sense of the confabulatory stories told by people with dementia. (Of course, designating a story as 'confabulatory' already involves a value judgment in relation to 'real-life' referents.) In deciphering the 'underlying message or metaphoric meaning' of her mother's stories, Crisp uses her extensive knowledge of her mother's life. Rather than abandoning 'referentiality' entirely, Crisp instead temporarily brackets it in an attempt to make sense of her mother's stories. At the same time, Crisp notes how confabulation is generally 'very disconcerting to caregivers who know enough about the teller's past life or present circumstances to realize how fantastic many of the claims made in them actually are' (133). Since confabulation presents a major impediment to intersubjective understanding,

Crisp's strategies for meaning-making are vital. Similar strategies—paying attention to what the story aims to do in the world and bringing in autobiographical knowledge where relevant—can be used in the context of reading the narratives in *Tell Mrs Mill*.

However, drawing on autobiographical 'facts' in the context of interpreting stories told by people with dementia turns out to be a double-edged sword. McLean's coherence-seeking analysis of Mrs Fine's story represents a fine balancing act between drawing on biographical 'facts' and not overestimating the criterion of 'facticity.' She alerts the reader to an inherent power dynamic that the criterion of facticity sets up when external sources are used to either confirm or disconfirm an elder's story (175). In many cases external information can help make sense of a narrative and underscore the intelligibility of the storyteller's identity claims. Nevertheless, I query the editorial practice, in *Tell Mrs Mill*, of inserting 'factual' information in prefaces or footnotes, when the only function of these facts is to highlight the extent of that person's confusion and thereby undermine her authorial voice. Instead, it seems more productive to follow McLean's pragmatic suggestion to make use of the paratext when it helps elucidate the metaphoric, psychological, or emotional coherence of a narrative. What is at stake here, in short, is how to make sense of confabulatory and fragmented dementia narratives by acknowledging their use in the performance of identities in discourse.

Attending to recurrent or dominant themes, as Crisp suggests, provides another way of reading the narratives in *Tell Mrs Mill* as a means of identity construction ('self-making') and 'sense-making'[14] (Örulv and Hydén 2006). Sid's story, for example, revolves around his survivor's guilt, a deep admiration for his mother and an overwhelming sense of loss at his close friend Frankie's death during the war. In Sid's account, versions of key events in his life (his mother's death by drowning, various people being killed by a bayonet) contradict each other. However, each version highlights how his life was marked by violence and loss, how he continues to struggle with survivor's guilt, and how his love for both his mother and his friend Frankie persist. Similarly, Ann repeatedly laments the loss of her doll's house, which her mother gave away when she was a child. The strong emotion this memory evokes indicates how formative early childhood experiences can be, while also suggesting the extent to which earlier memories may come to dominate the present in dementia. However, in the terms set out in Crisp's study, the loss of the doll's house can also be seen as a metaphor expressing Ann's current experiences of loss.

Although much more could be said about the stories in this collection, I will elucidate how the ideas discussed thus far may be brought to bear on one specific example. I focus on Janet's story, not because it is representative, but to show how narrative identity is constructed in a comparatively fragmented, non-linear, and partly confabulatory narrative. Indeed, this text may not be considered 'narrative' at all if one applies strict criteria of causal linearity and logical coherence. Yet in the context of everyday storytelling, let alone collaboratively produced dementia narratives, such criteria rarely apply (see Hyvärinen et al. 2010, Ochs and Capps 2001). In the following discussion I elucidate how Janet's narrative, though partly confabulatory, functions as a counter-narrative. I engage with the difficult question as to how much context needs to be restored to make sense of her utterances—and what role the listener, editor, and reader play in constructing a 'coherent narrative' and possibly by extension a 'coherent identity' for and with Janet.

Janet's story: confabulation, continuity, and agency

Unlike most narratives, Janet's story is framed by some introductory information (distinguished from the narrative 'proper' through the use of italics). This states that she worked as a housekeeper for a large hotel for thirty years and has been living in a modern purpose-built care home for three months (189). The first part seems intended to help the reader make sense of what she says, while the second emphasises the extent of her dementia—since she is uncertain about how long she has been in the care home and whether she lives there permanently. Despite her confusion, her narrative nonetheless highlights how aware she is, both of her dementia and of her environment. As she blandly puts it, 'People sometimes think I'm not aware of what's happening but I am' (189). She describes how disconcerting the symptoms of dementia are: 'I feel like I'm out of my depth ... like I've been swimming along and suddenly I can't feel the bottom. That's the feeling. It's not my cup of tea at all' (191). Her account is rich in emotional appeal since it evokes her sense of frustration, struggle, and loss. Among other things, Janet is aghast at her loss of agency: 'I feel as if the rug's been pulled out from under my feet' (191), she states. Also she feels she has been 'shuffled about a bit,' 'inveigled' or 'hustled into' the care home by her family. Although Janet acknowledges that her children are trying to protect her from her own frailty she nevertheless states 'I'd much rather take the risk and stay at home' (191). Her account closes movingly with the words '... all my life has gone now ... all my memories are at home ... I'm sure all this is with the very best intentions' (191). Janet's evocative use of imagery and the insight she provides into her condition allow the reader to get a sense of what it might feel like to be losing all sense of certainty and agency. Her self-awareness clearly undermines the common presumption that people with dementia are 'mindless vegetables' unaware of what is going on either 'inside' or around them.

Janet's account also represents a counter-narrative in another, related sense. Her life experience of working in a hotel provides a framework for making sense of—and severely criticising—her care environment. So, for instance, she refers to a member of staff as a 'waitress' and to the other residents as 'guests.'

> The way that waitress talks to me ... she swears ... it's just not the thing. I told the lady last night that she didn't have to go just because they said

> it's time to go to bed. I don't understand it. They came to the lounge, got hold of my hand and tried to cart me off to bed. I said I don't want to go to bed. I can go to bed on my own, thank you very much.
>
> (189)

By applying the norms of social conduct of a hotel to her environment, Janet starkly highlights how radically social norms shift in the context of dementia care. While her account might be interpreted as a misapprehension of reality, the storyline she employs nevertheless exposes the forms of conduct in care homes as contrary to what is considered acceptable in other social contexts. Common courtesy, respect, and politeness all suddenly go out of the window:

> I think I irritate the staff sometimes but some of them are so rough that they scare me. I heard one of them say something to one of the guests the other day and I said, 'Please, you should say "please."' They looked at me as if I'd gone mad because I asked them to say please rather than just pull the lady out of her chair.
>
> (190)

In interpreting the care home as hotel Janet uses a dominant storyline from her life history. This storyline helps her make sense of her environment as well as assert her identity by linking the past to the present and by providing an evaluation of the current setting (Örulv and Hydén 2006). Janet's account illuminates how residents in care homes are infantilised and robbed of their autonomy in every conceivable instance—frequently unnecessarily. I find it remarkable that this aspect of her narrative, which could easily be dismissed as confusion, instead highlights the persistence of her social identity and provides a damning critique of this so-called 'home.'

Counter-narratives in context: the editor's role

Taken in context, Janet's narrative suggests more generally how the whole Trebus Project represents a multilayered and multifaceted counter-narrative to the dominant discourse on dementia—in large part because of the way Clegg frames the stories. Here, I briefly want to consider the editor's role in presenting these narratives and how this affects our reading of the stories in the collection.

The provocative title of the collection derives from what may be considered an exemplary counter-narrative—provided by Clegg himself. Clegg relates how Mrs Mill would camp out in front of the locked door to her residential unit because she wanted to get out to prepare tea for her husband—dead for twenty years. In order to keep her from obstructing the door the nursing staff would pretend her sister was on the phone. Clegg finds that 'repeatedly tricking a frail old woman and then hoping she would forget seemed so contrary to care, so mocking and so wrong' that he decides to tell her the truth about her husband's demise (11). Clegg relates how Mrs Mill, after some initial confusion, visibly relaxed at the thought that her husband was not in fact waiting for her. He manages to persuade the staff to tell her the truth in the future. The next day he finds a message on the notice board: TELL MRS MILL HER HUSBAND IS STILL DEAD. The reader is left to infer with how much sensitivity the staff is likely to have proceeded. Interestingly, when more than a hundred pages later we come to Mrs Mill's life story there is no mention of these events. Yet what is remarkable, for want of a better description, is how much of Mrs Mill is still there. She remembers her childhood and working life in detail and, notably, cherishes the opportunity to tell her life story: 'I'm so pleased to do this ... I never thought I was popular enough to write a biography' (157). Clegg advocates a change in the perception of dementia and the treatment of people with dementia, and offers his own work as one way such a change can be brought about.

Apart from this introductory anecdote, Clegg's strongest act of 'countering' resides in one of the narratives in which his work as editor is seemingly least pronounced. The middle section of the collection is entitled (again provocatively) 'Fun and Games.' This section is distinguished from the rest by being printed on harder, egg-shell coloured paper and framed by a stripy cover. It includes another introduction by Clegg in which he describes the opportunity to revisit three of his storytellers after a break of five years. Clegg here takes a much more ethnographic approach: describing and transcribing the background details; the date; time of day; and the words, actions, and gestures of both the residents and their caregivers. Although Clegg here takes *less* licence in editing out sections of the interaction, and therefore, arguably, has less of a shaping influence on the counter-narrative, I consider this section the most powerful counter-narrative of the collection—fittingly placed at its heart. In his transcriptions, Clegg provides context for what may otherwise seem meaningless or incoherent behaviour. Importantly, the detailed description reveals how callously—and sometimes brutally—the care staff respond to the patients in their care. For instance, Clegg queries the enforced cropping of Daisy's long hair—long hair which had previously been a great source of pride. Although her distress is evident in her words—'look at what they have done to me' (XXXVI)—Clegg's additional description leaves no doubt as to the meaning of her utterance: '(*She tugs violently at her cropped hair.*)' (XXXVI). The image of cropped or shaved hair is in turn reminiscent of other outrages against humanity. In evoking and underlining this image, Clegg highlights the brutality of acts of supposed 'care' which instead humiliate and dehumanise the person receiving care.

Conclusion

The question of the relation between narrative and identity remains an open one. In this chapter, I have argued that narrative identity is crucial to people with dementia, particularly in the context of dementia life writing. Rather than focusing on the ontological question of whether selfhood is constituted through narrative, I have suggested that narrative is a tool, a means of constructing and negotiating identity in the social world. Writing dementia autopathographies represents one means of making identity claims. In the context of collaborative dementia life writing, narrative is similarly a means of claiming identity, both locally in the context of interactions within the nursing home and more globally through the publication and dissemination of these texts to a wider audience. In turn, in order to be able to make sense of these narratives and understand their function, we need to expand the notion of 'coherence.' In the light of ideas from conversation analysis, ethnographic approaches to narrative and previous research on storytelling in dementia, the narratives in *Tell Mrs Mill* can be read as 'emotionally/ psychologically,' 'thematically,' or 'metaphorically' coherent. Further, the creation of coherence involves a collaboration among the storytellers, editors, and readers.

Coherence, in fact, is the contested backbone around which both identity narratives and counter-narratives are built. Recent work in narrative studies premised on the view that coherence is an interactional achievement opens up new avenues of thought for considering how coherence is constructed in collaborative dementia life writing. The operative terms then become positioning and performance rather than referentiality and factuality. People with dementia continue to make coherent, that is intelligible, identity claims. Whether their claims are recognised or not depends, however, less on the formal criteria of their identity narratives than on the willingness and ability of the people around them to engage with these claims.

By showing how coherence is achieved through a two-way process that involves the coherence-creating capacity of the listener or reader, I have aimed to underline two issues: One, narratives by people with dementia present an ethical demand or *ought to* for the listener/reader, who is prompted actively to engage with these attempts at meaning-making rather than disregard them as 'incoherent'—even if this attempt entails the risk of over-reading or misinterpreting certain narratives. Two, not only narrative but identity is interactively and intersubjectively constructed, frequently *through* the exchange of narratives. Dementia life writing, especially collaborative life writing projects, acknowledges our interdependent nature—that we are socially constituted beings—thereby refuting the myth of the self as autonomous agent. Narrative is one means of creating and shaping a social environment ('world-making'), claiming and negotiating identity ('self-making'), and making sense of one's environment and one's position in the world ('sense-making') (Örulv and Hydén 2006)—providing the answer to such questions as 'What is this? Who am I? How did I get here?' Broadening the conception of narrative coherence, we can attend to the actual ways people with dementia use narrative and the moves they make in social interactions to position themselves more favourably.

Further, I aimed to address the question to what extent life narratives by people with dementia represent counter-narratives to the dominant cultural construction of dementia as 'loss of self' and 'death before death.' My analysis of dementia autopathographies suggests that the authors of these texts criticise the stigma attached to Alzheimer's; they reclaim a sense of agency for themselves by becoming writers, advice givers, and dementia advocates (Ryan, Bannister, and Anas 2009), and they revise the view that dementia entails a tragic progression of losses by suggesting ways in which the disease has changed them for the better. But does this really mean they serve as counter-narratives vis-à-vis the dominant discourse on dementia?

By and large, illness narratives by people with dementia represent ambiguous and unsettling examples of counter-narratives. On the one hand, their authors frequently use the same dehumanising metaphors that circulate in the cultural imaginary to describe those in the later stages of the disease—including their prospective selves. They thereby confirm the dominant trope of dementia as 'living death' (see Davis 1989, DeBaggio 2002). On the other hand, these memoirs represent remarkably lucid, coherent, and rhetorically powerful narratives about dementia (see, in particular, Bryden 2005, DeBaggio 2002, McGowin 1994). There is a risk here that countering is understood only in terms of resistance and opposition—in the sense of offering a counter-image to the dominant one.[15] In the case of dementia life writing, there is an inherent risk that by (re)positioning—and therefore valuing—the storyteller with dementia as an autonomous, able-minded, coherent, linguistically expressive person, as many of the above mentioned life narratives do, authors and readers alike continue to stigmatise the dependent, cognitively impaired persons that people with dementia increasingly become. Together with disability critics I therefore query whether it is appropriate to use this form of life writing in rights-based movements in the context of neurodegenerative diseases.[16]

By writing about their stigmatised diseases these authors entail certain risks. As Einat Avrahami has noted,

> in a society where health is upheld, paradoxically, both as a normative, regulating category and as an ideal state of personal utopia, the decision to disclose a seriously debilitating illness is itself transgressive, verging on admittance to a state of sin.
>
> (Avrahami 2007: 76)

The authors of dementia autopathographies are well aware of such risks. In some cases, by positioning themselves as 'able-minded' in their narratives, these authors may therefore be seen as attempting to curtail the risk of associating with dementia. Such a move will necessarily be double-edged.

In any case, neither the narratives nor the identities that these narratives project are untouched by the dominant and overly negative cultural construction of dementia. This can be seen, for instance, in the reduced levels of self-esteem experienced by most narrators due to the cultural meaning attached to dementia. Even this expression of lowered self-esteem, however, can in itself be considered an act of countering, in that it alerts the reader to the negative impact of the cultural construction of dementia. Countering is never a simple act, and reading counter-narratives depends as much on authorial intent as it does on the perspective and values of the reader.

Reading the collaborative life stories in *Tell Mrs Mill* we find that any given narrative may counter a different *strand* of the dominant discourse on dementia. Counter-narratives are also constructed at different *levels*: by the storyteller(s) in the original interaction; by the listener and interlocutor David Clegg; by the editors of the stories; by the general reader; and by this reader and researcher, myself. My own research agenda will, of course, significantly shape the counter-narratives I construct (Jones 2004). In the final analysis, counter-narratives—in general and about the experience of dementia in particular—represent a subjective category that depends on the convictions and agenda of all involved, including the beliefs and goals of the researcher studying these stories. What is the story that I myself want to hear? Could it be that I herald certain narratives as counter-narratives because I need reassuring narratives of resilience in the face of cognitive decline (see also Herskovits 1995)? Am I thereby continuing to ignore the essential vulnerability of human life—preferring to 'erase' the presence of decline and death in what is already a death-denying society? On the flip side, by criticising the authors of dementia memoirs for using the same devastating metaphors for dementia as are current in popular culture, and by claiming that these narratives on this account partially fail as counter-narratives, am I not denying these authors the right to express their fears about their illness through the means they find most pertinent?[17] The problem remains too, that by highlighting how people with dementia continue to use narrative to make identity claims, I leave untouched the pernicious effects of the narrative constitution view—that is, the view that identity is not just negotiated but constituted by stories—for those who are no longer able to tell even these minimally coherent narratives. I therefore do not purport to provide here a definitive account of what counter-narratives in dementia look like. Instead, I hope to have opened the floor for further debate about how we think about—and act towards—people living with dementia.

The question of how to represent late-stage dementia remains. While current dehumanising tropes in the media increase fear and anxiety in the population as a whole and increase the stigma attached to the disease, there is also a responsibility to engage with our shared vulnerability. Therefore, *not* to represent people in the later stages is equally problematic. Eliding the later stages or 'putting a positive twist' on them, furthermore, risks denying the reality of the disease, and may also undermine needs-based advocacy movements that aim to increase funding for this care sector. How can we represent people with advanced symptoms of dementia without othering them? Couser (2004) suggests drawing on contemporary ethics of ethnography, and based on his framework I argue that collaborative life writing projects, although clearly not exempt from ethical pitfalls, provide one productive means to attempt to represent dementia, as much from the 'inside out' as possible. Whether this view may be able to counter the stigma attached to dementia or not will depend to a large extent on the reader.

Collaborative life story work pays due attention to the interdependent and intersubjective nature of our lives and identities. Maybe the most vital counter-narrative is not the one that asserts agency and autonomy in cases where we no longer expect it but the one that draws attention to our vulnerability and interdependency—in practical matters as well as in matters of identity. The ability to express one's subjectivity, to tell an identity narrative, is not solely dependent on the individual but is rather a function of a communicative situation, which is co-created. Our identities rely on the willingness of others to engage with us and listen.

Notes

1 For a historico-literary overview see Oksenberg Rorty (2000). For studies that consider personhood and personal identity specifically in dementia from psychiatric and philosophical perspectives, see Hughes (2011) and Hughes, Louw and Sabat (2006).
2 For an exploration of the relation between philosophical approaches to the 'good life' and old age see Small (2007).
3 Compare Oliver Sacks' claim: 'It might be said that each of us constructs and lives a "narrative," and that this narrative *is* us—our identities' (Sacks [1985] 2015: 110; original emphasis).
4 This is not to say that dementia does not damage the capacity to tell (life) stories.
5 Taylor's essays were initially published as blog posts. The comments on the advantages of sequential writing can be extended to blogging, since blogging is comparable to journaling in its ad-hoc everyday nature.
6 From psychoanalysis to contemporary 'narrative' or 'scriptotherapy,' there is a long line of thought which suggests that telling or writing about one's life may have a beneficial effect on psychological well-being. Without entering into a debate about the pros and cons of these therapeutic interventions, I see no reason to challenge the anecdotal evidence provided by the autobiographers discussed here that writing had a therapeutic benefit. Beyond anecdotal evidence, see Klein (2003) for a review of how creating narratives about stressful events may lead to health benefits and an improvement in cognitive functioning.
7 This move is similar to the one that Leibing and Cohen (2006) describe in the context of gerontology: by way of distinctions between the 'young old' and the 'old old,' the stigma attached to old age is shifted to the frail elderly. In a second move, this stigma becomes attached to those affected by a deteriorating mind. In the final move, described above, people with early-onset dementia (or at an earlier stage in the disease) distinguish themselves from the severely impaired, by asserting their continuing competencies. The end stages of dementia, in this paradigm, continue to be considered a stage of meaningless existence, a 'death before death.'
8 Helga Rohra, for instance, includes scanned images of her notes, what she terms her symptom diary ('Symptomtagebuch'), in her published account (Rohra 2011: 19, 27). In her introduction she also explicitly addresses the process of working with a writing assistant, stressing that it was important to her not to use a

ghostwriter which would have masked her need for assistance in creating such a coherent account (Rohra 2011: 11, see also Zimmermann 2017: 112). Bryden similarly recounts how she made a habit of bringing brain scans to her talks in order to counter any challenges as to the validity of her diagnosis.

9 I use the terms 'incoherent' and 'broken' advisedly, since collaborative storytelling is always an 'interactional achievement' (Ochs and Capps 2001) and the seemingly 'whole' stories published as autopathographies are themselves the product of shared literary conventions. Narrative coherence is, hence, to be understood as a graded quality. In other contexts, the term 'broken' is frequently used to indicate a psychological rift or traumatic experience in life rather than, or in addition to, referring to characteristics of a given life narrative.
10 See the project website for further information: www.trebusprojects.org/.
11 Abbreviated henceforth as *Tell Mrs Mill*.
12 Lyman (1989) cites infantilisation as one of the negative outcomes of the current disease construct. People with dementia are deemed incompetent and irrational, when competence is in fact a local phenomenon and should be assessed case by case. Globally denying people with dementia agency in their lives may lead to excess disability since, as Stokes and Goudie argue, 'people can become de-skilled if their needs are automatically met by others' (Stokes and Goudie 2002: 5–6).
13 The ellipses are part of the original manuscript. They suggest hesitation in the storyteller's speech.
14 See also Herman (2013) for an account of narrative as an instrument of mind and a sense-making practice.
15 In the context of disability life writing, Couser similarly highlights the harmful depiction of disabled people as 'supercrips' (Couser 2005). Seemingly 'positive' representations according to the norms of the culture do little to question dominant values and may place excessive burden on people who fall outside these norms to nonetheless live up to cultural expectations.
16 Moreover, autopathography tends to be a white middle-class endeavour not representative of other sections of society. While collaborative life writing is more diverse in terms of class and race it runs into similar ethical problems, concerning the power dynamics of representation, as ethnography.
17 Compare the problem of 'triumph narratives' as models for telling about serious illness (Conway 2007). Conway suggests that the triumph plot type suppresses some authors' need and ability to express the calamity illness may present.

4 Relational identity in (filial) caregivers' memoirs

As the number of people living with dementia increases, so does the number of people affected by this condition at one remove. While many people with dementia are cared for in institutions, the larger part of care still takes place within the community (Innes 2009: 40). Family members then find themselves becoming care partners: primary caregivers,[1] living with a spouse with dementia, or secondary caregivers—as describes the situation of many filial caregivers who may not be there on a daily basis but are nonetheless involved in organising and providing care for their parents. An ever-growing number of caregivers' memoirs is motivated by the need to work through the experience of living alongside someone with dementia. In this chapter, I continue my concern with genres of life writing and the ways in which these relate to questions of identity in dementia. I investigate what caregivers' memoirs contribute to an understanding of relational identity in dementia, and how genre and gender may modulate this understanding of relational identity. What is at stake in writing about a family member with dementia? Can caregivers' memoirs contribute to a more nuanced understanding of what exactly is lost and what, in fact, remains?

To answer these questions, I situate the subgenre of filial dementia memoirs in the wider political and literary context of a fast-growing number of dementia caregivers' memoirs. Genre, as Couser points out, 'is not about mere literary form; it's about force—what a narrative's purpose is, what impact it seeks to have on the world' (Couser 2012: 9). In investigating caregivers' memoir as a genre and sketching out a number of subgenres, my intention is to highlight their particular political force as well as to explore the ethical issues raised by dementia life writing. I then move on to a close analysis of select examples of filial caregivers' memoirs to address the impact of gender, genre, and medium on relational identity: Jonathan Franzen's autobiographical essay 'My Father's Brain' (2002), Judith Levine's memoir *Do You Remember Me?* (2004), and Sarah Leavitt's graphic memoir *Tangles* (2010).

The aesthetics, ethics, and politics of caregivers' memoirs

Caregivers' memoirs are by far the most common type of dementia narrative. These autobiographical texts are written by spouses or adult children[2] involved in caring for a family member with dementia. In detailing the progress of the disease, they form part of a group of narratives of illness and disability that have emerged within the context of the 'memoir boom' of the last few decades (Smith and Watson 2010). The memoirs often deal with the first occurrence of minor symptoms of dementia, the difficult process from denial to diagnosis, and a critique of the failures of the care system, thereby drawing on some of the staple components of the 'master plot' of illness narratives (see Avrahami 2007: 75). At the same time, caregivers' memoirs are paradigmatic examples of what have been termed *relational autobiographies* (Couser 2012, Eakin 1998, 1999, Smith and Watson 2010). It has become a critical commonplace in life writing studies that all autobiography necessarily includes the lives of others and therefore is more properly described as 'auto/biography' or 'heterobiography' (Couser 2004: x). Caregivers' memoirs, however, not only include the shared life history of caregiver and the family member with dementia, but often focus on the family member's past to an extent that other auto/biography does not.

Caregivers' memoirs are frequently born out of an impulse to memorialise the parent or spouse,[3] as well as out of the need to make sense of the devastating experience of watching a loved person die (see also Couser 2009: 223).[4] Indeed, authors frequently comment on the therapeutic quality of writing, both during caregiving and after the family member's death (see also Zimmermann 2017: 34). In a first step, a diary or journal may provide a coping mechanism: an outlet for negative emotions that arise in the course of caregiving. Later, reworking these diary entries into a coherent memoir is, as Couser notes, 'a way of grieving, of achieving—or at least approaching—emotional closure on a painful chapter of one's own life' (Couser 2009: 228). The intellectual pursuit of researching and writing about dementia might also be therapeutic because it provides a means of distancing oneself from the emotional rawness of caregiving encounters.[5] Zimmermann comments to caregiving can present a coping mechanism (2017: 34). In her aim to provide a history of dementia life writing, she particularly stresses the closeness of earlier caregivers' accounts to advice literature and argues that these texts filled a much needed gap—given that in the 1980s and early 1990s when these authors had been living alongside dementia there had been little literature available on dementia care (34). Researching the social, psychological, neurological, and economic factors that constitute the experience of dementia, as many writers in the new millennium do, further seems to provide family members with a meaningful activity in the face of a neurodegenerative disease that is *prima facie* meaning-defying. In many cases, the memoirs allow their authors to maintain a relationship to a declining and finally absent family member, by reconstructing and at times revising or re-envisioning their previous relationship.

At the same time, the status and skill of these memoirists has implications for the political force of their narratives. In the spirit of the second-wave feminist slogan 'the personal is political,' professional writers[6] use their personal struggle with caregiving to engage the wider public in a debate about the ethics and politics of dementia care. Not unlike autopathographies by people with dementia, relational memoirs challenge the stigma attached to dementia, criticise the current health-care system, and seek to raise awareness for the financial, practical, emotional, and ethical problems attendant on this condition. The writers of caregivers' memoirs also aim to provide solace, support, and advice for people who find themselves in a similar situation. As Arthur W. Frank has argued in relation to illness narratives in general, these stories are *for* the other. Frank sees such stories as living up to the moral duty of bearing witness (Frank 1995: 17). However, such texts are not without certain ethical risks themselves.

In fact, Couser identifies intimate life writing—that done within families, couples, or close relationships—as particularly prone to ethical pitfalls: 'The closer the relationship between writer and subject, and the greater the vulnerability or dependency of the subject, the higher the ethical stakes, and the more urgent the need for ethical scrutiny,' he writes (Couser 2004: xii). People with dementia, according to Couser, represent 'vulnerable subjects.' He defines vulnerable subjects as 'persons who are liable to exposure by someone with whom they are involved in an intimate or trust-based relationship but are unable to represent themselves in writing or to offer meaningful consent to their representation by someone else' (Couser 2004: xii). Indeed, according to Couser, dementia makes a person doubly vulnerable: subject to harm (abuse and exploitation) in their life and, in the context of life writing, vulnerable to being misrepresented (Couser 2004: x)—at times, in such exposing media as film[7] or photography.[8] Furthermore, since people with dementia depend on others for tasks of daily living, their caregivers have access to intimate details of their lives. These may be moments of confusion, hallucination, or loss of control over bodily functions. When such intimate moments are exposed in relational autobiographies, these texts violate the privacy of the person with dementia.

Nancy K. Miller picks up on this sense of violation when she claims that writing about a parent's death necessarily entails some form of betrayal (Miller 1996). The authors of filial caregivers' memoirs frequently experience a sense of transgression. Mary Gordon, in describing her mother's bodily disintegration, notably feels like Ham, 'the son of Noah, the betraying son' (Gordon 2007: 216). Deliberating on the conflicting demands of witnessing (and bearing witness in writing) and the injunction not to expose others, Gordon decides that she has made the most dishonourable choice: 'to speak and then to confess one's own (superior) knowledge of the dishonour of speaking' (Gordon 2007: 217). The writers of caregivers' memoirs struggle over the conflicting demands of their own need to tell, on the one hand, and the ethical imperative not to harm the person with dementia, on the other hand. This conflict becomes particularly pronounced when the narrative reveals transgressions that involve disclosing intimate details that the subject has specifically asked not to be revealed, or when the person with dementia is defined as a private and reticent person—as, for instance, in Jonathan Franzen's description of his father Earl: 'My father was an intensely private person, and privacy for him had the connotation of keeping the shameful content of one's inner life out of public sight. Could there have been a worse disease for him than Alzheimer's?' (Franzen 2002: 24). The reader may wonder instead whether there could have been a worse fate than being exposed posthumously by the son's writing.

The possible misrepresentation of people with dementia might not only be harmful to the individual, or the individual person's memory, but also to other people suffering from the condition, in that a gruesome or dehumanising representation might reinforce the stigma attached to dementia (see Couser 2004: 31). As Couser notes, we need to recognise that 'groups, and not just individuals, may have interests, if not rights, and those interests may be harmed by representation' (2005: 20). In this connection, it is important to distinguish between the *mimetic* and the *political* dimension of representation (Couser 2004: x). The mimetic dimension of representation raises questions about faithfulness to 'reality.' Here the issue of infringing on another person's privacy and dignity, or to put it another way, the problem of voyeurism, is weighed against the writer's need to provide a full account of his or her experience: for therapeutic reasons, because this constitutes part of the writer's own story, or because the writer wants to raise awareness for aspects of dementia care that are silenced by powerful taboos. As Couser points out, 'memoirists assume two types of obligations: one to the historical or biographical record and another to the people they depict' (Couser 2012: 10). At times these obligations may indeed be diametrically opposed.

Representation in the political sense refers to the notion that in writing *about* certain groups or conditions, writers may actually be attempting to speak *for* those groups, that is, advocate for their rights and interests. A large number of dementia narratives by caregivers, explicitly or implicitly, engage with the politics of care: the insufficiency of care provisions, the callousness or ignorance of care professionals in relation to people with dementia, and the need for better, more sustainable and affordable dementia care. In pursuing better care provisions, writers simultaneously advocate for people with dementia and their caregivers. The question remains, who has the right to speak for a certain group; and what conditions or relationships, if any, confer surrogacy in life writing (Couser 2004: xi).

The hybrid nature of relational life writing makes it difficult to decide to whom a life or life story belongs. Thinking about life narratives in terms of property highlights that telling another person's life may represent an appropriation of that person's story. Paul J. Eakin has foregrounded the importance of 'the story of the story' (Eakin 1998) when evaluating the extent to which a life narrative represents an appropriation of another's story. Forewords and acknowledgements might discuss the process of production as well as self-reflexive passages in the narrative itself. In David Sieveking's documentary, additional material on the DVD discusses the process of production, and elucidates the viewer about the critical reflection on what to show (as well as why and how) that writer and producer engaged in. The documentary also provides a case in point, in that 'the story of the story' in this additional material underscores that the process of filming was beneficial to the 'object' of the film herself: Gretel, according to Sieveking, enjoyed the attention that the production of the film accorded her and became more animated and lively when engaging with Sieveking and the crew. Of course, one could also argue that any person with dementia should ideally be able to receive such loving attention and care without having to be objectified through a camera lens. Nevertheless, the hard fact remains that the funds Sieveking gained for producing the film provided him with the time and the financial resources to spend extended periods with his mother.

In his discussion of 'the story of the story,' Eakin is primarily concerned with memoirs that claim to incorporate their subjects 'own' autobiography, such as 'as told-to' narratives by former slaves or indigenous people in the US. The memoirs I am concerned with rarely, if ever, claim to be telling the story from the point of view of the subject with dementia. However, narrative strategies allow for varying degrees of self-representation, or for the 'voice' or perspective of the person with dementia to shine through. I am thinking here, for instance, of the potential of documentary film in contrast to written representations. As discussed in Chapter 1, documentary allows for the words and gestures of the person with dementia to be recorded and retransmitted verbatim. Although editing still raises the possibility of overwriting or changing the meaning through recontextualisation, the words and gestures of the person with dementia as well as their caregiver at least remain unchanged, and the caregiver, too, is exposed to public scrutiny.[9] Caregivers' memoirs generally represent dialogue with the person with dementia, the person's behaviour, or even attempts at conveying their thoughts, fears, or attitudes. By doing so, they risk overwriting, misreading, or misrepresenting the subjectivity of the person with dementia. However, the writers of caregivers' memoirs acknowledge the problem of appropriation and of misrepresentation, admitting also the limits of their own faulty memory. Rachel Hadas, in the prologue to her memoir cum poetry about her husband's early-onset dementia, notes:

> This story, if it is a story, lacks both a clear beginning and a final resolution. Within the cloudy confines of those years ... I tried to keep track; I tried to tell the truth. Nevertheless, it is largely a one-sided truth ... I can't claim to be telling the story from his point of view. For better or worse, *this is my story*.
>
> (Hadas 2011: xi; my emphasis)

Caregivers' memoirs are frequently hedged by such disclaimers. Authors subscribe to an ethics of 'truth-telling' while they simultaneously acknowledge the impossibility of realising such an agenda. At the same time, these memoirs become the stories of their authors not only because they outlive their subjects but also because of their urgent need to tell, as Sue Miller highlights in her memoir about her father:

> This is the way I have to tell this story, moving from these details into my parents' lives, my father's history. Into *how it was* for us. And all the while I feel behind me, over my right shoulder and my left, the sense of both my parents, of how differently they would tell it ... Of how my representation itself makes the story mine, not hers or his. But uneasy and unsure as I sometimes feel as I call up the memories and the words to cast them in, I am the one who has the need to do it.
> (Miller 2003: 48; original emphasis)

Such disclaimers and moments of self-reflection can be seen to represent 'the story of the story' and play into the readers' evaluation of the ethics of the life narrative.

Caregivers' memoirs also raise *aesthetic* questions entangled with their ethics: how much poetic licence can one take with another person's life? Does truthfulness to the biographical record outweigh aesthetic considerations of beauty and balance, on the linguistic and structural plane? Does the shock aesthetic of voyeurism, providing insight into intimate moments of bodily decline and dysfunction (at times going so far as to describe the actual moment of death) gratuitously violate the other person's privacy and dignity? And how does one create a coherent story out of dementia, provide closure in the face of the open-endedness of life? Couser has addressed some of these questions under the heading of the *poetics* of illness narratives (Couser 1997: 13–4). He particularly points to the intertextual nature of illness narratives, asking what genres, conventions, and formulas they employ and how these influence the way we interpret a memoir (Couser 2012: 38).

Caregivers' memoirs can be classified into a number of subgenres based on the type of literary genre(s) and media they draw on. Often this choice reflects the kind of audience the author aims to engage. Memoirs aimed primarily at other caregivers may be closer to advice literature or self-help books (see Alterra 1999). Zimmermann suggests a historical development and attitudinal shift in dementia life writing, in that earlier memoirs in the 1980s and 1990s are supposedly more guide-like in nature while more recent memoirs have become more autobiographical (2017: 35–6). While this timeline might not hold in all cases, form and function clearly do go together in dementia life writing. Those engaged in dementia advocacy frequently employ a journalistic style presenting current research into the condition— including demographics, drug research, the history of the disease, and philosophical inquiry (see Gillies 2010, Levine 2004, Magnusson 2014). Caregivers' memoirs may also draw on literary genres such as testimony, apology, conversion narrative, elegy, or the *bildungsroman*.[10] In the latter case, the memoir might enact the author's journey of discovery into the ways in which the potential for relationships and love remains, despite an initially bleak outlook based on the cultural script of inexorable decline. Filial narratives, in addressing the difficult ethical issues of exposing their parents' lives, frequently draw on confessional life writing genres—not to be judged (and forgiven) by God but by their (secular) readers. Finally, these memoirs also often act as a *memento mori*, a reflection on the author's own inevitable decline and death.

Drawing attention to the aesthetic, mimetic, and political aspects of representation should not lead to the erroneous conclusion that these are neatly segregated dimensions. On the contrary, instances of misrepresentation by the standards of the individual with dementia may in fact be a fairly accurate representation of the effects of the disease, and necessary for political advocacy. And yet, an overly negative or dehumanising representation of people with dementia may reinforce the stigma of the disease and thereby disincline the reader or audience towards engaging with people with dementia—thus indirectly harming the interests of all people suffering from the disease syndrome. Conversely, and somewhat paradoxically, a positive picture of dementia might equally be harmful for the community of people living dementia. Highlighting the persistence of personhood and the ability of people with dementia to contribute to society and engage in relationships risks eliding the difficulties both of caregiving and of living with dementia, thereby potentially undermining urgent calls for more support (see Magnusson 2014).

It is important to note that caregivers' memoirs are situated also in the wider politics of cultural representation which affects whose life gets written (or published) in the first place, and whose story gets read or achieves critical acclaim. There are political (and demographic) reasons, for instance, to support a gender-sensitive approach to caregivers' memoirs. The provision of care remains, globally, 'woman's work' (see World Health Organization 2012: 69). Furthermore, the correlation between old age and dementia coupled with greater longevity in women means that, overall, more women than men are affected by the disease. More mother-daughter pairs, consequently, are engaged in the giving and receiving of dementia care. And yet, the only article to date to address filial caregivers' memoirs notes a 'significant disparity between the demographics of the epidemic as a whole (and its representation in *all* published life writing) and the demographics of what might be called its *literary* representation' (Couser 2009: 226; original emphasis). Couser remarks that despite a preponderance of women both as subjects and as narrators of dementia memoirs, the most 'visible' memoirs, that is, those 'published by a mainstream press and recognized by mainstream reviewers' (226), concern male subjects (and/or are written by male authors). While his analysis seems a fairly apt description of the North American context at the time—although Couser omits available examples of female authorship and female subjects that fall within the domain of 'literary' memoirs (see Appignanesi 1999, Cooney 2003, Gordon 2007)[11]—the situation is somewhat different on the other side of the Atlantic. One of the earliest British dementia memoirs is Linda Grant's *Remind Me Who I Am, Again* about her mother's multi-infarct dementia.[12] [13] The title insistently calls attention to the relational component of identity construction. Equally, the last two memoirs to have achieved wide dissemination and to have won critical awards in the UK were both by and about female subjects (Gillies 2010, Magnusson 2014). I aim to redress this critical oversight of literary mother-daughter memoirs, by including a case study of Sarah Leavitt's graphic memoir *Tangles*, while also emphasising the complex role of relational identity in any form of dementia life writing.[14]

However, there are also socio-economic reasons for why certain narratives get published and reach wider audiences. My study of mainly white, middle-class caregivers' memoirs may then be seen to contribute to a 'white medical humanities,' in the same way as Chris Bell speaks about 'white disability studies' (Bell 2010). While this study focuses on Western case studies, from the US, Canada, the UK, continental Europe, and Australia, this has nothing to do with the prevalence of Alzheimer's worldwide. Contrary to Martina Zimmermann's assertion that 'dementia, in general, and Alzheimer's disease, in particular, continue to belong, first and foremost, to the developed world' (Zimmermann 2017: 15), dementia poses a global health issue (World Health Organisation 2012). Instead, my focus on Western culture is motivated by the aim to explore the particular problem of neurodegenerative diseases within a hypercognitive society in which selfhood is seen to depend on cognitive functioning alone. However, in this study the lack of non-white and non-middle-class caregivers' memoirs from within Western societies is based on a lack of visible memoirs by more-or-less mainstream presses. Collaborative life writing as discussed in Chapter 3 redresses, to a certain extent, the focus on largely middle-class sections of society. This blind spot with regard to caregiving experiences could also be remedied by exploring more self-published memoirs and blogs. These genres certainly warrant future research. Nonetheless, hard economic facts, such as lack of leisure time to devote to a life writing project in the first place, will continue to play a role in the representation and experience of dementia caregiving across different sections of society.

Beside questions of gender and class, the nature of the relationship to the person with dementia has important implications for the representation of the disease. If life writing can be seen as making identity claims, then one question to consider is what kind of claims are made in relational memoirs for both subjects involved. Are caregivers primarily concerned with the diseased person's loss of social roles—their role as parent or spouse or their professional identity—or are they concerned with the loss of certain characteristics of the person? Do they affirm the relationship and focus on what remains, or do they focus on what is lost? Do they help to preserve the individuality of the person with dementia in contrast to a medical perspective that tends to conceive of people with dementia as a homogeneous group, or do they accede to the cultural script of dementia as dehumanising 'death before death'? And how is the caregiver's identity affected by the family member's dementia?

With regard to these questions, dementia in a parent might have different effects on a caregiver's sense of self than if a life partner is losing his or her memory. Filial narratives often comment on the sense that roles have been inverted: parents have become children. And yet they simultaneously assert a continuing need for the parents to act as parents. Female authors writing about their mothers more often seem to identify strongly with them; compare Annie Ernaux's stark claim 'I am "her"' (Ernaux 1999: 17).[15] Of course, there are also counter-examples such as Roz Chast's attitude to her mother in her graphic memoir *Can't We Talk About Something More Pleasant* (2014). In general, gender affiliations may not unfold as expected. John Thorndike, in assuming the role of caregiver for his father, sees himself as taking his mother's role. He also identifies more strongly with his mother with respect to his temperament and his need for physical intimacy. Franzen, according to Couser (2009: 230), aligns himself with his father against his mother's materialism and insensitivity. And yet, in emphasising his father's intensely reserved nature, Franzen, as a writer of autobiography, may also be seen as diametrically opposed to his father. Like many other filial memoirs, Franzen underscores the importance of his father's role in his life: 'I was inclined to interpolate across my father's silences and mental absences and to persist in seeing him as the same old wholly whole Earl Franzen. *I still needed him to be an actor in my story of myself'* (2002: 15; my emphasis). In considering relationality then, one can ask a number of questions: What is the nature of the relationship between the author and the person with dementia? How is it affected, both positively and negatively by the disease and the process of caregiving and care-writing? What effect, if any, does gender have on relational identity? How does the narrative reconstruct, revise, or perform relational identity?

Indeed, memoirs can be viewed as enacting a form of relational identity, which is both particularly pertinent and particularly troubled in the context of neurodegenerative disease. Originally proposed as a concept to capture the unique development of female identity in both life and life writing—in opposition to Gusdorfian notions of the autobiographical self as autonomous agent (Gusdorf 1980)—relational identity is now recognised as central to both male and female identity construction (Eakin 1998, Miller 1994, Parker 2004, Peaches 2006). Since our identities are constituted through interactions with others (Sabat and Harré 1992), relational identity, and the 'telling' of another person's life narrative, may present a reparative move to counter the loss of identity in dementia. Significant others, such as family members, are then called on to continue to tell the life story of their loved one (Radden and Fordyce 2006). However, relational identity is a two-way system. Lucy Burke points out that reading dementia narratives highlights 'the degree to which the task of sustaining another's identity is problematized by the rupturing of mutual recognition' (Burke 2014: 45). Burke questions facile recourses to 'intersubjectivity' and 'narrative identity' as a means of sustaining personhood in dementia. While she acknowledges the importance of 'telling another's story,' she nevertheless cautions that 'such a task is more complex and potentially more difficult than a simple evocation of intersubjectivity implies' (45–6). Caregivers' memoirs bear out the point that the caregivers' own identity is significantly affected by the onset of dementia in a parent or spouse and that intersubjective understanding is no easy feat. Furthermore, narrativising the other's life story, while serving the important function of memorialising the other, can never do justice entirely to the subjectivity of a person with dementia. Caregivers' memoirs explore this complex interplay of memory, narrative, and relational identity.

What happens, then, when the person with dementia loses the ability to recognise significant others? Lucy Burke explores this breakdown of intersubjectivity in dementia, somewhat incongruously, through a close reading of a *novel*: Michael Ignatieff's *Scar Tissue*. Burke suggests that the narrator loses his self when his mother fails to recognise him. Since life writing is about claiming and performing identities, I propose that we need, instead, to attend more closely to how the breakdown or, alternatively, the reparative potential of relational and narrative identity play out in contemporary dementia *memoirs*. Lack of recognition may severely impact the caregiver's sense of self, irrespective of gender, or the nature of the relationship. At the same time, the authors of caregivers' memoirs may develop new and various forms of intersubjective understanding in engaging with their family member. Their narratives bear witness to the importance not only of recognition of historical roles (as parent or spouse) but also of recognition of the evolving personality of the person with dementia, revealing the need for family care partners to find new ways of acknowledging the other's continuing subjectivity.

Gender, genre, and the self: rethinking relational identity in dementia

The question of self, or loss of self, is without doubt the central concern of most, if not all, discussions of dementia. Unsurprisingly then, it is also at the forefront of a number of memoirs—as expressed in the subtitle to Judith Levine's memoir: *'a Search for the Self.'* In these memoirs, caregivers explore the question of how pathology and personality interact. The authors also explore how their own identity is affected by their family members' dementia and throw new light on how relational identity plays out in this context. They find that everyday encounters with the person with dementia throw up challenges to previously held beliefs—both about the disease and about the nature of the self. Many authors consequently work towards a new understanding of the disease syndrome: they trace the history of the biomedicalisation of dementia, integrate recent neuroscientific findings, and incorporate critiques of the current model of dementia. In tracking their authors' development towards a more accepting position and a greater sensitivity towards the needs of people with dementia, these memoirs provide a model trajectory for the reader. Part *bildungsroman*, part advice literature (but in a more self-reflective mode), these memoirs fulfil important pedagogical functions. Even if their authors' attitudes (and behaviour) are frequently less than 'model' in the moral sense, these texts register conflicting attitudes towards the question of selfhood in dementia and may therefore spark debate about the complex nature of identity. This is not an insubstantial contribution in a culture where rights-based ethics predominate, and where cognitivist notions of personhood underpin the recognition of these rights.

My Father's Brain

Jonathan Franzen's essay *My Father's Brain* (2002) provides a miniature case study of the effect of cultural scripts, gender, and genre on questions of selfhood in dementia.[16] The essay also highlights some of the ethical pitfalls of writing about a family member with dementia. As the title suggests, the essay explores the nature of the relationship between neurology, memory, and identity. It also touches on some of the staples of dementia narratives, such as the history of the disease, the insidious onset of Alzheimer's, and the family's subsequent slow road towards recognition. Franzen sees his unwillingness to recognise his father's dementia at least partially as 'a way of protecting the specificity of Earl Franzen from the generality of a nameable condition' (Franzen 2002: 19). His attitude also reflects his scepticism of the biomedical model that turns people into patients. Franzen is particularly concerned about the way biomedicine currently holds primacy in explaining human behaviour:

> Conditions have symptoms; symptoms point to the organic basis of everything we are. They point to the brain as meat. And, where I ought to recognize that, yes, the brain is meat, I seem instead to maintain a blind spot across which I then interpolate stories that emphasize the more soul-like aspects of the self. Seeing my afflicted father as a set of organic symptoms would invite me to understand the healthy Earl Franzen (and the healthy me) in symptomatic terms as well – to reduce our beloved personalities to finite sets of neurochemical coordinates. Who wants a story of life like that?
>
> (2002: 19–20, original emphasis)

Franzen, instead, counters the dominant biomedical explanation of dementia by telling stories of his father's life and of sections where their lives overlapped, and, significantly, by reflecting on the stories we tell about Alzheimer's in our society.

Franzen, for instance, is concerned that scientific research literalises and reinforces the 'Alzheimer's patient as child' metaphor. According to this research, the disease progression mirrors in reversed order the developmental achievements of a child. David Shenk (2001) has suggested that there may be some redeeming aspects to the reversion to a state comparable with infancy in that it provides a release from responsibility with the concomitant ability to live in—and potentially savour—the present. Franzen invokes the metaphor of 'second childishness,' only to assert his father's individuality and reclaim his identity from the homogenising effect of the disease label. Indeed, Franzen suggests that his father's drive for adult independence is gendered—part and parcel of his male identity:

> Unlike the female inmates, who at one moment were wailing like babies and at the next moment glowing with pleasure while someone fed them ice cream, I never saw my father cry, and the pleasure he took in ice cream never ceased to look like an adult's.
> (Franzen 2002: 28)[17]

In a similar fashion Franzen sees the persistence of his father's 'will' as a symbol for the continuing 'essence' of his father's personality. In his son's interpretation, Earl's death from starvation is not a symptom of dementia—in the course of the disease any patient who lives long enough will lose the ability to swallow—but a conscious decision to put an end to his life. Similarly, Franzen sees his father's sudden breakdown on entering hospital not as a common experience shared by Alzheimer's patients confronted with an alienating and unfamiliar environment, but as an expression of his father's will to 'crash' (30). Or rather, as Franzen suggests, his sudden deterioration represents 'a relinquishment of that will, a letting-go, an embrace of madness in the face of unbearable emotion' (30). In other words, Franzen asserts the individuality of his father against a neurochemical understanding of how behaviour is affected by neuronal breakdown.

And yet, Franzen acknowledges that this interpretation of his father's behaviour is a product of his own needs: 'what I want (stories of my father's brain that are not about meat) is integral to what I choose to remember and retell' (31). In the end, Franzen remains undecided on the question of selfhood in dementia. While Franzen sees his father's will, and therefore essence, as persisting until the very last moment, this selfhood is always also dependent on the son's perception—or even on his creation. The self arises from the process of 'seeing a whole where there are only fragments,' of 'fashion[ing] stories ... of a man whose will remained intact enough to avert his face when I tried to clear his mouth out with a moist foam swab' (36). Franzen's view is perhaps excessively social constructivist; his father's identity relies on being constructed in the words of his family. In response to his mother's view 'I see now ... that when you're dead you're really dead,' Franzen proclaims

But, in the slow-motion way of Alzheimer's, my father wasn't much deader now than he'd been two hours or two weeks or two months ago. We'd simply lost the last parts out of which we could fashion a living whole.

(37–8)[18]

However, reflecting on the commonplace trope of Alzheimer's that its 'particular sadness and horror stem from the sufferer's loss of his or her "self" long before the body dies' Franzen wonders 'whether memory and consciousness have such secure title, after all, to the seat of selfhood.' Franzen concludes, 'I can't stop looking for meaning in the two years that followed his loss of his supposed "self," and I can't stop finding it' (30).

Franzen subscribes to a number of dehumanising and infantilising conceptualisations of Alzheimer's, such as using the trope of 'death before death,' invoking the image of his father as 'an unstrung marionette, eyes mad and staring, mouth sagging' (28), comparing his father to a one-year old (28), and his state to an 'unwanted second childhood' (35). And yet he recognises and celebrates lucid moments, comments on verbal and non-verbal forms of communication, and continues to 'find meaning' until the very end of his father's life. Indeed, as in other descriptions of dementia, the disease at times seems to make his father more like himself, as when his inability to communicate exacerbates his former characteristic unwillingness to communicate. Significantly, much of the meaning Franzen detects rests in, or is communicated through, the body. He speaks, for instance, of 'some bodily remnant of self-discipline' (30) and recognises the importance of bodily identity:

Hour after hour, my father worked his way toward death; but when he yawned, the yawn was his. And his body, wasted though it was, was likewise still radiantly his. Even as the surviving parts of his self grew smaller and more fragmented, I persisted in seeing a whole. I still loved, specifically and individually, the man who was yawning in that bed.

(36)

Somewhat ironically, while Franzen is bent on upholding an individualistic, self-disciplined, and mature version of his father's self, his essay bears witness to the fundamentally relational and interdependent aspects of identity. Relationships are fundamental in reconstituting and recognising his father's identity. Relationality plays out negatively, in that his father's confusion and memory loss impact on his mother's sense of self (25), but also positively, in that his father long continues to perform his role and loving duty as grandfather. Further, despite losing the specific knowledge of their relationship, Franzen's father never fails to recognise his son 'as someone he was happy to see' (27).

In many ways, Franzen's ambivalence about the effects of dementia on his father's identity is representative of most caregivers' memoirs. Many memoirs seem to simultaneously assert and deny the persistence of identity in dementia. By taking into account the autobiographical, relational, and embodied aspects of selfhood, Franzen helps the reader understand the complex ways in which the self is constituted and the ways in which it may persist. Franzen criticises overly materialist views of identity—resisting the view that 'reduce[s] our beloved personalities to finite sets of neurochemical coordinates' (20). That said, he oscillates between conceding that 'the brain *is* meat' (19; my emphasis) and offering the reader stories that challenge neuroscientific understandings of dementia. Franzen's essay both enacts and reflects on the driving motivation of illness narratives to return 'the voice of the patient to the world of medicine, a world where that voice is too rarely heard, [by asserting] the phenomenological, the subjective, and the experiential side of illness' (Hawkins 1993: 12). Franzen stresses the need to assert the personal dimensions of illness, not only for the person suffering from a disease but also for their immediate family members.

As already mentioned, 'My Father's Brain' raises serious concerns about the ethics of recounting events involving a person whom the author himself describes as 'intensely private' (24). Is he, as Nancy K. Miller claims about Art Spiegelman's and Philip Roth's memoirs about their fathers, flaunting 'the artist's power to override paternal authority' (Miller 1996: 13)? 'Invariably,' Miller notes, 'children's right to produce these representations of their parents raises an ethical problem. The dead instantly lose their entitlement to privacy' (13).[19] What is more, Franzen exposes not only his father, but also his mother by criticising her behaviour and publicly proclaiming his parents' marriage an unhappy one. He even quotes his mother's letters at length, in a bid to retrace his father's decline. In doing so, he makes a private communication public, and exposes her feelings, views, and personal style to public scrutiny. As with other memoirs, one is tempted to ask, is there some ethical pay-off for this intrusion on another person's right to privacy?

On a first reading I was tempted to answer such a question in the negative. The author seems to be using his father's disease and demise mainly to pursue an intellectual activity: namely, exploring the link between memory, neurology, and selfhood. Furthermore, the relative brevity of the essay, and consequently its focus on a small set of issues, seems to undermine the primary function of many other memoirs to memorialise a family member. Of course, this is not a necessary consequence of the essay genre per se, but a consequence of the choice of focus. There is too little 'history,' too little of his father's as well as their joint history, for the reader to develop more than a cursory sense of who Earl Franzen was. The essay cannot, therefore, provide the kind of compensation for intrusion that the inscription of 'a lasting, if not permanent, account of a life and personality' may bring (Couser 2009: 229). Unlike other caregivers' memoirs, Franzen's essay does not represent an exploration of the dilemmas of caregiving either. This may be due to the author's relation to his father, not as primary caregiver but as a son visiting only intermittently. While the essay touches on his father's unhappiness about being institutionalised, it lacks many of the topoi of caregivers' memoirs, such as incontinence, worries about letting a person with dementia continue to drive, or concern about placement in a nursing home (Couser 2009: 230). It does not function as either advocacy, testimony, or advice literature. However, while essayistic narratives are typically brief, in narrowing the focus they may also become more accessible to a wider audience. Franzen's essay is, no doubt, one of the more 'visible' memoirs (Couser 2009), read also by memoirists who have written after Franzen. Its main 'pay-off' may therefore lie in its potential to spark debate about the nature of the self, the role of relationships in maintaining identity, and the types of stories we want and need to tell about dementia.

Do You Remember Me? A Father, a Daughter, and a Search for the Self

Judith Levine's memoir *Do You Remember Me?* (2004) provides an excellent example of how the topics raised in Franzen's essay may be elaborated in the context of a fully fledged memoir. Levine's research on the disease is representative of a number of recent memoirs that aim to investigate the social, historical, neurological, and philosophical underpinnings of dementia. The effect is both to inform the reader and to tie in abstract concerns—about autonomy, the self, memory, and identity—with the concrete experience of one family living with dementia. The individualised portrait of Levine's family is set against the backdrop of dominant values and attitudes in contemporary American society. In fact, Levine's family's 'reverence for the rational' is entirely in line with contemporary American values: 'we value, and dread, what our whole culture does,' Levine writes (30). Levine, who is from a secular, Jewish New Yorker background, describes herself and her family as 'hyper-hypercognitive' (36). However, by engaging with the work of the ethicist Stephen G. Post, she comes to reconsider her own and her culture's values. Levine is concerned that in today's 'hypercognitive' society (Post 2000), personhood, and with it full moral and legal consideration, is granted only to 'one kind of person—the rational autonomous kind' (30). She traces how her father, Stan, risks losing the status of personhood and how his needs are progressively disregarded as he becomes de-individualised by the Alzheimer's script.

The Levine family values critical thinking above feelings and emotions, and the members of the family pride themselves on their intellectual prowess. This is particularly true of Levine's father himself, a former school psychologist, who throughout his career pretended to have a doctorate he had not earned. Prior to her father's dementia, Levine's relationship to him was defined by the strength of their intellectual disagreements. As her father begins to lose the ability to engage in verbal disputes, his dementia offers Levine unexpected opportunities to become closer to him—to discover new, non-antagonistic ways of engaging with her father. The memoir tells the story of the growing love of a daughter for her father, and how that love allows Levine to revise and repair her former relationship.[20]

By contrast, Levine's mother's relationship to her husband undergoes a converse development. As Stan loses the ability to engage in coherent conversation with his wife, she, in turn, finds it harder to maintain a relationship with him. Not unsympathetic to her mother's predicament, Levine nevertheless finds herself turning into her father's advocate over the question of whether to place him in a home. Levine believes that institutionalising him would lead to him 'decompensate' (184), as the professional jargon has it, since his attention-seeking personality would not be satisfied in a nursing home environment. Furthermore, Levine comes to challenge what she calls the 'official Alzheimer's story' (119) rehearsed in support groups. This story casts the caregiver both as hero and as a victim in the relationship. On the one hand, her mother feels that Alzheimer's is exacerbating her husband's difficult personality traits to such an extent that she cannot deal with him anymore. On the other hand, she takes consolation in the caregivers' mantra that it's not his fault, it's his brain (119). Finally, based on this reductionist neurological view, her mother comes to claim that her husband is 'not even a human being anymore' (167). Levine believes that the caregiver support group narrative strips people with dementia of their humanity, turning them into 'creature[s] without ordinary perception or emotion' (167):

> *I am no longer his wife. Now I am his caregiver.* ... to transform him from husband to Alzheimer's patient, Mom is divesting Dad of his former self, even of his capacity for happiness.
> (Levine 2004: 168; original emphasis)

Levine's interpretation is, of course, influenced by the pain of seeing her mother leave her father when she herself is slowly beginning to have a closer relationship with him. However, her analysis does underscore that the narratives we tell about dementia may serve the emotional needs of caregivers, and society at large, better than people with dementia.

In her mother's case, Levine believes that stripping her father of his former self allows her mother, to some extent, to divest herself of her guilt at leaving him. Furthermore, as Levine puts it,

> The anguish described by many caregivers arises from the persistence of the old self and the old relationship. The new self-free identity of the patient can ease some of that anguish. A creature hollowed out of traits both beloved and reviled, the person with Alzheimer's enters the

caregiver's life afresh. Historic ties to the old self dictate obligation, which is of course a kind of relationship. But now that relationship can be cleansed of the sadness of perpetual loss. The "endless funeral" is over.

(168)

Levine's analysis resonates with a widespread perception that while family caregivers perhaps are more capable of providing individualised care, they may nonetheless not always be ideal caregivers. Professional carers may be better able to provide competent care since they are not burdened by the same emotional anguish family members experience. Also, professional carers are not influenced by negative relational patterns that may make the family caregiver more resentful, less patient, or otherwise less empathetic towards the needs of the person with dementia. As Levine's analysis shows, acknowledging the ways dementia may change a person, even going so far as redefining the relationship only in terms of caregiver and care-receiver, rather than husband and wife or parent and child, represents a coping mechanism. For all Levine's criticism of this approach, it is by no means clear that a reappraisal of the other's identity necessarily leads to a worse care relationship. What does seem crucial, though, is to acknowledge that the person with dementia is not 'self-free' but remains a person with unique characteristics, needs, and emotions.

Contrary to Levine's view that family caregivers may strip the person with dementia of their identity, Fontana and Smith (1989), by contrast, see family caregivers as engaged in unduly 'reconstructing' selfhood. In their words, which reflect the stereotype of people with dementia as 'selfless shells,'

> The self has slowly unravelled and "unbecome" a self, but the caregivers ... assume that there is a person behind the largely unwitting presentation of self of the victims, albeit in reality there is less and less, until where once there was a unique individual there is but emptiness.
> (Fontana and Smith 1989: 45, qtd. in Herskovits 1995: 158)

While contesting the point that there can ever be mere 'emptiness' in a sentient human being, I agree with Herskovits tentative suggestion that 'perhaps by re-visioning the self in Alzheimer's,' in reaction to this dehumanising view, 'we (as a society and as individuals) can feel better about being and becoming old' (Herskovits 1995: 148). The writers of caregivers' memoirs may be partly motivated to assert their family members' continuing identity to assuage fears about their own mortality. Indeed, my own reading of these memoirs—foregrounding the ways selfhood persists in dementia—may in fact be an expression of our shared cultural unease with the prospect of losing one's cognitive functions and of our inability to face up to decline and death. Also, while welcoming the sea change in conceptualising dementia that Tom Kitwood's work has brought about, I remain uneasy, as does Herskovits, about reconceptualising dementia as 'exemplary model' of how to be human (Kitwood and Bredin 1992: 286, qtd. in Herskovits 1995: 157)—since doing so risks obfuscating the pain and suffering this disease inflicts on both family members and people with dementia.

In any case, in providing a detailed description of her father's life world and his behaviour, Levine's memoir contributes to a more nuanced understanding of how dementia affects the self. Snatches of dialogue bring home how, while not strictly rational and coherent, her father's utterances are nevertheless meaningful and to the point, such as when in a struggle with his wife over getting dressed her father laments his loss of independence: '"I can't do anything," he yells at her. *I have no boat. I have no money*' (116; original emphasis). Furthermore, Levine emphasises the persistence of embodied memory, and with it embodied identity: 'His personality perseveres in his body: the literally in-your-face aggression, the Catskills comedian shrug, the pipe-smoking intellectual's eyebrow raise' (133). It persists in activities, such as rowing, which he continues to be able to do, even as his language skills disintegrate. Above all, however, Levine explores the body's potential to convey emotion. The latter can not only be seen in instances of aggression—that convey her father's anger and frustration—but also in his bodily response to music: using his fingers, arms, feet, and rhythm to express the emotional cadences of a Beethoven sonata, from coquettish frivolity to grave sadness (171).[21]

Levine's memoir also functions as a counter-narrative to the reductionist neurological view of dementia. For instance, Levine challenges a nurse aide's neurochemical view of behaviour when the latter expresses her surprise that Stan apologised for hitting an aide: 'Something in his brain must have done something, and he kept apologizing after that.' Levine wryly replies, 'Yeah ... Like anyone, he feels remorse' (178). Levine attests to the many ways in which her father remains the same, underlining the persistence of—not necessarily positive—attributes in her father that constitute his personal identity. And yet, she also acknowledges the many ways her father is changed and the emotional and practical challenges this transformation poses.

Perhaps the most important contribution her narrative makes is to recognise the many ways relationships constitute identity. Her parents' relationship reveals how gender may influence the ways spousal relationships change in dementia. Social science research suggests that female caregivers are more adversely affected by their partner's decline; perhaps because the necessary prerequisites for intimacy differ between men and women, so that the impact of the disease on communication, for instance, is more likely to deter women from engaging in physical intimacy with their partners than men (Hayes, Boylstein, and Zimmerman 2009).[22] 'Dementia clearly makes the difference for Mom,' Levine writes. 'She cannot have relations with someone who can't have a rational conversation. The man in the body she knows almost as well as her own had become alien, infantile, an untouchable baby' (149–50). His desexualisation and verbal impotence has the opposite effect on his daughter. Caring for her father's body involves a reappraisal of Levine's relationship with her father and allows her a new kind of physical intimacy: 'He feels like neither a child, nor a flirt, nor a threat. He feels only like a father. And I feel not like a nurse, a mother, a wife, or a sex object. I just feel like his daughter' (147). In other words, although he can no longer recognise her as his daughter, his dementia, and the fact that she no longer feels threatened by him, allows Levine to comfortably inhabit, for the first time, her role as daughter. This is not to say, however, that Levine embraces the paternalistic ethics according to which 'dutiful daughters' are to be expected to take care of their fathers (see Couser 2009).

Levine not only traces how her own relationship to her father improves in the course of her father's dementia, but also how new relationships outside the family circle develop. The professionals, hired to look after Stan in his own apartment, form lasting relationships with him. One of the male caregivers comes to assume the role of 'younger brother' and, as Levine views it, her father's 'nastiness toward Ernesto becomes the time-honored abuse of younger brothers, competitive but affectionate, even protective' (259). The relationship to his female live-in Argentine caregiver, Nilda, not only approximates a spousal relationship, but, in Levine's interpretation, fulfils her father's need for the 'unconditional love' that his own mother could not provide. In what amounts almost to a panegyric of the professional caregiver, Levine states,

> Nilda answers Dad's every need without needs of her own, she loves him openly and without judgment, she neither competes with nor criticizes him, is always there, and (as far as he knows) will never leave him. She lavishes on my father the love sought to no avail from every woman since his tight-hearted mother ... "I was a little, little boy, all alone." With Nilda in his life, this plaint has ceased. At the age of eighty-three, as the layers of his adult self curl away, Dad has finally been granted his infantile wish ... And besides Dear, Darling, and sometimes Lil, he has another name for her, which he calls out, almost without guile: "Ma-ma!" ... Finally, my father has a good mother.
>
> (261–2)

Contrary to Franzen, Levine interprets her father's seeming return to childhood as in line with his adult personality and his lifelong, deep-seated need for affection. At the same time, she recognises his current state as an opportunity to heal childhood wounds. While making a person with dementia feel safe and loved is of the highest priority, the question arises how such seemingly selfless caregiving can be realised for everyone. The question arises also whether it is fair to expect low-wage professional female caregivers, frequently with an immigrant background, to provide such care 'without needs of their own.' In her memoir, Levine raises these uncomfortable issues of social justice—or rather of prevalent gender, race, and class inequality in the care sector (see Innes 2009, Kittay 1999)—while acknowledging her own complicity in the perpetuation of the current care system.

Indeed, contrary to Levine's eulogy of the professional carer, the socially and economically precarious position of (frequently immigrant) labourers in the care sector is more likely to lead to insufficient than to optimal care. Shortness in staffing, lack of adequate remuneration, training and support mean that the lofty or, as Innes calls them, 'utopian' ideals of patient-centred care are unlikely to be put into practice (Innes 2009: 45). On the contrary, Innes points out how problematic it may be that care workers, often in a marginalised and powerless position in society, end up in a position of power over those they care for (42). This situation, she seems to suggest, may lead or at least contribute to cases of verbal, emotional, and physical abuse of people with dementia in institutional settings. Rather than seeing such instances of abuse as personal failings and attributable to 'rogue' employees in the care sector, Lucy Bure argues that instances of violence and abuse must be seen as fuelled by both the 'symbolic violence encoded in language' and the 'systemic violence' that may be seen to underpin the current economic and ideological state of the care sector (Burke 2016: 597, 599). Further, Burke demonstrates the way 'care' has been reconstituted as both a 'burden' and 'discontinuous with normative familial and emotional relationships' (602), on the one hand, and a matter of market economy and state interventions, on the other hand, in which the person receiving care is constituted as passive and vulnerable other. This reconfiguration of care, she argues, has contributed to the connection between care and abuse, may even be said to have led to an expectation of abuse in care settings. Clearly, wider social, economic, and institutional parameters need to be addressed when it comes to evaluating care or attempting to implement respectful, patient-centred dementia care. While Levine's memoir only hints at some of these factors, her narrative nonetheless functions as a thoughtful critique of certain care practices and the ethics of dementia care.

Levine's discussion of nursing homes and of her father's specific needs, for instance, is interwoven with philosophical reflection on how the question of selfhood in dementia directly impacts on the ethics of caregiving. Caregiving dilemmas include how to adhere to advance directives, and the question whether or not the 'then-self' before dementia can know what is in the best interest of the 'now-self' (Francis 2001). Discussing the bioethical principles of autonomy, beneficence, and justice, Levine laments that autonomy, and the ability to recognise one's best interests, is not established on a case-by-case basis: *'Doesn't know best interest when standing in traffic; knows best interest when refusing to go to a nursing home'* (216; original emphasis). Levine rehearses the current bioethical debate over whether 'critical interests' or 'experiential interests' of a person with dementia should take precedence in determining treatment options at the end of life (Dresser 1995 vs. Dworkin 1993). While critical interests relate to one's values in life, experiential interests relate to experiencing pleasure or avoiding pain. Ronald Dworkin (1993) uses the distinction between the two in order to argue that critical interests should override experiential interests when making the decision on whether to act on an advance directive. Levine not only offers up a condensed summary of these difficult debates, through the lens of her reflections on her father's situation, but also a narrative approach to understanding these ethical dilemmas. While not offering a definitive answer, the narrative of her father's life suggests that not only experiential interests but also values may change. Her father of the past, whom she describes as strictly Cartesian and terrified of mental decline, appears in his dementia to be relatively content—provided he receives enough attention—and, as Levine puts it, is 'in no hurry to leave this world' (225).

Levine's account highlights that how we assess and recognise selfhood directly impacts on caregiving decisions. Relational identity can protect and support the identity of the person with dementia and lead to sensitive caregiving decisions. But it can equally lead to the denial of selfhood in the context of a deteriorating relationship. The burden to sustain identity, in the face of a myriad of substantial changes, can become too heavy: 'In losing his memory, the person with Alzheimer's allows his caregiver to lose her memories too,' Levine writes (168). Levine's account, like others, calls attention to both the negative impact of a 'malignant social psychology' (Kitwood 1997) on people with dementia and the continuing positive potential for relationality.

Tangles: A Story about Alzheimer's, My Mother, and Me

Sarah Leavitt's graphic memoir *Tangles* (2010)[23] is a relational memoir *par excellence*. It explores the ways that the lives and identities of mother and daughter are 'entangled.' The title takes its name not only from the characteristic plaques and tangles that define Alzheimer's disease on the neurological level, but also from the tangles of curly black hair that characterise the Leavitt family. On one level, then, tangled curly hair signals Leavitt's ethnic roots and genetic ties to her family. In the course of the memoir, however, tangled hair comes to represent the emotional ties, the changing but persisting relationship between mother and daughter. Untangling Midge's hair during the later stages of the disease is an act of loving care but also evokes memories of her mother's fierce protectiveness of her daughter as a young girl. Leavitt later collects her mother's and her own hair, shelving it in boxes above her bed. The presence of the boxes comes to function almost as a surrogate mother, soothing her to sleep. Insofar as they include Leavitt's own hair, the boxes also hint at the ways their relationship has been incorporated into her own identity and will help her thrive even after her mother's death. The metaphorical use of 'tangles' therefore provides a guide to the key patterns of relationality in the text.

While Leavitt underscores the importance of the mother-daughter bond in her life, she also identifies herself in opposition to others, representing herself as autonomous human subject. Leavitt's singular subject position is brought out, for instance, in an image that positions Leavitt's individualised avatar against a featureless groups of others huddled in the opposite corner of the panel: 'Hannah and I weren't a unit like my Mom and her sisters. In my mind, there was me and then there was the rest of my family, who I missed and felt liberated from at the same time' (15). This sense of alterity or singularity is at least partly due to the author's homosexuality. However, as in other memoirs, the very production of the text, modulated by the self-reflexive perspective and voice of the author, even as it includes others' views and memories, in itself underlines the author's singular consciousness. Even in relational autobiographies, then, authors make sense of their life by employing the Gusdorfian strategy of 'looking-back-over-the-personal-past' (Freeman 2007: 122). What differentiates relational memoirs from the Gusdorfian model, though, is their insistence on foregrounding the (life) story of a significant other, or rather a segment of two lives intertwined. While the author 'counts,' so does the other, and instead of merely bearing witness to herself, the author of a relational memoir also bears witness to the other. Notably, of course, the notion of what aspects of lived experience are worth relating has shifted remarkably since the 1950s, so that, contrary to Gusdorf's view, narratives of caregiving, and not just the life experiences of 'great men,' are nowadays considered 'significant to the world' (Gusdorf 1980: 29). Overall, Leavitt's memoir exemplifies that both the formation and representation of female identity cannot be subsumed under the concept of relationality. Furthermore, it exemplifies that reading female autobiography solely through the lens of relational theory forecloses relevant analytical inroads to women's autobiography (see also Henry 2006: 18).

To date, Leavitt's graphic memoir is one of only a handful of full-length explorations of Alzheimer's disease presented in comics format.[24] It is situated, however, in a fairly extensive history of autographics,[25] and, like these, *Tangles* bears witness to the potential of the medium to provide informative and moving accounts of what it's like to be living with a medical condition (Chute 2007: 414). Though doodle-like in style, Leavitt's simple black and white drawings attest to the effectiveness of combining word and image to engage with the experience of illness, whether one's own or another's. The images sometimes provide evocative illustrations of her sparse prose. In other cases, they serve to undercut the narrative voice-over, adding a layer of ambiguity or irony to the narrative. Finally, the style of the images conveys much of the emotional tone, potentially going beyond what can be portrayed in words, or at least opening up a larger spectrum of possible interpretations and emotional responses to the reader.[26]

Leavitt's memoir sits squarely within the genre of filial caregivers' memoirs and raises similar ethical issues in relation to the politics of representation. Leavitt grapples with the guilt that attends her writing project, her sense of feeling 'like a vulture hovering and waiting for [her mother] to say or do something [she] could record and preserve' (7). Leavitt relates how her mother at times physically resisted her daughter's project, pulling the paper and pen away from her. It remains open to interpretation whether Midge did this to gain her daughter's attention or out of an impulse expressing unease at being recorded in this fashion. Although critically acclaimed autographics such as Spiegelman's *Maus* and Marjane Satrapi's *Persepolis* have established the comics format as an appropriate medium for 'serious' autobiographical writing, the form nevertheless raises a number of ethical issues particular to its representational mode, as I shall discuss later.

Leavitt clearly wants to memorialise her mother: 'to remember her as she was before she got sick, but also to remember her as she was during her illness, the ways in which she was transformed and the ways in which parts of her endured' (7). Like other memoirs, Leavitt simultaneously affirms and denies her mother's persisting identity. Significantly, both the introduction and the text as a whole bear witness to the importance of relational identity and the complex ways in which it is affected by dementia. As Leavitt states, 'As my mother changed, I changed too, forced to reconsider my own identity as a daughter and as an adult and to recreate my relationship with my mother' (7). Even in the way the memoir is framed paratextually, showing mother and daughter holding hands or in close embrace, the images on the dust jacket and title pages insistently draw attention to the intimate nature of the mother-daughter relationship. The first chapter underlines the strength of the mother-daughter bond while also foreshadowing how their relationship will become perturbed by the disease: 'My mother was floating away from me,' Leavitt writes about a dream; 'I woke up crying but she wasn't there' (11). While the text never explicitly invokes the common trope of an inverted parent-child relationship, it does highlight Leavitt's continuing child-like dependence on her mother in adulthood, and suggests that the pattern of dependence and care is finally reversed by the disease.

Other graphic memoirs are more explicit about the role reversal in dementia between parents and adult children. These texts explore the difficulty of becoming one's parent's caregiver. Former roles, behavioural patterns, and power relations interfere with the transition from parent and child to caregiver and care-receiver. Roz Chast's graphic memoir *Can't We Talk About Something More Pleasant?* (2014) indeed suggests that the roles of daughter and caregiver are incompatible. The memoir humorously exploits the conventions of the popular, educational comics genre 'Gallant and Goofus'— intended to teach children social mores (2014: 146). Chast opposes the ideal daughter/caregiver ('Gallant') with a supposedly more realistic version of what the author feels about her new role ('Goofus'). Two columns represent the opposing attitudes of the ideal caregiver with the conflicted daughter's view, whereby the 'Gallant' column is headed by the avatar of Chast smiling with a halo above her head. The images of her as 'Goofus' depicts her seething with anger (a black squiggle above her head and aggressive facial expression) and with devil's horns. While Gallant has 'forgiven her parents,' 'treasures the time' spent with them, and doesn't 'worry about money because she would be *thrilled* to have them come live with her!' (146, emphasis original), Goofus, on the contrary, 'is still seething with resentment about crap that happened forty years ago,' cannot stand being with her parents for any length of time, and has veiled suicidal thoughts at the prospect of them moving in with her (146). Her humorous approach allows Chast to address the internal conflicts that the new caregiving role produces in her. By drawing on a moralising and at the same time starkly manicheistic genre, Chast also highlights (and questions) the cultural and societal expectations that arise within the context of familial caregiving.

In his graphic memoir *Heavy Snow* (1998), John Haugse similarly captures this difficult aspect of filial dementia care in the chapter title panel 'Who gets Dad?' (31, see Figure 4.1). The image shows the artist interrupted in his work of drawing a nude, while a miniature version of his Dad that barely reaches the doorknob but is nevertheless dressed in the formal wear, hat, glasses, and the ubiquitous collar of a minister steps through the door and into his life. The image, by returning the father to the size of a pre-schooler while nevertheless retaining the characteristics of professional adult attire, brilliantly evokes the fundamental conflict that may arise when 'parenting' a parent.

Haugse and Chast explore the problems as well as opportunities that arise within conflicted parent-child relations when dementia comes to affect a parent. While Leavitt and her mother have a close and supportive relationship compared to what Haugse or Chast describe, *Tangles* nonetheless similarly tracks the ways Alzheimer's affects the mother-daughter dyad. On visits home, Leavitt finds herself becoming increasingly involved in her

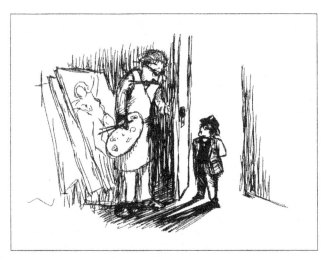

Who Gets Dad?

Figure 4.1 The problem of inverted child-parent relations in Haugse (1998: 31) by permission of the author illustrator John Haugse.

mother's personal care. This new dependence in her mother impacts on Leavitt's sense of self. Having to look after a mother, whom she finds bathing in her own excrement, leads Leavitt to 'feel a new loneliness and a new strength' (60). The change of roles is also expressed in her momentary sense of herself as 'the calmest, most capable nurse' (110). However, the affirmative image of Leavitt, smiling in a nurse's uniform, is immediately countered by an image of herself doubled over by nausea and her acknowledgment that she frequently felt unable to cope with the demands of caregiving.

Furthermore, Leavitt's account stresses how her mother's identity is affected by becoming a care-*receiver*. Leavitt notes, 'It gets hard to see someone as a person when they've become a list of needs: BATH, CLOTHES, BRUSH TEETH, WALK, FOOD ETC' (85). The exigencies of care can, then, in themselves contribute to the dehumanisation of people with dementia, as highlighted in the work of Tom Kitwood. Kitwood (1997) invokes Martin Buber's philosophy of dialogue to elucidate this process of dehumanisation. The Jewish philosopher Buber distinguishes between two ways of relating to another person: the *I-It* and the *I-Thou* relationship (Buber [1923] 1958: 15). 'Relating in the I-It mode,' Kitwood writes, 'implies coolness, detachment, instrumentality. It is a way of maintaining a safe distance, of avoiding risks; there is no danger of vulnerabilities being exposed' (Kitwood 1997: 10). As Leavitt points out, reducing her mother to a list of needs provides her with a means of coping: 'If you just think about that list, then you're not as sad' (85). However, Buber emphasises the cost of this attitude for both sides of the *I-It* dyad. The 'I,' Buber maintains, does not exist outside these two ways of relating. And since the 'I' is only present in its entire being in the *I-Thou* encounter, arguably not only the Other but also the self is diminished by interacting in the *I-It* mode (see Buber 1958: 15–6; 52). Leavitt's account brings out the ambivalent effects of these two modes of relating. She describes how her mother's behaviour, playfully pretending to be a monster while being given pills, prompts Leavitt to snap out of her instrumentalised attitude towards her: 'And she's a person again and you don't only love her, you like her' (85). Here Leavitt highlights not only her filial love but her appreciation of her mother's personality. However, the disturbing images of her parents' despair that conclude this section underline how entering into an empathetic relationship increases not only her sense of her parents' suffering but also her own distress.

Leavitt's account also addresses one of the potentially most painful moments in the progression of the disease for the family member: the moment when a parent no longer recognises a child, or a spouse his or her lifelong partner. Early on in the narrative, Leavitt establishes her mother's love of nature, animals, and children as central to her identity. This finds expression in her 'undying love' (66) for her cat. Her mother's obsession with this rather aloof pet grates on Leavitt's nerves as she experiences a sense of injustice that the cat is so dearly, but undeservedly, cherished. Most importantly, Leavitt recounts, 'She recognized and talked about Lucy [the cat] even when she seemed confused about who I was' (66). In contrast to the characteristically understated plain sentences of her narrative voice-over, the graphics express the emotional resonances of this situation in Leavitt's downcast look and resigned and protective pose in the first panel and in her puerile expression of annoyance at the cat in the second panel—sticking out her tongue and her middle figure at the back of her mother's cat. 'Is it weird to be jealous of a cat?,' Leavitt self-reflectively asks herself and the reader (66).

Similarly, in the one instance where Midge actually *asks* her daughter who she is, the images, rather than the verbal track, come to express Leavitt's as well as her mother's emotional reaction. With a quizzical, surprised look on her face Leavitt replies 'Your daughter. Sarah.' The next panel describes her mother's reaction, but not her own: 'My answer seemed to stress her out. She turned away and started mumbling and breathing heavily.' The image of Leavitt included in the panel, however, registers and communicates her pain: in the grieved expression on her face, in her deflated body posture with her arms cradling her stomach, and in her firmly closed eyes—possibly expressing an attempt to block out the reality of the situation (102, see Figure 4.2).

Leavitt makes use of the expressive potential of the body by depicting posture, gesture, and facial expression (Eisner 2008). But she also exploits the potential of visual metaphors, background, typeset, panel size, panel boundaries, and other elements of graphic narratives to communicate the emotional tone of her experiences. Leavitt diverges from the otherwise fairly 'realist' mode of representation—within the limitations of the medium and her own drawing style—in moments of intense emotions, such as when her anger at a homophobic attack on her and her mother turns her avatar into a raging monster who explodes across panel boundaries (77). Equally, in describing the difficult decision of placing her mother in a nursing home, she uses evocative surrealist imagery to underline (and convince both herself and the reader of) the necessity of the move (116) (see Figure 5.4: 173).

Overall, then, the visual track of the graphic narrative opens up a number of communicative and aesthetic opportunities for the dementia autographer. It allows Leavitt to emphasise the importance of nonverbal communication in the later stages of dementia (see also Killick and Allan 2001) and also to

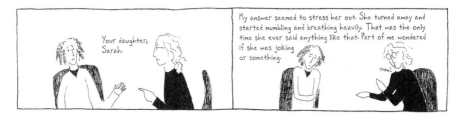

Figure 4.2 Facial expression and gesture indicate emotional distress in Leavitt (2010: 102). Image courtesy of Sarah Leavitt.

foreground the physical closeness that she craves and continues to enjoy with her mother. However, the visual form of representation also raises a number of ethical issues. For one thing, the simplification inherent in the cartoon form, while narratively effective and economical, risks turning representation into dehumanising caricature. Leavitt's depiction of her mother with unkempt hair or without eyes behind her glasses is a case in point. Leavitt uses the lack of eyes as metaphor for the increasing sense of her mother's 'absence.' While this metaphor speaks to the author's emotions, it may enforce stereotypes of people with dementia as 'living dead' and oversimplify the issue of (self-)awareness in Alzheimer's disease. Furthermore, the risk of invading the privacy of the person with dementia, inherent in all caregivers' memoirs, seems particularly pronounced in the graphic depiction (in both senses of the word) of her mother's nudity, body hair, and bodily dysfunctions. However, while 'graphic,' the comics format ultimately screens her mother from more direct—although still mediated—exposure (as, for instance, in documentary film or photography) and arguably makes it possible for Leavitt to address the complex ethical issues that arise around personal care. Leavitt does not gratuitously expose her mother to public scrutiny but explores the risks inherent in caregiving of invading another person's privacy—a point I explore in more detail in Chapter 5.

Sarah Leavitt's *Tangles* deals with how Alzheimer's disease affects both the individual and the family. The narrative shares with other memoirs about dementia an emphasis on issues of diagnosis, treatment and caregiving, institutionalisation, death, and mourning. It raises the complex issue of selfhood in people with dementia, and it addresses the painful losses that dementia entails. But foremost it asserts on every page the continuing relationship between the author and her mother, their love, and the positive influence of that love—even beyond the grave. The memoir is a testament to the primary force of relationality in both shaping and maintaining identity.

Conclusion

In this chapter, I explored the effect of gender, genre, and medium on the notion of relational identity; that is, I asked, to what extent the identity of the person with dementia is maintained through relationships and, on a different plane, through relational life writing. What aspects of identity do relational memoirs highlight, and what conclusions do these memoirs reach about the persistence of selfhood in dementia? How do formal aspects influence the representation of dementia? And also, how is the caregiver's identity affected by dementia in a close family member? Although dementia caregivers' memoirs represent a growing genre across different media and national literatures, and thus require further exploration, the present chapter has sought to answer questions like the ones just listed through a close reading of three filial dementia caregivers' memoirs (and also briefer glosses of other relevant texts): Jonathan Franzen's autobiographical essay 'My Father's Brain,' Judith Levine's memoir *Do You Remember Me?*, and Sarah Leavitt's graphic memoir *Tangles*.

In considering gender as a central feature of dementia life writing, my intention has not been to essentialise gender, nor indeed to use gender as an all-purpose 'hermeneutic key' (Peterson 1993: 81, qtd. in Eakin 1998: 67). Indeed, I would dispute the claim that gender necessarily influences or constrains the formal means chosen to represent an illness or the experience of caregiving (see Zimmermann 2017). That said, although debates continue over the relationship between life and art in autobiography, I second Eakin's view that 'autobiography is nothing if not a referential art' (Eakin 1992: 2). In that sense, real-life and re-presented gender dynamics merit close attention when it comes to examining how relationality is constructed in the context of dementia caregivers' memoirs. As previously mentioned, there are demographic as well as political reasons for considering gender as an important aspect of contemporary dementia care, and consequently caregivers' life writing. At the same time, an in-depth study of the aesthetics or 'poetics' (Couser 1997) of caregivers' memoirs is crucial, since genre, medium, and other formal aspects crucially shape the way dementia is constructed in relational life writing. Caregivers' memoirs about dementia, in fact, incorporate a wide range of literary subgenres and draw on a variety media. The thematic focus and political force of these life narratives depends on formal choices, on the nature of the caregiving relationship (spousal, filial, primary or secondary caregiver, previous history, and personal characteristics), as well as on the author's and subject's gender and professional status. All these factors affect both the ethical difficulties that writing about dementia raises and the tentative conclusions these texts arrive at in relation to the question of selfhood in dementia. In the next chapter, I continue my exploration of the ethics of caregivers' memoirs, but with a focus on what these texts suggest about the project of developing a new practice of dementia care.

As the present chapter indicates, caregivers' memoirs bear witness to the importance of relationships. They are inspired by the writer's relationship to a significant other, and they highlight the continuing potential and need for relationships in people with dementia. Human beings are relational animals that depend on recognition by others. As these memoirs attest, dementia changes many things, but not this.

Notes

1 In recent dementia advocacy there has been a call to recognise that people with dementia are not merely the receivers of care and that so-called care*givers* are therefore better described as care partners. While I find it important to acknowledge that relationships in dementia, despite certain changes, remain reciprocal, I refrain from using scare quotes to indicate the problematic nature of the terms caregiver and care-receiver in my analysis. I retain the terms not only for ease of reading and disambiguation, but also because I argue that caregivers' memoirs

have become an established genre in dementia life writing. Nevertheless, in some cases I also use the term care partner to highlight the reciprocal nature of care relations.
2. Occasionally they may be written by a long-standing family friend (see Heywood 1994) or an in-law (see Gillies 2010).
3. Memoirs may serve the double function of memorialising a parent and providing an extended family memoir, such as Grant (1998) on her Eastern European Jewish heritage, Appignanesi (1999) on her Jewish family's history during the Holocaust in Poland, or Gordon (2007) on her mid-century American Catholic working-class background.
4. Less frequently, caregivers' memoirs may aim to settle old scores. When written in a vindictive mood, or when gratuitously exposing the dead or dying person, caregivers' memoirs are considered particularly ethically suspect. The reception of Tilman Jens' (2009) memoir about his father Walter Jens, a well-known German intellectual, provides a case in point. In the UK, John Bayley was equally criticised for publishing his memoir *Elegy for Iris* (1999) about his wife, the writer and philosopher Iris Murdoch, while she was still alive but too advanced in her disease to challenge his representation.
5. Graham (1997) suggests that writing can provide a distancing effect and thereby a means of coping with illness since it allows the author to remain an authorative agent in one domain of her life. Although his analysis is concerned only with autopathographies written by the person affected by the disease, it can be seen to apply equally to caregivers' memoirs.
6. Authors discussed here are fiction and memoir writers, poets, or work in professions such as journalism, broadcasting, or literary criticism.
7. See Tony Harrison's (1993) film-poem *Black Daisies for the Bride* which, while winning a number of awards, was greeted with mixed responses—as can be gleaned from the reaction of one reviewer (Pitt 1993) as well as Burke's discussion of the work (Burke 2007b). The film poem or musical docudrama displays, alongside actors, the patients of a closed mental ward. These patients were unable to provide meaningful consent at the relative stages of their disease and their representation in the film raises uncomfortable questions with regard to the 'ethics of spectatorship' (Burke 2007b: 62). While caregivers' documentaries certainly raise complex ethical issues, they tend to be fairly thoughtful and at least offer self-reflexive engagements with the problem of voyeurism. Contemporary 'footage' of people with dementia aired on YouTube, without notions of consent or the critical process that a professional production might offer, is certainly highly problematic with regard to violating the affected person's privacy.
8. The poet John Killick's collaboration with the photographer Cordonnier (Killick and Cordonnier 2000), which includes images of people with dementia, raises similar issues with regard to the ethics of representation. Zimmermann (2017) also discusses a number of photographical memoirs by family member, such as Carol Wolf Konek's father-daughter memoir *Daddyboy* (1991) and Judith Fox's spousal memoir *I Still Do: Loving and Living with Alzheimer's* (2009). While Zimmermann judges the latter 'devoid of any voyeurism' (2017: 37) and grounds her appraisal in the beauty of the photographic style, on the one hand, and the nature of a loving spousal relationship, on the other, questions remain as to the nature and content of the images, as well as the metaphors of fading away, darkness, and decline that they evoke.
9. See on this point Couser's discussion of Oliver Sack's television documentaries (Couser 2004).
10. See also Hartung (2016) on dementia narratives as *bildungsroman*.

11 A definitive inventory of such a fast-growing genre as filial dementia memoirs lies beyond the scope of this chapter.
12 Grant's memoir was preceded by Heywood's *Caring for Maria* (1994), a relatively unusual case of non-spousal male caregiving.
13 Compare also the works of the French author Annie Ernaux (1987, 1999).
14 The limited focus here on white, middle-class Anglophone life writing needs to be expanded to take into account life narratives from other cultures and sections of society. A more extensive study would also address 'on-line' and 'new media' acts of self-representation (see Smith and Watson 2009).
15 Burke (2014: 29) argues that Ernaux's identification with her mother and exposure of painful and undignified experiences in both their lives leads to a reproduction of violence on the narrative plane.
16 See also Krüger-Fürhoff (2015). I differ from her interpretations of this text as a 'joint narration between father and son' (99). Further, there is little critical reflection in her essay on Franzen's interpretation of his father's behaviour as a heroic act of asserting his will.
17 Franzen here repeats long-standing gender stereotypes, which cast childish behaviour as 'female.'
18 While Franzen's view risks dehumanising people with dementia, casting them as the 'living dead,' it also points to the kind of pre-death grieving many caregivers experience. Noyes and his collaborators (2010) make the case that the magnitude of stress caused by ongoing caregiver grief is equal to, or even greater than postdeath grieving. Franzen's mother, contrary to her son, makes a clear-cut distinction between the actual death and the metaphorical death of a person. Similarly, Sue Miller, present at her father's death, recalls the feeling that 'he was suddenly, palpably, *absent*' (2003: 153; original emphasis).
19 Couser argues that death entails 'maximum vulnerability' (Couser 2004: 16) and, rather than releasing authors from ethical obligations, writing about deceased subjects remains open to ethical scrutiny. I agree with Couser, although I believe the type of harm that can be caused to a person after his or her death is qualitatively different from any potential harm he or she may experience while alive. In the context of dementia life writing, the representation may have the most detrimental effect, not on the particular person portrayed but on people with dementia as a group.
20 Haugse's graphic memoir (1998) similarly traces how the father-son relationship improves in the course of his father's dementia as they develop new ways of being together.
21 Music has impressive potential to engage people with dementia: as a therapeutic tool, to improve memory and cognitive functioning, and as a means of interacting with others and expressing one's inner life-world. See Chapter 5 for a further exploration of this topic.
22 A cursory comparison of male and female authored spousal caregivers' memoirs seems to support the view that female spousal caregivers are more adversely affected; or rather that the relationship is more adversely affected when the caregiver is female (Alterra 1999, Bayley 1999, Hadas 2011). That said, caution is necessary when making such generalising claims about the impact of gender configurations. In these cases, as in the sociological research just cited, cultural expectation may cause male caregivers to mask their distress—leading to a skewed representation. Further, in the three memoirs just cited, the age at onset of the spouse's dementia may have had a greater impact on the ability to accept the disease than gender, since life course expectations are more radically challenged by early-onset dementia, by which Hadas's husband was affected. By contrast, June and Brian Hennell's life as related in Lucy Whitman's (2016: 146–55) collection of stories

by people with dementia may be considered to provide counter evidence to generalising claims about the impact of gender on care relations. The contribution discusses marital problems due to symptoms of early-onset frontotemporal dementia but also bears witness to the strength of the couple's relationship.
23 Currently being adapted into an animated film by Giant Ant. See http://tanglesthefilm.com/.
24 For further autographics—autobiographical graphic novels or memoirs—that deal with dementia see Chast (2014), Demetris (2016), Farmer (2010), Haugse (1998) and Husband (2014). For a more explicitly fictional graphic novel outside the English-speaking world see Roca's award-winning *Arrugas* (*Wrinkles*) (2007), which has also been turned into an animated film.
25 For a history of the genre of autographics see Gardner (2008).
26 See McCloud (1994) for the argument that the less fleshed-out the drawing of a character, the more latitude there is for readers to project their own situations or responses onto that character.

Part III
Narrating dementia/ rethinking care

5 Care-writing reconsidered

Towards a new practice of dementia care

To date a cure for most forms of dementia remains elusive. Therefore, a key question to address is how people with Alzheimer's or related disorders can best be cared for and how their care partners can best be supported. Practitioners have developed a range of approaches to improve the delivery of dementia care and to help people with dementia thrive.[1] Current research in the social sciences focusses on unpicking the factors that contribute to the 'burden' of caregiving, with the aim of relieving caregiver stress and preventing burn out.[2] Since there is an urgent need for humane and sustainable care, which can only exist if caregivers themselves are supported, such research is timely. Nonetheless, the methods of social science research—such as questionnaires or semi-structured interviews—leave some vital questions about dementia care unanswered. In general, they also focus on the caregiver rather than the caregiver–care-receiver dyad,[3] or indeed the needs of the person with dementia.[4] In this chapter, I argue that caregivers' memoirs are able to complement research on caregiving, by addressing problems that may lie outside the scope of social science methodologies. Further, I argue that 'care-writing' can be understood as a form of caregiving in itself. On the one hand, care-writers are changed by the process of living alongside and writing about the disease in ways that may have strengthened their capacity to provide care locally. On the other hand, by providing insight into the experience of caregiving, these memoirs can contribute to the investigation and development of dementia care generally. The aim of this chapter is not only to extract from these narratives an understanding of the context of dementia care, but also to outline how strategies for improving such care can be developed on the basis of studying care-writing in a broad sense.[5]

Caregivers' memoirs explore the dilemmas involved in caring for someone with progressive cognitive impairment. They thereby provide a means for readers to vicariously live through—and think through—difficult issues and complex scenarios. Further, the authors of these memoirs imagine and develop alternative treatment and care options which could be adapted to other contexts. And finally, because they have lived alongside the person with dementia, familial caregivers are ideally placed to identify that person's evolving needs and to advocate for them when those needs are not being met—whether in the community or in institutional care. These authors are thus well-positioned to articulate strategies for addressing the needs of people with dementia, and of their care partners, more holistically.

Such representations are, however, aesthetically mediated. This chapter therefore examines how the form and medium of a given narrative shape the reader's experience of living through (Rosenblatt [1938] 1995: 33, 38) and responding to the challenges and dilemmas of dementia care as represented in these memoirs. Let me clarify that this notion of 'living through' an aesthetically shaped representation of dementia care does not refer primarily to a sense of reader identification or vicarious experience—although reading caregivers' memoirs is likely to involve some such element. Rather the notion developed by Louise Rosenblatt underlines how the experience of reading a literary work is shaped by how it has been crafted. Attending to a work's ethical, social, or political impact therefore necessitates paying attention to its form.

Exploring caregivers' dilemmas

Dementia caregivers are faced with an array of complex and, due to the progressive nature of the disease, constantly shifting care-decisions. Many of the caregiving dilemmas can be framed as problems of coercion or paternalism (in relation to social behaviour; in relation to practical concerns over personal care such as dressing, feeding, and toileting; in relation to the difficult decision of when, how, and where to place a person in institutional care; and finally, in relation to medical treatment, both during the course of the disease and when it comes to end-of-life decisions). Although there may be some overlap with strategies for giving care to persons with other conditions, the care-decisions discussed below are particularly salient in the context of caring for someone with progressive cognitive impairment. They involve assessing the extent of the impairment, and the capacity for choice, agency, and responsibility in the person with dementia.

This section explores how the authors of caregivers' memoirs encounter, frame, and attempt to resolve some of the above-mentioned caregiving dilemmas. Caregivers' memoirs not only provide insight into the caregiver's predicament but may also indirectly benefit others living with or alongside this condition. These texts model empathetic ways of engaging with people with dementia and of resolving certain caregiving dilemmas, without necessarily representing 'model' caregivers. Indeed, the fact that these caregivers frequently fall short of any ideal (or idealised) standard of care makes their accounts a productive tool for thinking through care practices. In their failure to find resolutions or in describing the 'bad choices' their authors faced in their roles as caregivers, these memoirs have the potential to provoke debate about what constitutes ethically sound dementia care and what aspects of care urgently need to be addressed by society at large—from policymakers to care managers to taxpayers helping to support care systems.

The most challenging ethical dilemmas in dementia care, no doubt, arise out of the conflicting need to respect the person's autonomy while also protecting the person from harm and fulfilling his or her most basic care needs. In the case of parent-child relationships, the adult children of people with dementia frequently feel as if roles have been reversed, with the children becoming guardians of their own parents. And with this reversal they enter the quagmire of ethical decisions about the extent of autonomy in dementia. As Sally Magnusson succinctly puts it in her memoir, addressed throughout to her mother:

> Ours was the same problem that besets every family trying to look after someone with dementia whom they want to allow to be themselves for as long as possible; how to keep your independent spirit flying and help you feel like a free agent capable of decisions, when the decisions you made were so often disastrous (like insisting on walking out on a road shiny with ice) and the decisions you increasingly could not make (to get up, to dress, to eat) were so fundamental.
>
> (2014: 148)

This section draws on a number of memoirs which represent not only different genres and media (print, film, and graphic memoir) but also different caregiving relations and gender configurations, to explore how the authors of these narratives grapple with the difficult issues of coercion and paternalism. Given that genre conventions as well as the properties of storytelling media can significantly shape the representation of caregiving, I explore issues of (sub)genre or medium when they bear on the 'point' the narrative makes about caregiving dilemmas. By paying due attention to how the narrative form shapes what these authors have to say about the experience of caregiving, I aim to redress the problem of previous approaches to illness narratives that frequently treated these narratives as a 'transparent medium for the investigation of something else' (Mattingly 1998: 12, see also Woods 2011). David Sieveking's documentary *Vergiss Mein Nicht* (2012) and John Thorndike's memoir *The Last of His Mind* (2009) deal with the question of coercion in relation to feeding and 'activating' the person with dementia. Sarah Leavitt's graphic memoir *Tangles* (2010) elucidates infractions in the realm of personal care, while also hinting at aspects of physical coercion. Both Leavitt and Rachel Hadas in her memoir *Strange Relation* (2011) address the difficult issue of placing a family member or spouse in institutional care while also exploring the 'tipping point' at which home care becomes no longer feasible.

Care or coercion? Autonomy in dementia

A number of memoirs explore the issue of autonomy in dementia. In Thorndike's memoir *The Last of His Mind* (2009), for instance, the question of coercion is a recurrent theme. As primary, cohabitating caregiver, Thorndike repeatedly finds that pressurising his father into doing things which he is initially disinclined to do actually helps to improve his father's mood and well-being. Nevertheless, Thorndike remains undecided over when and whether his acts of care—to feed his father, motivate him to go out, and get him out of bed—may represent unwarranted instances of overriding the latter's wishes. Thorndike explores the moral obligation to feed another who is seemingly unable to remember to feed himself—or who has, on Thorndike's alternative interpretation, consciously decided to forego eating. Evoking the case of an elderly lady who 'was tired and infirm and didn't care about eating,' he quips that, for the caregivers around her, 'food was gospel and eating her duty' (85). Thorndike's choice of words suggests that there is something inherently ludicrous in this demand that the younger and healthier generation places on the old and infirm—to eat, to move, and to be active. Thorndike wonders whether showing little interest in food might not be his father's way out, a wish to 'crash for good' (85) as he puts it. However, he doubts his own ability to act on such a view: 'I consider this, but I doubt it will be long before I slide another plate in front of him. It's the habit of care, and the assumption that everyone must eat. Though I question this, I am tied to the wheel myself' (85–6). The ethical imperative to keep a dependent person alive here overrides the conflicting demand to honour this person's (apparent) wishes.

Indeed, Thorndike here taps into the complex debate about patient autonomy in dementia. This debate usually focuses on the question of advance directives and whether these still hold when the person affected no longer shares the same values or outlook on life as when these directives where formulated. Here Ronald Dworkin's distinction between 'critical interests' and 'experiential interests' comes into play (1993). While critical interests relate to one's values in life, experiential interests refer to both more immediate and more general categories such as experiencing pleasure or avoiding pain. According to Dworkin, critical interests should override experiential interests when making the decision on whether to act on an advance directive. That is, if the patient specified that all life-sustaining measures (including antibiotics) be withheld once past a certain stage in the illness, it does not matter whether that person still experiences pleasure and satisfaction in the present moment and may benefit from antibiotics in order to sustain her current (quality of) life. Rebecca Dresser (1995) takes the opposite view. She argues that experiential interests should take precedence in such cases. Whereas Judith Levine's memoir, discussed in Chapter 4, reviews this debate—arguing that autonomy should be assessed on a case-by-case basis—Thorndike's memoir offers another tack. In the absence of any advance directives, Thorndike is presented with a set of dilemmas: how can he reliably know what his father wants? How does he balance his father's apparent wish for autonomy and his own wish to respect his father's preferences with his moral duty to care for him? Can his father's seeming disinterest in food be understood as a genuine choice or is he simply too forgetful to remember to eat food? In which case, would honouring his father's apparent wishes not represent an instance of inhumane care, of starving a dependent person? And indeed, whose needs do the practices of caregiving actually fulfil—the (so-called) caregiver's or the (so-called) care-receiver's?

Thorndike's memoir offers a case study, a practical experiment centred on these difficult caregiving dilemmas. One day, Thorndike undertakes to discover his father's wishes by letting him decide not only whether to get up but also whether to have food at all: 'all offers are coercive and for once I'm not making any' (100). The narrative then moves through the day—torturously, it seems—for the author (and reader) while Thorndike's father shows no interest in getting up or eating. The use of mainly one-word, end-stopped phrases for time specifications at the beginning of each paragraph (e.g. 'Noon.' 'Three o'clock.' 'Five-thirty.') underlines how slowly time seems to be passing for the author. In addition, Thorndike's agony and insecurity are reflected in the number of rhetorical questions he asks. Thorndike finally aborts his plan to wait for his father to initiate any act of care, without having discovered what the right stance towards coercing a person with dementia might be:

> Should I return to my jaunty self tomorrow morning and make him take a shower, make him change his clothes, invite him to sit down to his breakfast and morning medications, urge him to walk to the mailbox, insist on driving him to the ocean, hound him about drinking more fluids? At what point should I let him do what he chose to do today: lie in bed without talking or moving.
>
> (102)

Based on his experience Thorndike is inclined to think that coercion might be a necessary part of caregiving. 'On the day I give him completely free rein, he winds up with no shower, no breakfast, no lunch, no time outdoors and no conversation. He's passed *what seems to me* a lost and unhappy day, stretched on his bed' (102; my emphasis). While the anaphoric use of 'no' in the first sentence emphasises the seemingly disastrous effects of his experiment, his phrasing in the next sentence is significant in that it introduces the possibility of doubt. The wording 'what seems to me' underscores that this is Thorndike's interpretation of the quality of the day, not his father's, and leaves open the possibility that to the latter this might have been a satisfying, restful way to spend the day. Chillingly, the passage concludes, 'And I have to ask: how much did I do this because I wanted a break myself, a day without responsibilities?' (102). Here and elsewhere, Thorndike repeatedly asks to what extent caregiving (or the absence of providing care) may fulfil the needs of the person providing care rather than the needs of the person with dementia.

Thorndike's narrative provides a framework in which the question of coercion is debated, both on the story level and on the discourse level. While the reader is presented with intellectual arguments, the rhetorically arranged 'argument' of the story has an affective impact that provides the reader with a sense of 'what it's like' to face the ethical quandaries of dementia care. What is lacking from this narrative, unfortunately, is a clear sense of what the person with dementia wants or needs. As the situation is presented from the caregiver's point of view, the reader, with Thorndike, is left in the dark about how his father experiences the presence, or indeed absence, of coercion.

In his documentary *Vergiss Mein Nicht* (2012), David Sieveking similarly struggles with the problem that caring for his mother Gretel necessarily involves many instances of overriding her wishes. This issue is brought out in a number of scenes in which health professionals, David himself, or his father all try to coax Gretel into participating in activities, avowedly for her own good. An encounter with a physiotherapist with a Slavic accent in which Gretel staunchly refuses to do anything takes on an almost comic character. The mood is signalled by Sieveking's voice-over narration: 'Even professional therapists try their luck with Gretel' [15:12].[6] Sieveking seems to want to highlight the absurdity of these therapeutic interventions in cutting to a scene in which a woman sounds a singing bowl, while Gretel lies on her bed, either asleep or staunchly ignoring her. Although the narrator doesn't explicitly comment on the value of these therapeutic interventions, Sieveking's humorous tone in the previous scene is likely to shape viewers' responses. The viewer is left to wonder why older people lose their right to be left alone when they express a wish for peace and quiet. Such a reaction is also borne out in a post-performance discussion included in the additional material on the DVD. Here an audience member remarks in relation to these therapeutic interventions whether it would not have been kinder to leave Gretel in peace when she clearly communicated her unwillingness to be engaged.[7] And yet, as the quotation from Magnusson above underlines, people with dementia may become unable to make the 'fundamental' decisions necessary for life. The ethics of care demands that others prompt, help, or even coerce them into activities that can improve their health and quality of life.

Sieveking initially takes a humorous stance in relation to all activities aimed at engaging his mother. As the narrative progresses, however, Sieveking increasingly finds himself in the role of coaxer, prompter, and coercer. As he is faced with the question of when coercion becomes unethical, the documentary in turn puts the same question to the audience. Compared to verbally mediated accounts of coercion in other caregivers' memoirs, the direct representation of Gretel's expressions of disinterest, or even discomfort and fear, arguably has a stronger emotional impact on the viewer. Responses of this sort are perhaps most obvious in a scene where David takes his mother to the swimming pool in an attempt to recapture the joy she previously experienced while swimming. His hopes are disappointed as his mother refuses to enter the water. She shields her face with her hands and then turns to the camera, a look of fear on her face, and asks the camera man: 'Can we go sit somewhere where we don't die?' [30:59].[8] The semantics of death make sense in this context and clearly express Gretel's fear of the water. More to the point, her facial expression, gestures, and bodily movements provide access to her current state of mind to a degree that cannot easily be ignored—and in contrast with the way written memoirs such as Thorndike's may occlude or omit the reactions of the person receiving care. Here the use of a close-up shot of Gretel's face directs viewers' attention to her facial expression and arguably reinforces the emotional appeal of her plea. Viewers are implicated in her plea as her direct gaze at the cameraman, although mediated, is experienced as a direct gaze at the viewer.

Being confronted so directly with Gretel's obvious fear and discomfort led to an animated post-viewing discussion between audience members and Sieveking himself (see also Zimmermann 2017: 124).[9] While acknowledging that his attempts to get his mother to swim may in retrospect have been considered ill-advised, he relates how only months before his mother had greatly enjoyed swimming once he had coaxed her into the water. Nevertheless, he concludes that his experience of caring for his mother taught him that it was more productive to abandon the approach of trying to recapture or reanimate past or lost capacities and instead meet his mother where she was. Sieveking's documentary does not offer up a definitive answer to the question of whether coercion is a necessary—and beneficial—aspect of caregiving, and at what point it represents an instance of disrespect or perhaps even potential harm to the person with dementia. The viewer is left to arbitrate case by case, based on the ways that Sieveking frames his material (by scene selection, voice-over narration, and use of film music) and also based on the bodily and verbal reactions Gretel manifests—be they of joy, pleasure, annoyance, or fear.

Both narratives confront their readers and viewers with the difficulty of ascertaining the limits of autonomy and the legitimacy of coercive caregiving in dementia. They do this by representing complex yet specific situations within the shared life world of caregiver and care-receiver. By providing rich contextual detail and by aesthetically shaping their lived experience, both narratives allow a 'living through' (Rosenblatt 1995) of the complexity of day-to-day caregiving decisions and practices. While Thorndike's narrative incorporates to a larger extent his own thoughts, reasoning, and emotional responses to these ethical dilemmas, Sieveking's narrative relies more on the process of 'showing' the effects of caregiving decisions, rather than overt reflection or commentary. By representing his mother's disinclination or fear, Sieveking's film evokes emotions of pity and empathy in the viewer. This emotion, as post-performance discussions of the film highlight, also triggers viewers to reflect on the ethical problems of coercing a person with dementia, even when it is aimed at promoting their own good. Thorndike's narrative, by contrast, aligns the reader with the point of view of the narrator. We become privy to the caregiver's conflicting thoughts and emotions, are invited to share his anxiety about doing right by his father, and speculate with him about his father's wishes and needs. Neither narrative achieves a comfortable solution to the caregiving dilemmas they pose. But it is this lack of closure, or lack of clear instructions (in contrast to advice literature), that has the potential to spark debate about ethically sound dementia care practices.

'Bad grooming': intimate care in dementia

While Thorndike and Sieveking cover a variety of caregiving dilemmas, there are two areas in which they are less instructive—with regard to personal care and to the question of institutionalisation. The latter issue barely arises in these narratives since the parents are cared for in their own homes—except for a brief period in Gretel's life. With regard to personal care, Sieveking's narrative is extremely reticent. Sieveking's reticence may be because documentary film is perceived as more 'immediate' and therefore more starkly exposing.[10] It is obvious from interviews that Sieveking worried about violating his mother's privacy.[11] The documentary, consequently, only alludes to toilet issues metonymically—for instance, by filming Sieveking's father wiping the floor after an incident of incontinence. Thorndike, by contrast, almost seems to revel in a kind of shock aesthetic in exposing his father's bodily decline. Thorndike, it seems, uses the stark description of his father's naked, ageing body in order to confront his own fears of mortality and in order to desensitise himself with regard to his anxiety over providing intimate care for his father. In line with Burke's arguments (2016), such representations might be considered acts of symbolic violence towards the person with dementia. Indeed, Burke wonders

> whether any other condition but dementia could give rise to such forensic descriptions of bodily decline, as if dementia as a condition somehow gives permission to describe intimate care in a manner that is not seen to be appropriate or necessary in the representation of other ways of dying.
>
> (2016: 598)

Sarah Leavitt's graphic memoir *Tangles* (2010) addresses head-on the challenges and ethical dilemmas of both personal care and institutionalisation. On her visits home, Leavitt finds herself taking on an increasing range of 'hands-on' care tasks for her mother Midge. Leavitt's graphic (in both senses of the word) depiction of bodily decline, nudity, and problems with personal hygiene transgresses a number of powerful cultural taboos. In the chapter 'Good grooming,' for instance, Leavitt reflects on the taboo of grooming an increasingly less able-bodied and able-minded mother. Leavitt notices that as her mother's disease progresses, she becomes more docile and easily submits to being physically cared for. In an attempt to make it easier to keep their mother clean, Sarah and her sister Hannah decide to trim their mother's pubic hair (see Figure 5.1a).[12]

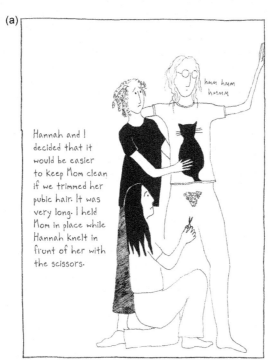
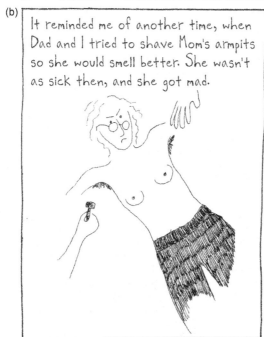

Figure 5.1 (a, b) 'Good grooming': Ethical issues in personal care in Leavitt (2010: 110). Images courtesy of Sarah Leavitt.

The narrative then moves on to a flashback of a similar instance earlier in the disease processes: 'It reminded me of another time,' the narrative voice-over reads, 'when Dad and I tried to shave Mom's armpits so she would smell better. She wasn't as sick then, and she got mad' (111). The image is evocative. It represents Midge's angry facial expression. The image suggests a physical struggle insofar as Midge's glasses are askew, while two depersonified hands reach out towards her—one with a razor, the other seemingly holding her down (see Figure 5.1b). Leavitt clearly feels distressed by the event as the next panel shows her running from the scene while she considers how the 'secret intimacy' between her parents had been 'breached forever' (111). She then reflects on how, due to her own homosexual orientation, administering personal care to her mother takes on a particular poignancy and evokes concern over 'being accused of perversion' (111). There is a parallel here between the culturally ingrained notion that it is inappropriate for men to care for women, due to concerns over sexual decency (Kittay 1999).

However, the main point is that, irrespective of the particular caregiving relation, instances of personal care necessarily (or sometimes unnecessarily) involve violations of privacy. When other family members judge the act of trimming their mother's pubic hair to have been superfluous, Leavitt and her sister come to reassess the situation: 'We felt bad then' (111). Moreover, the whole experience leads Leavitt to conclude, 'You get sick and your body is no longer private. Even if none of your caretakers ever hurts you, some basic dignity is lost' (111).[13]

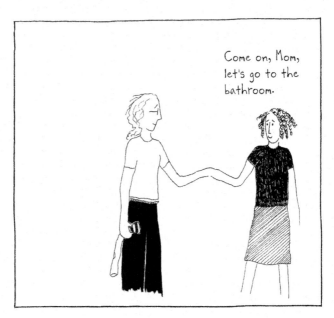

Figure 5.2 Care as connection in Leavitt (2010: 111). Image courtesy of Sarah Leavitt.

Despite these comments about the negative impact of certain acts of caregiving, however, the panel that follows suggests that care can also provide a means of connection. It repeats the image from the front cover of the memoir: Leavitt and her mother are holding hands and gently smiling at each other (see Figure 5.2). Only at this point in the narrative does it become clear that this image represents an instance of Leavitt providing personal care for her mother. Care can then also be a form of connection.

'No good choices': institutionalisation in dementia

Like many other caregivers' accounts, Leavitt's also addresses a particularly salient dilemma: that is, the question of whether, when, or where to place a person with dementia in institutional care. In her memoir *Death in Slow Motion* (2003), Eleanor Cooney evocatively describes the painful process of moving her mother first from her own home into her daughter's and from there into a series of institutions. Cooney describes the nightmare of negotiating a public health system that invariably represents a number of Catch-22s. Her anguish grows out of her inability to keep caring for her mother at home while having to acknowledge that 'there is only one drug in the world that can keep my mother calm and centred, and I am that drug' (174). However, in taking the reader into the nightmarish world of impossible choices which induce guilt, depression, and alcoholism in the author, the narrative may leave its readers feeling overwhelmed or even paralysed when it comes to contemplating the prospect of looking after a family member with dementia. Cooney's memoir is seemingly trapped within the immediacy of overwhelming caregiving dilemmas. Her memoir then raises the question of how much refashioning of a life is necessary for a caregiver's memoir to turn into care-writing.[14] Although other memoirs do not present 'solutions' for caregiving dilemmas, they provide a working through of these dilemmas, for the authors and their readers, that lead to a place other than despair: acceptance, on the one hand, and the will to look for productive, liveable solutions, on the other.

To represent and reflect on the decision-making process involved in placing her mother in a care home, Leavitt mines the potential of the visual track in graphic memoir as a meaning-making device. The physical and emotional effects of caregiving, for instance, are depicted visually without, necessarily, addressing the issue verbally (see Figures 5.3 a,b,c). Leavitt draws on the potential of facial expressions, body postures, and gestures to evoke the emotional reactions and physical exhaustion due to caring for a family member with dementia. She also exploits the potential for non-realist, metaphorical imagery to convey the intensity of certain emotions (see Figures 5.3c and 5.4). The skeleton-like monster with Leavitt's signature curls represents how the strain and anxiety of caregiving has made her emotionally unbalanced and difficult to live with for her partner.

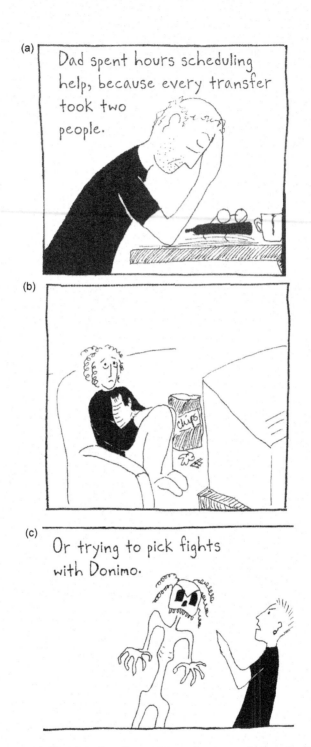

Figure 5.3 (a, b, c) Figuring the effects of caregiver stress in Leavitt (2010: 116–7). Images courtesy of Sarah Leavitt.

Further, Leavitt effectively employs surrealist images in her narrative in recounting the difficult decision of placing Midge in a care home. The matter-of-fact description of how her father hurt his back helping his wife off the couch is accompanied by two black, tortured, hairless figures, reminiscent of Picasso's *Guernica* or some of Dali's contorted human figures. Every element of these figures spells out the agony of their experience: their emaciated state, their impossible postures, and their oversized hands grasping at thin air. The next panel contains only the words: 'Neither of them could live like this' (116)—adding an air of finality to Leavitt's conclusion. While falling short of any claim to representational 'truth-telling,' this image transmits something of the agony of the experience. Importantly, it is strategically employed to justify (or possibly to persuade Leavitt herself of) the rightness of the decision to place Midge in a nursing home.

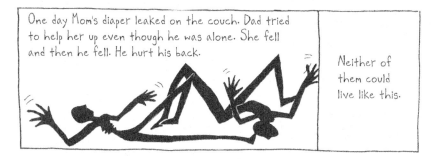

Figure 5.4 Drawing style as part of narrative rhetoric in Leavitt (2010: 116). Image courtesy of Sarah Leavitt.

If Leavitt's artistic representation makes sense of and justifies her family's decision to place her mother in a care home, Rachel Hadas' memoir, in contrast, highlights how the caregiver can struggle with a distinct lack of clarity about when to move a spouse into an institution. In *Strange Relation* (2011), a memoir which incorporates the author's poetry, Hadas explores the tipping point, different in every caregiving relation, at which home care becomes no longer feasible. In her case, this tipping point is not linked to the physical unmanageability of the disease but to the emotional 'cost'[15] of living in a near-state of silence: 'If there was one reason I decided that I could no longer live with George, that coordinating his care had gone from arduous and unrewarding routine to unbearable pain,' she states, 'that reason was the grinding loneliness imposed by his silence' (133). The emphasis is on how both the decision-making process and the consequent guilt entailed by the decision become a lonely burden for the care partner to carry. At the same time, Hadas finds solace in poetry, myth, and Greek tragedy, which, unlike caregiving literature that shies away from addressing the 'salient truth' (142) of how difficult institutionalisation is, offers up its own versions of unpalatable dilemmas. As Hadas points out, 'when it comes to scooping someone out of the house where they have lived for thirty years and inserting them [into institutional care]—when it comes to doing this, *there are no good choices*' (142; my emphasis). However, the poetry of others as well as her own helps her make sense of certain aspects of her experience that might otherwise remain incomprehensible, or at least intractable. Poems, in her words, 'get to eat their cake and have it too' (24) in their ability to exploit the ambiguous and plurivalent nature of language—and hence describe the ambiguous and conflicting experience of caregiving, or of handing over the care of a family member to others.

All these caregivers' memoirs put the dilemmas that dementia care raises in the context of a particular social, cultural, and familial configuration. By doing so the reader is immersed in the specifics of each case and can, in Rosenblatt's terms, 'live through' the caregiving experience in an aesthetically mediated form. And yet, these case studies also offer up generalisable problems—the conflict between autonomy and paternalism in making care-decisions, the fine line caregivers must tread between safekeeping and infantilising, respect for autonomy and neglect. The narrativisation of caregiving dilemmas highlights the complexity of dementia care and the lack of easy solutions. But by giving meaning to particular cases, by making use of the affordances of particular media (be it the audiovisual in film, the visual in graphic memoir, or the many possibilities of the written word), caregivers' memoirs structure these dilemmas for their readers and signpost pathways towards acknowledging—and perhaps solving—difficult ethical issues in dementia care. At the same time, as my analysis has shown, this representation is not neutral. It pushes readers and viewers to come to certain conclusions. This form of emotional and rhetorical 'manipulation' of the reader can no doubt be employed for pedagogical purposes. And yet, it is important to note that these aesthetic choices might equally close down other ways of seeing or reacting to dementia caregiving dilemmas.

Imagining alternative approaches in dementia care

Greenhalgh and Hurwitz (1999) suggest that illness narratives provide a framework for approaching patients' difficulties holistically, and that attending to illness narratives may aid with diagnosis as well as with discovering alternative treatment options (48). Along the same lines, moving on from the ethical dilemmas that dementia raises, I argue that caregivers' memoirs may contribute to dementia care—by questioning common care practices and by modelling alternative attitudes and responses. Caregivers' memoirs detail their authors' own journey towards discovering new ways of seeing and dealing with dementia and how, in the process, they developed alternative (therapeutic) responses to the person they cared for. My discussion will focus on several representative questions raised by these accounts, including how to respond to confabulation, how to meet the person with dementia in their own world, and how to enhance their well-being by using music (or other art-related interventions). However, the texts themselves contain a much larger repertoire of care practices and models. Contrary to care programmes where one method is made to fit all, narrative explorations underline the specificity of each person's care needs and describe responses that are designed to suit the situation and temperament of the person involved. At the same time, the memoirs gesture towards therapeutic interventions and everyday responses that may be beneficial for other people with dementia. They can therefore play an important role in educating readers about what the care needs of a person with dementia may look like while highlighting that care practices need to be adapted to each individual living with dementia.

Reconsidering confabulation

Reminiscence therapy and so-called 'orientation' exercises (reinforcing the day, time, season, and place) are frequently used in dementia care. However, practitioners have increasingly questioned the usefulness of such approaches, especially for people with more advanced dementia. They suggest that to challenge the way a person with dementia sees the world or to make them feel insufficient when they cannot recall certain facts does more harm than good. As the disease progresses, people with dementia often start confabulating. That is, they tell stories or make comments about a situation or a memory that do not align with the way others perceive or remember them. Confabulation is considered a typical symptom of dementia and can be defined as 'false narratives or statements about world and/or self due to some pathological mechanisms [usually memory problems], but with no intention of lying' (Örulv and Hydén 2006: 648). While confabulation may appear to be a relatively benign symptom of dementia, it has nevertheless been identified as a 'source of considerable distress to family members' (Örulv and Hydén 2006: 648). When people with dementia replace shared experiences with confabulated ones, caregivers may feel threatened in their own sense of self or struggle with how to respond to what seem to them fantastical statements. Both professional and family caregivers are frequently driven to challenge the confabulatory statement and insist, instead, on their own version of a situation. This insistence may distress the person with dementia and might lead to a communicative impasse. However, when caregivers try to enter the world of the person with dementia and 'go along' with his or her version of events they may also feel uncomfortable since they may consider such behaviour either patronising or deceitful vis-à-vis the person with dementia.

In *The Story of My Father* (2003), Sue Miller explores the conflicting feelings she experienced when confronted with her father's confabulation. 'My original impulses,' she writes, 'hadn't been to try and support my father's delusional life. I'd been fooled by my first few experiences with his hallucinations, when I'd been able to talk him out of them, to reason him back to reality' (Miller 2003: 119). As the disease advances, however, Miller recognises that her reasoning no longer produces the desired response, and she comes to question the effects of her own corrective remarks: 'It dawned on me that my insistence that what he saw wasn't "real," that what he heard was not what he thought it was, was making an insurmountable barrier between us, so I stopped' (120). She learns to accept his version of reality, to think of him 'as *having had* the experiences he reported' (120; original emphasis), and to commiserate with or be pleased for him accordingly. So much so that it begins to strike her as 'odd when others didn't or couldn't' (120). Miller openly criticises the nursing staff for their lack of empathy in this respect:

> When Dad spoke delusionally to them in my presence, they were openly dismissive. They reported his "mistakes" to me with contempt. This bothered me, more than a little. Had they had no training in the way these events seemed to occur to a delusional Alzheimer's patient? I wondered. Could they not flex their imagination a little bit? Their compassion?
> (120)

Indeed, Miller underlines how her father's confabulations potentially increased his sense of well-being in that they helped him to reconstitute his identity and reassert the patterns that had governed his scholarly life: the nursing home turns into a university, her father reports preparing or attending lectures, and—despite no longer being able to read—he reports on the reading he needs to do (121–2). She defends his solitary pursuits (or non-pursuits) and his unwillingness to join in the kind of activities offered at the nursing home, as a means of holding onto his personal identity. Defending her choice to 'lie' and go along with his 'mistakes' to the reader, she argues that his imaginary life actually made him 'feel happy and competent in some parallel universe' (123). In her view, supporting his confabulatory or delusional worldview constitutes a better approach than forcing him to take part in activities that she, at least, seems to perceive as mildly degrading. There is a sense, though, in which her acceptance of his confabulations is consoling to her own sense of what her father 'should' be: 'I was glad when he reported he'd done things—familiar Dad-like things—that I knew he hadn't done' (123). It could be that Miller's father does not inhabit a parallel universe in which he feels happy and competent, but his daughter's presence induces him to present this façade as a means of saving face.

In any case, Miller acknowledges that validation (Feil 1989, 1992, Feil and Altman 2004) of her father's confabulatory comments is not without problems. When her father's 'delusions' become painful rather than a source of pleasure, Miller is no longer able to empathise with his point of view. Following a night-time fire drill, her father believes that there has been an actual fire in which children have died. Miller finds it impossible to validate his claim and to act as upset as would be warranted in such a situation.

Her father, in turn, cannot understand his daughter's or the staff's unresponsiveness. He is appalled by her attempt to empathise with his feelings, rather than acknowledge the tragedy. In fact, the incident negatively impacts on their relationship, until her father eventually forgets about it. Miller is left with the gnawing question of whether she should have reacted differently, whether there was 'some lesson [she] could have learned from this' (125). Miller's question is rhetorical. She does not find a definite, ethically sound, and unambiguous solution to the question of how to respond to confabulation. But the fact that such a solution does not exist and that one's response to confabulation needs to be adapted over time and according to the situation and content of the confabulation is the very point of the narrative. Miller learns this lesson and finds a means to share this insight with her readers.

In *Where the Memories Go*, Sally Magnusson, by contrast, highlights mainly the constructive aspects of confabulation. By coming to see confabulation in a positive light, Magnusson also finds new ways of dealing with her mother's dementia. Confabulation is usually seen as fictitious and false—and therefore framed in terms of loss and deterioration on the part of the person confabulating. However, recent memory research stresses the extent to which all memory 'recall' is based on processes of narrativisation and confabulation (Brockmeier 2015, Fernyhough 2012). By engaging with some of this research, Magnusson comes to realise that her mother's confabulations 'are merely taking to excessive lengths the normal tendency of memory to reconstruct itself' (238). Memory, according to the research Charles Fernyhough brings together, is a product of the individual's present needs, created in the moment for the moment. In reconstructing memories, there is a conflict between *coherence* (internal and in relation to the present moment) and *correspondence* to reality: 'A coherent story about the past,' Fernyhough writes, 'can sometimes only be won at the expense of the memory's correspondence to reality' (Fernyhough 2012, qtd. in Magnusson 2014: 238). 'This helps me to understand,' Magnusson writes, 'the narrative fictions you have been crafting: your trip to the moon, your matey relationship with Attila the Hun and personal discovery of the New World' (238). Based on these insights from memory research, Magnusson comes to see her mother's confabulation not as a deficit but as a productive means of self-making and sense-making (see also Örulv and Hydén 2006). As Magnusson states of her mother, employing the second-person narration she uses throughout the memoir:

> So, you are doing what we all do, and what, as a matter of fact, I am doing right now. You are making sense of your experience by using narrative skills to stitch memory into a story. And you are doing it in the teeth of a strenuous assault on the delicate neural connections that make memory possible at all. I am, as so often, full of admiration.
> (239)

In fact, Magnusson sees her mother's confabulation not primarily as a symptom of the disease, but as an aspect of her mother's continuing identity. Creating 'a narrative path that makes sense of the moment ... from the memories that do manage to hack their way through the undergrowth' (223) is consistent with her personality:

> You are straining to take part in a conversation by appropriating whatever has presented itself to your imagination by way of a story once heard or a snippet of information absorbed. Delving into your own experience is what made you such an engaging conversationalist. You will not give up without a fight your right to keep saying, 'I did that, I saw that, I remember hearing, I was always struck by noticing, it reminds me of the time when....'
>
> (224)

Magnusson's interpretation of her mother's behaviour draws support from current research on dementia that posits confabulation as a productive means of making sense of the current situation ('sense-making'), maintaining personal identity in interaction with others ('self-making'), and organising and legitimising joint interaction in the world ('world-making') (Örulv and Hydén 2006: 647). Viewing confabulation in this light allows Magnusson to respond positively to her mother's narrative sense-making, to acknowledge its function, and to recognise in it her mother's persisting identity (see also Crisp 1995). In the process, Magnusson shapes the way we as readers understand confabulation, which, in turn, might perhaps lead to less dismissive reactions to this phenomenon when interacting with people with dementia.

The power of music

Rossato-Bennett's recent documentary *Alive Inside* (2014) has one aim: to demonstrate the power of music to engage people with dementia. One particularly moving example, that is widely circulated on the internet via YouTube and numerous other sites, highlights the transformative effect that listening to one's favourite music can have on people with dementia. Henry, a nursing home resident, who is described as 'almost unalive' (1:07:55) in the documentary, is shown sitting in a chair mute and unresponsive. However, when he is given an iPod with music from his favourite singer, he becomes animated and begins to sing along. This transformative effect lasts even after the music is switched off. Henry can talk articulately about his life, can respond to questions, and remembers the entire lyrics to his favourite song. Oliver Sacks, quoting Kant who once described music as the 'quickening art' concludes that Henry has been 'quickened,' has been 'brought to life' (08:21). Indeed, Sacks suggests that 'Henry is restored to himself, he has remembered who he is ... he has reacquired his identity for a while through the power of music' (10:28). The documentary abounds with examples of how the simple intervention of bringing meaningful music to people with dementia—tailored to their likes and drawing on their past—can have substantial positive effects on their well-being. However, the rhetoric of 'awakening' that the documentary invokes, including the very title 'alive inside,' which suggests a dead outer husk, is deeply problematic. Commentators such as Sacks who speak of people with dementia as 'almost unalive,' or 'being brought to life' reinforce the trope of people with dementia as living dead, zombies, or mere shells. And yet, what this documentary does show is that music is a powerful means for touching people with dementia, a means that can support or replace other forms of communication.

The idea to use music as therapeutic intervention is of course not new. Reviewing the current state of research, Samson and her collaborators call attention to 'the power of music and its nonverbal nature [as a] a privileged communication medium when language is diminished or abolished' (Samson et al. 2015: 250). However, the potential of music-based activities, and even the simple tool of using personalised music on iPods, is only slowly gaining ground in dementia care. These interventions have the potential to replace pharmaceutical interventions, such as the overuse of neuroleptics as tranquillisers, to target what are termed 'behavioural disorders'—such as wandering, excessive anxiety, lethargy, or aggression. There is a growing body of evidence that non-pharmaceutical interventions have a positive effect on emotional states in people with dementia, and that they can also reduce caregiver distress (see also Basting 2009). Importantly, unlike neuroleptics, they have no adverse iatrogenic effects.

Magnusson's *Where Memories Go* provides an excellent case study to illustrate the potential of music in dementia care. For one, Magnusson notices that words that have been learnt as part of a song remain accessible to people with dementia for longer. 'Long after your own words have begun to desert you in droves,' she writes to her mother 'familiar songs deliver an illusion of fluency' (275). The mnemonic effect of music is well-known and used productively in speech therapy. But Magnusson's memoir goes beyond this mnemonic effect to highlight the expressive and relational power of music. In a video on the website of her charity Playlist for Life, Magnusson describes how 'right until the very end almost of her life ... [her mother] was able to be brought back to a sense of her self, and crucially to us as well, by music.'[16] Singing, in particular, provides a means for her mother Mamie to contribute, in much the same way as she has done all her life:

> And it's instantaneous. Like a switch. Someone starts you on one of your favourites and suddenly you are *awake again, alive* and remembering who you are. Music, I begin to see, is what rescues you from silence and the bars of the prison-house.
>
> (276, my emphasis)

While Magnusson also uses the rhetoric of awakening here, she refrains from depicting her mother's less lively state as some kind of zombiedom. Being able to recognise her 'mother of old' as she sings familiar songs certainly has a positive effect on Magnusson. Importantly, however, singing is a joint activity, helping to strengthen their relationship as well as capable of breaking 'the monotony of a rainy Saturday afternoon' (275)—and, as Magnusson seems to imply, the monotony of life with dementia.[17]

Magnusson's memoir furthermore offers moving examples of how music can provide a therapeutic tool to lessen anxiety. Magnusson reveals how singing can have a soothing effect on the person with dementia when describing a particularly anxiety-inducing moment of intimate care, bathing:

> You emphatically did not want to get into this bath and I know for a fact that in a moment you won't want to get out either. You are upset and frightened by the transition from towel to water, this awful feeling of vulnerability. I start to hum 'It's a Lovely Day Tomorrow' and in a slightly quavery voice you join in ... You relax. The tension drains from your face. You shut your eyes. You let the water lap around your chin. You begin to smile. It really is a little bit like magic.
>
> (281)

Although neuroscientific research supports the view that music has a strong potential to engage people with severe memory loss and improve cognitive and motor functions, Samson and her collaborators caution against being misled by an 'exaggerated treatment effect' (Samson et al. 2015: 250). They suggest that the social interaction in itself, irrespective of the activity, is likely to contribute to improvements in emotional well-being in people with dementia (253). As the chief executive of Alzheimer's, Scotland has put it, 'human intervention is the chemotherapy for dementia' (Magnusson 2014: 282). In other words, while making music or listening to music may not work its 'magic' on every person with dementia, it is imperative to develop more ways (and make more time) to be with and finds ways to engage with people with severe memory loss. As Anne Davis Basting's overview (2009) so impressively demonstrates, such forms of engagement may be through touch, conversation, art-based activities, life history work, creative storytelling projects, intergenerational projects, song writing, theatre, or dance.

From control to letting go: being with vs. symptom management

Finally, Magnusson, like others before her, explores how, in trying to protect people with dementia from harm, caregivers may be limiting their family members' potential to thrive. Magnusson reflects on her mixed responses of guilt and shame when the address her mother gives at a funeral seems to go fatally wrong. A skilled conversationalist, Magnusson's mother Mamie delivers the talk with conviction and style, and it is well received by the funeral audience. However, due to her short-term memory loss, at the end of her speech Mamie proceeds to give the entire speech a second time. Magnusson is mortified for her mother's sake and worries about her own responsibility in leaving her mother open to such public humiliation. However, despite initially assessing the event as a failure of caring, Magnusson simultaneously tells another story. She describes how her mother 'revel[s] in the attention of dozens of friendly mourners' (149). The opportunity of giving one more public speech provides her with the 'the chance to be [herself] and feel the adrenaline of performance pumping through [her] veins again' (149). And as the congregation erupts 'in most unfuneral applause' her mother Mamie looks 'thrilled' (150). Initially, Magnusson reflects:

> I should have realised that embarrassment had flown to the same place as many of your social inhibitions. But as I steered you between these sympathetic faces, I felt sick with guilt. This was not how you should have left the public stage.
>
> (150)

Magnusson later realises, however, that in her ideas and expectations of her mother, she might be holding on to the wrong set of values. In other words, what matters to her—seeing her mother as a supremely competent public speaker who makes no mistakes—may no longer matter in the same way to her mother: 'Serenely unaware of gaffes and social expectations, you drank in only the appreciation. Perhaps it is my own embarrassment I am lamenting today' (152). Her experience leads her to realise that the social environment should be such as to support people with dementia in their current state of abilities, allowing them to flourish, rather than secluding them or restricting their activities for fear of humiliation. Magnusson here underlines that not just specialised health-care professionals but the community itself can 'bolster' (385) and support the person with dementia.

> My mother was able to revel in her public self again that day because a community held her in its arms. Imagine the difference if communities in general – churches, shops, offices, buses, hospitals, banks, theatres, schools – were well enough educated in what it means to have dementia (and, crucially, what it doesn't mean) to do the same for the mentally frail in their midst. No pressure then to hide away. No silly shame at a loved one's social solecisms. No stigma to bring out the cowards in us all.
>
> (384)

Magnusson reflects that letting go of her impulse to protect her mother from the risk of public humiliation proved, after all, a productive step.

In her graphic memoir *Tangles*, Sarah Leavitt provides a similar example of 'letting go.' One day, Leavitt, her sister Hannah, and their mother get caught out in a thunderstorm. The daughters' initial reaction is to run for cover, dragging their mother with them. However, once under the awning their mother Midge continues to lean forward into the rain. The image depicts the daughters quite forcefully holding on to their mother (indicated also by their mother's words "Ow! Stop it!"). When they let go, literally and figuratively, and follow their mother, who is tasting the rain on her tongue, this leads to a touching moment in which all three women stick out their tongue in the rain and then run home splashing happily in the rain (78, see Figure 5.5). Such moments of 'being-with' the person with dementia, silencing the ubiquitous drive in caregiving to be 'doing-to,' may lead to shared moments of appreciation and joy. Indeed, caregivers' memoirs can suggest that at times it may be better to let go of one's responsibilities as caregiver, to lose sight of one's task-focused care agenda, and instead to be led by the person with dementia and what matters to her in that moment.

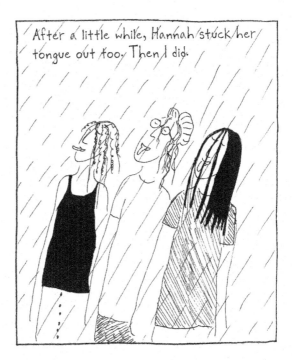

Figure 5.5 Letting go and being with in Leavitt (2010: 78). Image courtesy of Sarah Leavitt.

Challenging care practice

Caregivers' memoirs—though to varying degrees—function as vehicles of patient advocacy. In criticising the current care system, they raise awareness about dementia as a complex and urgent health priority and may, ultimately, be able to contribute to improvements in the care system. By dint of their form as well as their content, caregivers' memoirs speak not only for people with dementia but advocate on behalf of familial caregivers. They criticise the lack of support for caregivers, and the insufficiency of health-care policies in the US and public health care in the UK. Many of the issues discussed so far can be seen in the light of challenging current health-care practices. Instead of reiterating these critiques, or indeed exploring the full range of possible relations between these narratives and advocacy work, I limit my discussion to some of the details from Magnusson's memoir that explicitly challenge current care practice.

Magnusson's memoir provides a searing critique of the inability of institutions to cater to the needs of confused, elderly patients. The smooth running of the institution constitutes the prerogative of nurses and other professional caregivers—often to the detriment of the people in their care. If institutional care is depersonalised, inflexible, and often debilitating (in that patients are often discouraged from doing things they could well still achieve on their own), it is also hostile to intrusions from the outside world.[18] Family caregivers are seen to disrupt routines and are made to feel unwelcome. After her mother is admitted to hospital due to a broken hip, Magnusson describes her family's sense of helplessness and outrage when they are not allowed to spend the night with her. She describes her mother's ordeal of waiting several days for an operation (all the while not being allowed to eat for long stretches in anticipation of surgery) and the toll this takes on her mother's grip on reality. In the process, Magnusson questions hospital policies in relation to frail elderly people:

> Leaving you to face the night alone in a strange, noisy place, frightened and achingly vulnerable, is like abandoning a scared child. No parent would do it. No parent would be expected to. Can anybody tell me the difference?
>
> (162)

Indeed, the unfamiliar environment brings on a state of delirium in her mother. Once their mother is move to a rehabilitation centre, Magnusson and her sisters have to fight daily to be allowed to stay with her beyond visiting hours, and are criticised by care staff for 'traipsing in all the time' (175)—despite the fact that the care staff itself is overstretched and unable to monitor the movements of a mentally fragile person recovering from hip surgery. Magnusson and her sisters defy institutional routines and thereby protect their mother from the worst effects of institutional neglect.

However, during her mother's temporary stay in hospital and a rehabilitation centre, Magnusson witnesses up close how other patients are treated in institutional settings. While Magnusson acknowledges that nursing staff work hard, she reveals how ignorance, power games, and lack of empathy can result in dehumanising treatment of people with cognitive impairments and physical disabilities. Of course, rather than focusing on the failings of individuals, systemic failings such as long working hours, shortness in staffing, inadequate remuneration, training, and support for professional care workers need to be addressed if dementia care is to improve for all involved (Innes 2009).

Magnusson's critique does not limit itself to the nursing staff, but also flags up how doctors often lack the skills needed to communicate with a person with dementia. She criticises a doctor for reading out all the potential hazards of the impending hip operation to her mother: 'There is no use abandoning the does-she-take-sugar approach of talking over a patient's head,' she writes, 'if instead medics simply read the rulebook to someone whose speciality is missing the point' (167). Furthermore, like many caregivers before her, she emphatically questions the rationale of the Mini-Mental State Exam to assess memory impairment—given that the test entails no therapeutic benefits and given that, after it is used to establish her mother's mental impairment, 'no-one takes the slightest account of [her] dementia at all':

> asking questions a person is doomed to get wrong is a strangely heartless way to establish someone's cognitive ability in an alien place when she is already confused and uncertain. It seems almost as mean to measure bafflement in this way as it would be to confirm a weak heart by giving someone an almighty shock. Boo! Yes, as we suspected, heart failure.
> (173)

Magnusson's memoir is outspoken about the failings of the current care system. Compared to other memoirs her advocacy aims are also clearer. Especially in the afterword to the second edition of her memoir, she delineates the many ways she hopes to make an impact on dementia care. She outlines care paths and practices based on both her own and her readers' experiences as caregivers. For one thing, she calls for consistent care in dementia, a professional care manager to support familial care workers and oversee all aspects of health care. Such a role, in her view, would not require 'more money but more organisation' (393). She also explores various approaches to 'integrated dementia care'—institutions that imitate family homes and small-scale community models.[19] And finally, she advocates to use music—personalised playlists on iPods instead of antipsychotic drugs—to engage and soothe people struggling with the effects of dementia. Magnusson therefore moves from localised criticism of individuals and institutions to larger systemic failings—of the NHS and of communities—to suggest how individuals as well as society at large can contribute to better dementia care. Challenging care practice in a first step, these memoirs also move beyond criticism to explore new ways of delivering dementia care.

Conclusion

Caregivers' memoirs provide valuable resources for developing better dementia care—that is, care practices that fulfil the needs both of the caregiver and of the care-receiver. Indeed, the process of 'care-writing' in itself frequently helped improve the level of care that authors were able to provide for their family members. Discovering new ways of seeing dementia, through research and self-reflection, shaped the ways these authors responded to their family members and may also have enabled caregivers to cope better with the changes that dementia wrought. However, caregivers' memoirs act on more than just a local level. Caregiving grows out of concern for the other, and the authors of caregivers' memoirs frequently aim to enlarge that concern to include others outside the family circle by contributing a powerful voice to dementia advocacy. They pinpoint failings in institutions, communities, and society. They challenge current care practices and attitudes towards dementia which suggest that a person with dementia is already 'gone,' has nothing to contribute, and no longer deserves or is likely to benefit from respectful engagement. If these texts rail against the multiple ways the 'system' fails people with dementia and their caregivers, they move beyond mere critique by offering up productive new ways of thinking about and delivering dementia care.

Caregivers' memoirs differ in important ways from medical case studies, social science reports, or advice literature. Much useful information can be gleaned from these sources. Nonetheless, advice literature, for instance, can feel overly prescriptive and fail to address the ethical issues inherent in dementia care. The narrativisation of lived experience in its complexity, through the eyes of a self-critical and accomplished writer, provides a number of advantages over other sources of information on caregiving. A significant advantage is that these memoirs and documentaries have an aesthetic appeal to them, and as I argue more fully in the next chapter, aesthetically pleasing narrative may make topics like dementia care more palatable. That is, readers may engage with topics they otherwise shy away from when they are embedded in a literary narrative (see also Keen 2007, Nussbaum 1990).[20] Literature's capacity to appeal to its readers' emotions, to instruct and delight, distinguishes literary narrative (among other art forms) from medical case studies and social science reports. While these memoirs clearly share some of the affordances of imaginative literature, I explore in the following chapter how fictional narrative, free from referential (and arguably, also certain moral) constraints, may provide an even more radical 'thinking through' of the implications of the current construction of dementia for caregiving practices.

And yet, despite certain similarities between literary memoir and literary fiction, the differences between these two genres are also what give caregivers' accounts their ethical and political force (Couser 2004). It is the fact that the authors of caregivers' memoirs speak from a place of first-hand experience that makes their narratives such powerful tools in dementia advocacy. These memoirs are able to expand the horizon of current research agendas on dementia care by opening up questions that previous research never thought to ask. Among these is the realisation that although dementia creates pressing care needs, living with dementia offers up many opportunities for moments of joy and fulfilment—for both family members, professional carers, and people with dementia.

Indeed, contrary to Burke's analysis of current dementia life writing as infused by the 'language and logic of the market' (2016: 603), in which authors proclaim 'my mother's dementia ruined my life' (603), many of these narratives underscore the continuing relationality and positive experience of mutual obligation that inhere in personal relationships. Also, rather than focusing merely on dementia as personal tragedy—although these narratives clearly function as means to work through their authors' grief and unresolved feelings towards their dead partners or parents—these texts do, in fact, reach out to others with the aim of developing, as Burke demands, a 'collective societal framework with which to support people with dementia and those that provide their care' (Burke 2016: 600). *Pace* Burke, then, subjective and personal narratives do not necessarily undermine or stand in opposition to collective, political action.

Another advantage of memoir over social science and advice literature is that caregivers' memoirs are likely to reach a much wider audience. (Sales reports even suggest that memoir has nowadays surpassed fiction in marketability.) Swinnen (2012), similarly, argues that documentary may contribute to the personhood movement in dementia since it reaches wider audiences than scholarly work (122). Since dementia calls for changes on a societal scale, it is important that the question of dementia care is raised both within and outside specialised contexts. As one of Magnusson's readers says, these texts should constitute compulsory reading for a whole range of people, from 'the highest government minister in the land to the humblest care assistant' (Magnusson 2014: 381). They should be read not because they present ideal or 'model' caregiving, but because, in allowing readers to live through the complexity and ethical murkiness of dementia care, these memoirs stimulate profound debate about the possibilities and problems of looking after people with progressive cognitive impairment. They suggest a panoply of treatment options and stress the importance of flexible care tailored to the needs of individuals, families, and communities. And yet, as Swinnen (2012) also points out, it is necessary to scrutinise the ethics of representation in caregivers' memoirs—as well as documentaries, novels, or films—when they are employed as educational tools in health-care settings. As mentioned before, these narratives are not 'neutral' in the ways they frame dementia care for their readers or viewers, but use the tools of storytelling for their own needs, as well as for moral and political effect.

For all their criticism of the current care system, caregivers' memoirs are of course not beyond criticism themselves. In exposing the lives of vulnerable subjects they may become ethically suspect. As hinted at in the examples above and discussed more fully in Chapter 4, the writers of caregivers' memoirs may harm people with dementia by breaching their right to privacy. They may represent acts of symbolic violence towards people with dementia (Burke 2016: 599). They may also inadvertently contribute to the stigma attached to the disease. As Magnusson discusses in her afterword, the question of misrepresentation remains complex in dementia. Advocates have long painted a bleak picture of the disease in order to garner more support. Although their aim is laudable, by perpetuating a negative representation of dementia they also stoke fear of the disease. Conversely, while Magnusson welcomes the change in attitude towards people with dementia—acknowledging what people with dementia can still do, rather than focusing on their deficits—she also warns that this new way of seeing dementia may lead to a 'revisionist airbrushing of the suffering dementia causes' (385). What I have argued in this chapter is that some of the apparent shortcomings of caregivers' memoirs can actually provide food for constructive thinking.

In considering the ethical problems of life writing about vulnerable subjects, Couser asks whether there are any pay-offs which justify or balance out the ethical infractions such writing commits. I suggest that the ethical thinking these texts promote, the imaginative treatment options they develop, and the challenge they pose to current societal responses to dementia care represent such pay-offs. These memoirs offer up multiple new avenues for seeing, responding to and living with dementia. Such avenues are well worth exploring in the light of the pressing need for humane and sustainable dementia care.

Notes

1 See, among others, Basting (2009), Basting and Killick (2003), Killick and Allan (2001), Kitwood (1997) and Stokes (2010).
2 See, among others, Akpınar, Küçükgüçlü, and Yener (2011), Chappell, Dujela, and Smith (2015), Krause, Grant, and Long (1999), Russell (2001), and Wennberg et al. (2015). Many literary approaches also focus on the 'burden' of caregiving, see, for instance, Zimmermann (2010).
3 For an exception that addresses the care dyad see Whitlatch et al. (2006).
4 Once again, I use the term caregiver and care-receiver advisedly as I am aware these terms might enforce the notion of people with dementia as passive recipients of care who have nothing to contribute to relationships or society at large.
5 Published memoirs written by educated, white, middle-class persons, often professional writers, do not provide a cross-sectionally representative description of dementia care. Compare Kittay (1999) and Innes (2009) for an analysis of the problems of social justice that arise within the care sector, especially in relation to gender and racial biases in this undervalued, underpaid, and under-financed

service sector. See the World Health Organization's report on dementia (2012) for a cross-cultural exploration of the link between gender roles and care for dependents.
6 'Auch professionelle Therapeuten versuchen ihr Glück mit Gretel.' All translations are my own.
7 This is not to say that alternative forms of therapy, such as music, arts, or physical therapy are not valuable resources in dementia care (Basting 2001, Basting and Killick 2003). Indeed, Sieveking's representation risks undermining the value of such interventions and may contribute to the ageist notion that treatment is futile in such cases and that old people, especially people with dementia, no longer merit medical and therapeutic effort.
8 'Können wir irgendwohin setzen wo wir nicht sterben?' [sic]
9 See additional material on the DVD 'Filmgespräch mit Andreas Dresen und David Sieveking' (Sieveking 2012).
10 The medial differences in representation here hark back to my discussion, in the previous chapter, of the ethics of representing vulnerable subjects (Couser 2004).
11 See the joint interview with producer Martin Heisler in the additional material on the DVD (Sieveking 2012).
12 As mentioned in Chapter 4, the metaphoric omission of Midge's eyes, to suggest her increasing loss of awareness, risks contributing to dehumanising conceptualisations of people with dementia as 'living dead' (see also Burke 2007b, Herskovits 1995). Although it may speak to Leavitt's sense of 'losing' her mother, it represents an oversimplification of the issue of self-awareness in Alzheimer's disease.
13 Arguably, this loss of dignity is perpetuated in dehumanising and exposing representations of the person with dementia by family caregivers. Although, with Burke (2016) and Couser (2004), I worry over the violation of a person's privacy and the symbolic violence inherent in fictional and non-fictional accounts of dementia, I find Leavitt does not gratuitously expose her mother. Although explicit, the narrative does not revel in the kind of revulsion and shock aesthetic mentioned in other accounts. Importantly, her mother's bodily decline does not lead to a turning away from caring, or indeed 'prompt' or 'justify' any form of abuse (see Burke 2016: 598). Though debatable, the narrative medium in its abstract, cartoon form might also be seen to provide a further screen to protect the privacy of the person with dementia. See my discussion in Chapter 5.
14 See also the discussion of the politics of caregivers' memoirs in Chapter 4. The overwhelmingly negative representation of caregiving in Cooney may represent an accurate picture of the phenomenology of unsupported family caregivers and, as a cry for help, may thereby feed into the agenda of the dementia advocacy movement to increase funding and support. However, Cooney's account does not offer a productive approach to dementia care and may deter people from finding liveable solutions by suggesting that only the death of the care-receiver can relieve the caregiver from her excessive 'burden.'
15 See Burke on how the language of economics has permeated caregiving relationships with significant implications for those 'who are unable to reciprocate according to the logic of this "contract"' (2015: 28).
16 Playlist for Life, a charity founded by Magnusson, aims to bring personalised music to people with dementia. For further information see www.playlistforlife.org.uk/.
17 In her memoir *Circling My Mother* (2007), Mary Gordon similarly highlights how singing remains one of the few activities she can do with her mother in the nursing home. In describing this beneficial interaction, Gordon also criticises excessive noise levels in nursing homes, emphasising the 'ever-present television' which makes it impossible for them to 'sing and hear [themselves]. In peace.'

(Gordon 2007: 51). Considering that dementia leads to processing difficulties, it seems ill-advised to expose people with dementia to numerous intrusive stimuli. Adapting nursing home environments, by breaking the habit of having the TV or radio run constantly, would represent a first step towards creating a more dementia-friendly environment. See Stokes (2010) for a range of illuminating case studies on how to adapt nursing home environments for people with dementia.
18 See http://johnscampaign.org.uk/#/, a UK-based campaign to make family caregivers of people with dementia more welcome in institutional settings.
19 The most well-known and elaborate community approach is the Dutch village Hogeweyk, an institution modelled entirely on village life for people with advanced dementia. See https://hogeweyk.dementiavillage.com/en/.
20 Keen and Nussbaum are concerned with fictional narratives. Nonetheless, Nussbaum does not rule out that sufficiently *literary* life writing that 'arouse[s] the relevant forms of imaginative activity' and 'promote[s] identification and sympathy in the reader' may function in a similar way as fiction—especially, she writes 'if [it] show[s] the effect of circumstances on the emotions and the inner world' (1995: 5). The caregivers' memoirs discussed in this chapter clearly fulfil Nussbaum's criteria.

6 Making readers care
Bioethics and the novel

When we read novels, we become immersed in complex storyworlds that may mimic as well as differ substantially from our own world. We make sense of these storyworlds based on our own life experiences, and, in some way or another, will relate our reading experiences back to our lives as embodied, embedded, and socially positioned individuals. In the medical humanities—variously described as a discipline, field, or meeting point[1]—literary fiction has been called upon to play a number of (perhaps surprising) roles. Foremost among them, narrative (fiction) has been called upon as a resource to promote empathy and better clinical skills in health-care practitioners (Charon 2006). In the present chapter, I aim to distinguish my own approach from the practice of narrative medicine, as developed by Rita Charon (2006).[2] I propose to widen the scope of Charon's argument in favour of an engagement with narrative in health-care settings to include audiences outside the immediate doctor-patient encounter. My approach differs from her work in that I am concerned primarily with the reception rather than the production of narratives, and here in particular with the reception of literary narratives. Furthermore, I am concerned with all readers—doctors, care home managers, literary scholars, and the general public alike. Of course, this does not exclude the possibility that the novels I discuss may speak in particular ways to health-care professionals and (family) caregivers, or that they may be used in medical education and training.

While the dividends of literary exploration are difficult to quantify or qualify since they lie in the encounter between particular texts and readers, I nonetheless suggest some ways in which dementia novels may engage their readers in considering bioethical questions that arise in contemporary Western care culture(s). I use the term bioethics as a way to describe how novels explore the question of 'how to live'—including the question of how, when, and where to die. In particular, I ask how fictional narratives raise questions concerning autonomy, quality of life, and suicide or euthanasia in dementia. Indeed, a reassessment of cost-benefit understandings of care which underlie discussions around quality of life and euthanasia is central to a number of the narratives I consider in this chapter.

While Charon's work emphasises the clinical benefits of doctors engaging with literary and non-literary narratives, it is imperative to assess whether literature necessarily plays the positive role it is assigned in the medical and health humanities. The medical humanities are generally considered to be driven by an 'ethical imperative' (Rees 2010, qtd. in Jones 2014). On such a view, there is something wrong with the current practice of health care, which needs to be redressed. The humanities and social sciences enter to provide a critique of the state of biomedicine and offer new, more ethically sound ways of providing health care. My introduction outlined problems inherent in the argument that the humanities may 'humanise' biomedical practice. What I am concerned with here, since I deal with narratives that raise issues about well-being and care, is the question whether literary narratives themselves may be seen as tools for 'the good' or driven by an ethical imperative to improve care, or whether they instead enforce common stereotypes of dementia and thereby contribute to the dehumanisation of people with dementia. That is, what ethical vision do these narratives develop? In a second step I then move on to consider other ways in which literary narratives engage readers in thinking through complex ethical issues, such as end-of-life decision-making in dementia care, without straightforwardly acting as moral compass or tools for the common good. Following Meretoja's exploration of the ethics of storytelling, I argue that fictional dementia narratives can function as a 'mode of ethical inquiry' and 'expand or diminish our sense of the possible' (Meretoja 2018: 89–90).

In considering how dementia is represented in narrative fiction, my approach resembles the drive in critical disability studies to outline and deconstruct the way that a 'disease' or 'disability' has been represented historically in a culture. Dementia, like other disabilities, has accrued a host of negative stereotypes and dehumanising tropes that circulate widely in the cultural imaginary (Behuniak 2011, Burke 2007b, Herskovits 1995). The fact that literary narratives promote these negative representations of dementia seriously undermines the notion that reading literary narratives may promote better doctors, more caring caregivers, or more ethical world citizens. Rather than acting, necessarily, as subversive counter-narratives to reductionist and dehumanising biomedical and popular conceptions of dementia, literary narratives in such cases compound the stigma attached to the disease. The question, then, is how particular fictional dementia narratives live up to, or fail to live up to, the ethico-political standard that the term counter-narrative suggests.

Rather than cataloguing numerous stereotypical representations of dementia in fiction—of which there are many—I approach the relation of bioethics and the novel through four case studies to reflect on the ways these novels raise ethical problems vis-à-vis questions of selfhood and norms of caring. In my first case study, Michael Ignatieff's *Scar Tissue* (1993), I ask to what extent dementia novels may act as counter-narratives to the dominant discourse on dementia as loss of self. In discussing Ignatieff's text, I briefly touch on how literary fiction addresses the doctor-patient encounter—long the focus of medical humanities research—and I consider how fictional narratives mediate the contrasting epistemologies of the life world approach vs. biomedicine. In my second case study, B. S. Johnson's *House, Mother, Normal* (1971), I explore the potential of narrative fiction to disturb its readers, in particular by upsetting moral values. How do polyphony and dialogism act as a route to questioning and rethinking dementia care practices? And how may fiction act both as a dangerous democratising force—though the use of polyphony and dialogism—and as a dangerous rhetorical force, in its ability to sway readers' views, emotions, and attitudes. The dangerous and disturbing aspects of narrative rhetoric, I argue, may be productive as well as destructive when harnessed to the ethical imperative of a medical humanities agenda.

In a second step, I explore what fictional dementia narratives bring to the table when thinking through bioethical issues concerning 'quality of life.' Judgments about the quality and value of a human life are inextricably linked with making end-of-life decisions. In thinking about the obligations we hold towards more vulnerable members of our society, dementia narratives open up difficult questions about care*giving* and *withholding* care. In the second section of this chapter, I address how different media and means of narrative presentation affect the process of bioethical decision-making that these narratives simulate for and perhaps evoke in their readers. To this end, I return to the film and novel version of *Still Alice*, and also to Margaret Forster's novel *Have the Men Had Enough?* (1989). These narratives offer the opportunity to 'live through' (Rosenblatt [1938] 1995: 33; 38) as well as 'think through' the bioethical dilemmas attendant on dementia care.[3] Drawing on Martha Nussbaum's argument that novels provide means of addressing the question of how to live, I explore what type of 'ethical work' (Nussbaum 1990: 47) these narratives may engender in the reader. How may these novels elicit certain responses, without offering pat solutions, to bioethical dilemmas concerning the end of a meaningful life?

Ethics and the novel: countering, stereotyping, and disturbing

In approaching the question of ethics from a literary angle, I draw on a range of scholars before me who have made questions of ethics a primary concern of their reading practice. My reading of dementia narratives engages with pragmatist and rhetorical ethics,[4] represented by such scholars as Martha Nussbaum, Wayne C. Booth and James Phelan, since this strand of narrative ethics is frequently invoked in medical humanities contexts. It also draws on and is strongly aligned with Hanna Meretoja's (2018) recent exploration of the ethics of storytelling. Although the work of moral philosopher Martha Nussbaum supports my thesis that novels provide means of exploring ethical questions and of acting as moral laboratory[5] for the reader, I also have some reservations with regard to her claims to the moral good of literary fiction. Most importantly, Nussbaum, in my view, does not pay sufficient attention to the way narrative technique structures the reader's ethical deliberation. As Meretoja argues, 'the way in which a narrative is told crucially affects what is being told as well as its ethical underpinnings' (2018: 27).

At the same time, 'the very act of reading' in the words of James Phelan always has 'an ethical dimension: reading involves doing things such as judging, desiring, emoting, actions that are linked to our values' (Phelan 2003: 132). Phelan and Wayne C. Booth (1988) before him show through close rhetorical analysis how literary devices 'construct value-effects and elicit the reader's ethical engagement' (Korthals Altes 2005: 142). Such a focus on the interplay between the author, narrative technique, and the reader emphasises the co-constructed nature of ethical reading practices, referred to by Booth as 'coduction' (Booth 1988: 70–5). This process of coduction, which includes discussion with others, is of particular value in the teaching of narrative medicine (see Charon 2006). It also implies, contrary to seeing literature as a form of moral education, as Booth originally proposed, that engagement with literature is open-ended and depends on the reader's moral stance and persuasion, as well as on the text's capacity to open up messy and complex ethical dilemmas that are not already solved for the reader within the space of the narrative. Coduction can furthermore be considered an integral part of literary criticism in that professional reading, as John Guillory (2000) argues, constitutes a communal practice. Indeed, in sharing my readings of the novels I discuss in the present chapter, I aim to contribute to a process of coduction which explicitly addresses the ethical dimensions of these texts in relation to dementia care.

Scar Tissue: *biomedicine and the hermeneutics of selfhood*

Michael Ignatieff's *Scar Tissue* (1993) can best be described as a fictional caregiver's memoir. Indeed, it is stylistically and thematically so close to memoir to be nearly indistinguishable from it. It is therefore perhaps unsurprising that Lucy Burke has recently used it as a paradigm case to discuss relational identity, or intersubjectivity in dementia caregivers' writing (Burke 2014). Nonetheless, although Ignatieff worked aspects of his own life experience, notably of his mother's dementia, into the story, the novel departs from the referential stance of autobiographical writing. So, for instance, Ignatieff is 'not the son who gave up everything to be with his mother,' like the narrator of the novel, but 'the brother at a distance' (Vassilas 2003: 443). This departure allows Ignatieff to take a certain licence with his lived experience and to explore other avenues than those derived from his real-life experiences.

Writing a fictional memoir further allows Ignatieff to take certain views and experiences to their extremes and to explore the polarity between science and the arts, philosophy and lived experience. Ignatieff contrasts the figure of the unnamed narrator, a lecturer in philosophy, with the figure of the narrator's neurologist brother. In order to explore the question of whether selfhood persists in dementia, Ignatieff almost schematically opposes characters to show how philosophy, neuroscience, the arts, and later religion afford different vantage points on the self. The novel describes the breakdown of the narrator's own identity and of his family relations, especially to his wife and children. As he becomes the 'parent' to his mother (Ignatieff 1993: 96) he begins to neglect his actual parental duties. *Scar Tissue* therefore complicates the view that relational identity is unequivocally reparative in the context of identity crises in dementia. While caregivers are frequently called upon to maintain the identity of their 'loved ones' by continuing to tell their stories for them (Radden and Fordyce 2006),[6] *Scar Tissue* highlights the extent to which the son's own identity is shattered when his mother no longer recognises him: 'It was as my brother had said: if she failed to recognise you, you ceased to exist. No longer her son, no longer anyone. Acknowledge that I exist. Acknowledge your son' (Ignatieff 1993: 163–4). In Lucy Burke's words, the narrative exposes 'the way in which the narrator's desire to sustain his mother's identity is disturbed by her inability to recognise and thus affirm his own sense of self' (Burke 2014: 45). According to Burke, the narrative thereby takes to their extremes 'the consequences of the erosion of reciprocal or mutual recognition upon which the concept of intersubjectivity is founded' (45). In other words, this novel suggests that dementia erodes the identity of close family members as well as of the person with dementia.

However, the threat to the narrator's identity is not only of a relational kind, deriving from his mother's lack of recognition. Since the narrator believes he has a genetic predisposition to develop the disease—he ironically calls it 'the family silver' (1)—he sees the threat to his own selfhood as emanating from the inside, from the supposed build-up of plaques and tangles in his brain. Indeed, the entire narrative is less a means for the narrator to come to terms with his mother's dementia than a means for the narrator to work through his own fears of living with this condition. The narrator self-consciously grapples with ways to confront his supposed 'fate'—for instance in developing a Stoic attitude rather than relying on the pervasive North American myth of self-help and positive thinking,[7] or in trying to persuade himself that 'selflessness' is in fact an enviable state. He develops the first view in a Rotary speech delivered in front of his parents, and the second in his 'manic treatise' (179) on selflessness in the wake of grieving his mother's death—only to partially reject both attitudes later. Towards the close of the novel, the narrator seems to be experiencing the first symptoms of dementia himself. There is some ambiguity, however, whether these symptoms are due to neurological processes or rather due to his intense depression and his self-willed isolation. The novel clearly challenges the perceived notion that relational identity constitutes an answer to the dismantling of identity in dementia.

Apart from focusing on the question of selfhood and relational identity, the novel shares several other themes with contemporary illness memoirs. Among these, as suggested by its character constellation, is the interrogation of the 'truth value' of various master narratives: particularly, philosophy and contemporary biomedicine. The novel challenges the predominance of the biomedical paradigm while also criticising the way health professionals view, and consequently treat, dementia patients. So, for instance, the narrator contrasts the family's view of dementia with the clinical perspective in what is a staple of most illness narratives: the scene of diagnosis.

During the consultation with a neurologist in which his mother's diagnosis is imparted, the narrator is ruffled by the neurologist's patronising language: the neurologist uses the first-person plural 'we' to ask about his mother's well-being, refers to 'Mother' rather than using her name, and talks about her in the third person in her presence.[8] From the neurologist's perspective the patient's behaviour can be explained through brain pathology: 'disinhibition begins with disintegration in the frontal lobes. Your mother's frontal lobes are not yet affected ... which would explain why she is continent and why she is gentle' (59–60). The narrator, on the contrary, insists that his mother's behaviour is meaningful and consistent with her personality: '"She's gentle," I say, "because that's the kind of person she is"' (60). Frustrated at the neurologist's clinical stance, he eventually blurts out: 'a lot depends on whether people like you treat her as a human being or not' (58). That is, the neurologist's clinical perspective comes across as both depersonalising and dehumanising.

Despite the narrator's attempts to recognise his mother's humanity and sustain her personhood, he nonetheless struggles to separate identity and disease, and to understand the relation between pathology and personality. Ignatieff explores embodiment both in terms of pathology and in terms of representing a remaining seat of selfhood. His narrator asks, for instance, what role his mother's continuing ability to paint plays in maintaining or expressing her identity. The novel thereby touches on complex questions about the relations among intentionality, representational art, and creativity as 'expressions' of selfhood.[9] Faced with the biomedical narrative of inexorable decline that the mother's neurologist insists on, the narrator struggles to convey his sense of how his mother's identity persists in her bodily habits:

> I want to say that my mother's true self remains intact, there at the surface of her being, like a feather resting on the surface tension of a glass of water, in the way she listens, nods, rests her hand on her cheek ... But I stumble along and just stop.
>
> (58)[10]

Using metaphor, the novel here develops a more complex vision of selfhood in dementia and opposes it to the reductionist biomedical understanding. The image of the self as feather suggests fragility, lightness, and effervescence as well as durability. But in locating this embodied form of selfhood at the 'surface,' the novel also draws on entrenched notions of an 'inner' and inaccessible subjectivity that is considered more valuable than 'outer' or supposedly superficial manifestations. In the context of the clinical encounter, in any case, the narrator's views on the ways his mother's selfhood is embodied remain unexpressed and the two ways of seeing dementia seem irreconcilable:

> It is pointless to go on and we both know it. The doctor looks at Mother's PET scans and sees a disease of memory function, with a stable name and a clear prognosis. I see an illness of selfhood, without a name or even a clear cause.
>
> (60)

If the narrator of *Scar Tissue* defines dementia as an 'illness of selfhood,' he nonetheless adopts conflicting attitudes towards whether selfhood persists in dementia or not. On the one hand, the narrator rants at his brother when the latter questions whether there is still any point in visiting their mother. He maintains that she is a 'person,' not a 'vegetable' (159) as exemplified by her habits, her way of speaking, and her expression of preferences and emotions. And yet, after listing all the attributes that make her a person, the narrator concludes his rant by noting that 'She has left her self behind. I sit with her, ... and I think: What's so good about a self?' (161). Further, although he feels the need to assert his mother's identity and acknowledge what remains, he simultaneously reverts to stereotypical representations of people with dementia as selfless beings, with 'vacant eyes' (5) that bespeak a lack of interiority. Finally, the narrator also tries to persuade himself that the loss of self is, in fact, something worth striving for. However, he describes the project of countering the Western 'obsession' with individualism as an errant, misguided project: using the terms 'lunatic' and 'manic' suggests that he feels embarrassed for even entertaining the idea that selflessness might be considered a good, a goal worth striving for. Importantly, as noted above, the narrative disturbs the view that relational identity is unequivocally restorative. His mother's lack of recognition leads to his own pathological breakdown of identity. Conversely, the narrator pronounces his mother's social and spiritual death at the very moment that she fails to be able to recognise him:

> This time I was sure that she neither knew me nor cared who I was. ... The eyes that do not see. The eyes that have no memory, the eyes that are dead. I had arrived at the moment, long foretold, hopelessly prepared for, when Mother took the step beyond her self and moved into the world of death with her eyes open.
>
> (166)

Scar Tissue here confirms the dominant trope of dementia as 'living death,' thereby undermining its status as counter-narrative. However, as suggested previously, counter-narratives are rarely straightforward constructs.

They are necessarily entangled in the dominant discourses they set out to subvert. Indeed, seeing counter-narratives as merely oppositional counter-images that rely on invoking the binary opposites of any dominant representation short-changes their potential to question received ideas. *Scar Tissue* challenges current care practices as well as the 'neurobiological materialism' (Waugh 2013: 18) which constitutes the dominant mode of understanding dementia, and arguably what it means to be human. And yet, *Scar Tissue* also promotes the masterplot of dementia as 'loss of self' and compounds stigma through the use of gothic and animalistic imagery. The text may also be seen to reinforce the notion that dementia is a fate worse than death, a dismantling of self and of family relationships. Reading dementia narratives consequently opens up two levels of critique: (1) the potential of the narratives themselves to provide a means to criticise certain aspects of society and (2) the role of the literary critic to elucidate and criticise how novels engage us in ways of viewing and responding to the world.

Narrative and neuroimaging: raising epistemological questions

The narrator of *Scar Tissue* is critical of both the epistemological validity and the practice of biomedicine. He draws attention to conflicting neuropathological evidence, in which the brains of symptomatically 'normal' elderly showed evidence of the plaques and tangles which are commonly held to be the underlying cause of dementia (54). And yet he wishfully envisions a future in which the 'fate' of Alzheimer's will have turned into a manageable disease, fully explained by medical science. Towards the end, the narrator seems to reject his own philosophical and narrativising attempts to make sense of his experience and instead endorses the biomedical understanding of dementia: 'Human identity is neurochemical' (193). In a narcissistic reverie he imagines witnessing his own neuropathological breakdown with the help of neuroimaging techniques. In an elaborate conceit he (ironically) states:

> I want to be done with metaphors. I want to see the thing itself. I want to see deep into the hippocampus, deep into the parietal and occipital, down into the brainstem itself to the places where the protein deposits are building up, millisecond by millisecond, forming plaques and tangles, shutting down neurotransmitters ... causing me to forget ... Lie back in the scanning room and watch your own neurons watching you, thinking your thoughts, being you, your own forgetting as digital squares of light on a video monitor.
>
> (194)

This passage is in direct contrast to an earlier 'actual' scene of neuroimaging the narrator describes: the PET scans his mother is subjected to in the process of diagnosis (55). The earlier scene is offered up as a critique of the humiliating and seemingly futile nature of diagnostic procedures. It also represents one of the moments in the narrative that hint at more basic and productive processes of intersubjectivity in dementia which do not depend on role recognition—that is, the recognition of the other as parent/child or spouse, respectively. Instead, the scene foregrounds how intersubjective understanding depends on our own embodiment and ability to read others' thoughts and emotions through their body language and facial expression (Ratcliffe 2007): here the mother's 'terrified glances' and legs as 'struggling gestures of fear' (55). Strategically placed after the exposition of current scientific uncertainty about the neurobiological underpinnings of dementia, the passage is one in which the narrator questions the validity of biomedical knowledge, the 'brightly coloured neural images of [his mother's] fear and dread' (55), and criticises the callousness of medical practice. The narrator's insight into his mother's feelings, based on an interpretation of her body language, is contrasted with the technically possible 'insight' into her brain, which only produces seemingly random colour patterns. According to contemporary advances in neuroscience, cerebral activity registered by neuroimaging techniques reflects our emotions. The narrative emphasises, however, that the gap between understanding (and responding to) these emotions and interpreting 'coloured neural images' remains immense. In this instance, *Scar Tissue* underlines how the interpretation of neuroimaging techniques is in itself a hermeneutic process, not a scientific tool that somehow holds a distinct truth value—even if the current neurobiological master narrative of dementia depends on privileging such a view.

What is telling about the narrator's turn towards biomedical explanations at the end of his narrative is that he sees himself as leaving the territory of figural language, moving from fiction to fact, from a hermeneutic process to some kind of 'definitive' form of understanding. Without going into a discussion of the philosophy of science (or indeed of the inevitably metaphoric nature of language), I here want to explore how the narrator's reflections on the purchase of metaphorical language echo current debates in the health humanities—since these debates about metaphor and discourse resonate, in turn, with the notion of counter-narratives. In *Illness as Metaphor* (1979) Susan Sontag discusses how metaphors that attach to particular illnesses have pernicious effects for those who suffer from these diseases—paradigmatically tuberculosis, cancer, and later, AIDS (Sontag 1989). Sontag vehemently resists the use of illness as metaphor and claims that 'the most truthful way of regarding illness—and the healthiest way of being ill—is one most purified of, most resistant to, metaphoric thinking' (1979: 3). She suggests that particular illnesses become synonymous with death. They become mystified, taboo words that can no longer be uttered, and when they are attached to a person this person is seen to be 'morally, if not literally contagious,' and consequently to be 'shunned' (6). Arguably, although strenuous efforts to demystify and destigmatise dementia are underway, this condition remains the 'dread' disease of the century. Since dementia is referred to as a 'living death' or 'funeral without end,' it is easy to see why Sontag's call for non-metaphoric thinking remains pertinent. Indeed, efforts to rename the disease syndrome due to the inherently stigmatising connotations of the term 'dementia' are underway.[11] In this context, critical disability scholarship, which traces and criticises the representation of a particular condition and the metaphoric meanings attached to it, presents a productive avenue of inquiry.

However, the claim that supposedly non-metaphoric approaches to illness are the best means forward has by no means gone uncontested. As David Morris (1998), in response to Sontag, points out,

> There is practical, therapeutic value in calming the imagination of patients gripped by harmful myths. Yet, in her intention to deprive it of harmful meaning, Sontag wants to reduce illness to a scientific, biological fact. Unfortunately, returning illness to science does not deprive it of meaning but simply leaves it in the grip of a reductive, positivist, biomedical narrative that focuses solely on bodily processes ... the effort to cleanse illness of all meaning discounts the therapeutic benefit that positive myths and meanings can supply.
>
> (Morris 1998: 269–70)

Indeed, the entire health humanities movement is to a large degree founded on the assumption that metaphoric thinking and narrative exploration have beneficial effects for the person living with serious illness. In Morris' words, the use of 'metaphor can be turned to good use as well as ill' (270). The question is, then, how metaphor and narrative are used in *Scar Tissue* and other narratives to counter or confirm the dominant construction of dementia as 'loss of self.' And what role does narrative play in making sense of the experience of dementia?

To take the last point first: the narrative project, writing a 'memoir' about his experience, provides the narrator with a means of recovering his mother's identity from before her illness, memorialising her as well as others in the family who suffered from dementia (see also Vassilas 2003: 443): 'Memory,' the narrator claims, 'is the only afterlife I have ever believed in. But the forgetting inside us cannot be stopped' (Ignatieff 1993: 4). He accordingly writes in order to defy the 'betrayal' his brain is 'programmed' to enact (4). The fictional memoir represents the narrator's attempts to create meaning out of his experience. As John Wiltshire holds, 'Illness is the stripping of meaning from both person and event' and this 'challenge of non-meaning' is 'perhaps most acutely represented when the patient suffers ... from a neurological condition' such as dementia (Wiltshire 2000: 413). However, the narrative also registers the many instances in which the attempt to create coherence or master one's 'fate,' as the narrator puts it, is doomed. His mother's death represents such a moment that defies, if not representation, then domestication:

> There is only one reason to tell you this, to present the scene. It is to say that what happens can never be anticipated. What happens escapes anything you can ever say about it. What happens cannot be redeemed. It can never be anything other than what it is. We tell stories as if to refuse the truth, as if to say that we make our fate, rather than simply endure it. We live, and we cannot shape life. It is much too great for us, too great for any words. ... there at last in her presence ... I knew that all my words could only be in vain, and that all I had feared and all I had anticipated could only be lived.
>
> (172)

Ironically, the novel is far from over after this admission of defeat in the face of representing illness and death through narrative.

Scar Tissue, in striving to create coherence and to find redemption, follows the overarching goals of most illness narratives. At the same time, the novel enacts the failure of such redemption. In Wiltshire's view, it even comes close to what Arthur Frank somewhat oxymoronically terms the *chaos narrative* of illness, demonstrating 'the breakdown of boundaries between self and other ... in pathological form' (Wiltshire 2000: 419). Although, in my view, Ignatieff's novel is a far cry from Frank's notion of chaos narrative, it does enact the breakdown of relationality. Importantly, the narrative thematises its own failure to create coherence and to provide satisfactory closure. The narrative strand is continuously interrupted by different types of discourses or genres: such as a speech delivered by the narrator, the beginnings of a philosophical tract, excerpts from *King Lear*, a newspaper clipping on suicide in dementia, and an exploration of De Kooning's artwork. These narrative disruptions also represent contradictory viewpoints that the narrator inhabits in relation to the question of selfhood in dementia. In registering the difficulty of arriving at a definitive account of what dementia entails, both for the person affected and for her caregivers, the novel may offer consolation to others who, as John Skelton argues, 'may welcome the release that literature brings. They may feel that their own power to express themselves has failed and that there is relief in the words of others and the possibility of saying "This is what I mean"' (Skelton 2003: 212)—even if in this case the 'meaning' would be that the experience of living with dementia or witnessing the death of a parent or spouse cannot be adequately put into words.

In *Scar Tissues*, the patchwork of discourses and the narrative trajectory which allows the representation of conflicting views represent a destabilising approach for the reader and ask the reader to join the narrator in his unsettling journey with (and possibly into) dementia. In the end, the novel allows only an imperfect sense of closure. While the narrator seems trapped within the dominant discourses on dementia, the novel as a whole reflects the difficult position dementia inhabits in our society and our minds. It opens up to debate the hermeneutic means—medical, philosophical, artistic, religious, or narrative—through which we might approach the questions dementia raises about what it means to be human.

House Mother Normal: *disturbing care*

B. S. Johnson's *House Mother Normal* ([1971] 2013) presents opportunities to further explore the ethical potential and dangers of storytelling, beyond the question to what extent narratives might enforce cultural stigma or present counter-narratives. In particular, the text highlights literary fiction's potential to disturb its readers. Martha Nussbaum has suggested that novels have the power to make readers see things differently. Fiction is heralded for its emotive appeal, for making readers feel deeply about characters and plot outcomes (Nussbaum 1990, 1995, 1997). Although Nussbaum acknowledges that fiction's ability to arouse strong emotions entails certain risks, she largely glosses over the dangers inherent in fiction's powerful rhetoric and emotive appeal. *House Mother Normal* can be used to explore these other, less salutary effects of the novel's rhetoric on readers. Such a project does not deny that the 'literary imagination' represents a moral 'good' (Nussbaum 1995), but it more closely delimits what this 'good' may be and contests the claim that reading fiction generally has the effect of morally improving the reader. As Keen argues, 'linking novel reading to a widely shared moral principle—caring—without demanding that fiction be about caring allows broad claims about the medium to exist without evaluating content' (Keen 2007: 20). Taking my cue from Keen, I suggest that both form and content need to be taken into account when evaluating the ethics or ethical potential of any given narrative, and particularly the narrative's relation to promoting an ethics of care.

With regard to how literary fiction may do ethical work, scholars note a number of characteristics of literary fiction, such as polyphony, dialogism, and ambivalence (see Korthals Altes 2006, Meretoja 2018). So, for instance, Astrid Erll (2008) describes how from a post-structuralist perspective the ethical value of literature is located in its ambiguity: the 'polyvalency of literary forms,' she writes, forces readers 'to acknowledge that reality is a construction' and that 'different, equally valid perspectives on the same thing are possible' (Erll 2008: n.p.). According to Erll this aspect of literature leads readers to learn respect for alterity. When these perspectives become multiplied, as in the insistently dialogic and polyphonic structure of *House Mother Normal*, the ethical effect of respecting alterity may be seen to be enhanced. The representation of the events in a care home through the minds of eight residents allows the reader to appreciate the different meanings each individual attaches to his or her experience. The reader is sensitised to how the house mother's behaviour impacts on each resident's well-being and sense of self. By inhabiting each character's mind in turn, one sees the world through that person's eyes, appreciates how memories of the past, and wishes for the present structure that persons experience.

Further, the patients' interior monologues support each other (by allowing the reader to piece together the events of the narrative), even as they represent different and sometimes conflicting experiential points of view. Importantly, the various interior monologues by the residents are accorded equal weight and value. So, for instance, despite the narrative trajectory from more cognitively able to less cognitively able minds, each monologue is accorded the exact same number of pages. In representing the consciousness of people with dementia—subjects frequently 'othered' in contemporary discourse—and then diversifying this representation through multiple individualised portraits, Johnson seems to be working within or towards an ethics of alterity.

However, some problems remain with interpreting the ethical effect of the novel's dialogic structure in such a way. For example, taking inspiration from branches of criticism such as feminist, postcolonial, or disability studies, one might argue that Johnson's representation constitutes a misrepresentation or usurpation of the subjectivity of the other. In Emmanuel Lévinas's terms the other is never fully knowable, and therefore attempting to inhabit the other's perspective represents an unethical act of appropriation or erasure (Lévinas 1961, 1979). Although it is important to bear the complexity of the problem of (mis)representation and appropriation in mind, Johnson partially circumvents becoming the target of such criticism by drawing attention to the constructed nature of his representation.

It remains a problem, too that assigning a particular ethical value to a particular literary technique, does not pay due attention to how the specific cultural, historical, and textual contexts of a given technique affect its reception. Literary forms do not carry ethical weight in themselves but contribute to the ethical potential of a narrative in a specific context (see also Erll 2008). *House Mother Normal* lends itself to post-structuralist readings, which value disruption, undecidability, ambiguity, and a resistance to closure. At the same time, the text also disrupts hypotheses about the ethical potential of certain literary structures, such as the use of frame narratives.

Further, if dialogism and democracy are inherently linked, the 'democratic' distribution of narrative space in this case is upset by the house mother's frame narrative. The house mother's story, her point of view, takes precedence over the other accounts on a number of levels. She is after all the eponymous heroine of the novel; by framing the patients' accounts, her narrative may be seen to determine the interpretive field of the narratives that follow. She is given the 'last word,' literally and figuratively. Her narrative also exceeds the number of pages accorded each patient narrative, as stressed by a significant moment of metalepsis: 'And here you see, friend, I am about to step [page 21] outside the convention, the framework of twenty-one pages per person [page 22].' That said, Johnson's narrative suggests that her view is not meant to go uncontested. Rather than promoting her views on how people with dementia had best be cared for, the narrative is set up to disturb and shock. As mentioned in my previous discussion of the novel, the house mother provides a number of dubious, humiliating, and harmful 'entertainments' for the people in her care. She enlists their labour in manufacturing fraudulent medication, enforces a wheelchair tournament with wet mops that causes at least one of the patients severe pain, and conducts a game of pass the parcel in which the prize is one of her dog's feces. Her final act of entertainment involves pornographic acts with her dog, ending in the 'climax' of her public orgasm. By progressively revealing the extent of the house mother's shocking behaviour, Johnson subverts the parameters of 'normalcy.'

However, even this reversal of norms and normality undergoes a further twist in the house mother's final address. Her discourse is full of contradictions. It exposes her cruelty, sardonic nature, and apparent megalomania. And yet, in the fashion of the court jester, the fool who also speaks truth, Johnson makes her a mouthpiece for criticising care home environments that are, in other ways, worse than or at least as bad as the one she manages. In contrast to the house mother's theatrically and 'over-the-top' immoral acts of 'care,' the deplorable conditions in other institutions, she describes, seem plausible, even likely. At once self-absorbed and selfish, the house mother at times seems to show a real interest in her charges. It thus becomes difficult not to be at least partially persuaded by her argument. She draws an image of mental homes in which people are 'put away ... simply because they are old' and where they are 'stripped of their spectacles, false teeth/ everything personal to them' (198). Her own 'care,' by contrast, provides her patients with 'constant occupation, and/most important, a framework within which to establish/ – indeed, to possess – their own special personalities' (198). However, her means of allowing these personalities expression consist in nurturing petty rivalries among the residents, or giving them reasons to complain.

If Johnson uses the house mother to criticise the reality of subhuman care conditions—evidenced nowadays by increasing reports of elder abuse—he also uses her to expose the hypocrisy of a certain 'discourse' that has evolved around care. Her rhetoric evokes the suave language of care home advertising, only to be contrasted immediately with her dismissive attitude: 'Here we respect their petty possessions, so important/to them but rubbish to us' (198). By showing the farcical and sardonic effects of what following the rule book of what nowadays is termed 'person-centred care' could look like, Johnson's novel invites us to reconsider the very parameters of these care discourses.

In *House Mother Normal* we are confronted with immoral behaviour which is subsequently rationalised and justified. While the reader is unlikely to accept her justifications *tout court*, the house mother's arguments nevertheless have an effect on the reader. For instance, when we get to the house mother's account of the game of 'pass the parcel,' she defends her rationale for using the dog's feces as prize:

> How disgusting you must be saying to yourself,
> friend, and I cannot but agree. But think a bit
> harder, friend: why do I disgust them?
> I disgust them in order that they might not be

> disgusted with themselves. I am disgusting to them
> in order to objectify their disgust, to direct it to
> something outside themselves, something harmless.
>
> (197)

The house mother goes on to argue that her diversion is intended to prevent a deeper spiritual crisis in her charges. This passage reveals a key ethical crux of the narrative. Johnson not only shocks or disturbs the reader in revealing the amoral behaviour of his protagonist, but also disturbs the very norms of what constitutes 'care.' We cannot easily assimilate the house mother's reasoning, but it is not that simple to dismiss her view, either. The logic of the text and the house mother's rhetoric powerfully destabilise the reader's view of what represents morally acceptable caregiving. So, for instance, the residents' monologues bear out the house mother's reasoning that her disgusting behaviour redirects the residents' attention from their own immediate misery. Also, in portraying the differing reactions to her activities, from the 'tournament' to her public masturbation, the narrative underlines the difficulty of pleasing or doing right by all. The novel thereby highlights the conflicts between the needs and rights of individuals. What causes one joy causes another pain, and what may arouse one person causes another disgust. Balancing these needs cannot ever be simple. What this novel upsets, then, are discourses of care that presume that certain forms of caregiving are uniformly good for all care-receivers. In contrast to a moralistic text, *House Mother Normal* does not suggest ideal solutions; rather, it shocks the reader by presenting the effects of a warped care ethic.

In her final address to the reader, the house mother further challenges preconceived notions about what old people or people with dementia may want for themselves: 'What you do not understand, I think,/friend is that what we imagine they want for them-/selves is not actually what they do want. I do/ not know what they want, either' (193). Although in the next sentence she seems to reject summarily the humanity of the people in her care ('But I do know/that they are certainly not as we are, and that/therefore by definition they do not want what we want' (193)), her reflections nonetheless point to a distinct ethical problem: 'How does anyone know/what anyone else really wants?' (193). And if we do know what someone wants, how do we balance these needs and wishes against those of others, including, in the context of care, the caregiver's? On my first reading, the house mother's reasoning seemed only to confirm her 'demented' state of mind—structurally contrasted with the supposedly 'dementing' but otherwise mentally 'sane' inmates for a particular stylistic and ethical effect: the novel counters the stigmatising notion that people with dementia are out of their minds. My sensibilities were duly shocked by her cruel behaviour and apparent lack of empathy. However, on my second reading I was more inclined to take her challenges seriously, to be partially persuaded, as I noted, by her logic or rhetoric. What do we, indeed, know about the needs and wishes of others?

How can we provide care for people with dementia? And how can we know which previously stated wishes to fulfil and proclivities to support, when, as the house mother states, these are affected by the 'diffusing effect of time' (193)? Dementia raises, perhaps more than any other condition, ethical dilemmas about advance medical directives and the question of whether we can adequately assess our future selves' needs and wishes.

The effect of staging 'uncaring care' and presenting 'unjust justifications' may be diverse. It may lead certain readers to be shocked and outraged—which in turn may draw attention to actual power imbalances within caregiving environments and highlight the essential vulnerability of those who receive care. It may also lead readers to reconsider dominant humanistic care ethics, to wonder about the rationale behind certain care practices, either to reject them or to re-assert them. What is unlikely, though, is that the narrative will leave its reader untouched. Johnson develops means for us to imagine the phenomenology of dementia and to consider our shared vulnerability as humans. The narrative is perhaps most ambiguous in its representation of the house mother. While Johnson portrays her as a somewhat reprehensible character, he also indicates her isolation, the lack of support she receives from the 'authorities.' Current debates about the chronically underfunded care sector and the woefully underpaid work of professional carers resonate with this text and add complexity to the house mother's character. Rather than seeing her as a *rogue* character—as Burke suggests frequently occurs in the context of actual cases of abuse by carers (Burke 2016: 596)—we are invited to consider also the systemic failings that may lead to such atrocious 'care.'

Significantly, Johnson puts into the house mother's mouth a lyric and yet melancholy invocation of the *carpe diem* motif.

> Still, I'll finish off for him [the author], about the sadness,
> the need to go farther better to appreciate the
> nearer, what you have now: if you are not like
> our friends, friend, laugh now, prepare, accept,
> worse times are a-coming, nothing is more sure.
>
> (204)

House Mother Normal functions as a *memento mori* for its readers. By evoking the complexity of care home settings, the individuality of people affected by dementia, the vulnerability of not only 'care-receivers' but all human beings, it provides food for thought about what it may be like to grow old with dementia, and how we might prepare, individually and collectively, for the increased dependency that this stage of life inevitably brings.

Exploring bioethics: 'living through' as 'thinking through'

In her introduction to *Love's Knowledge* (1990), Martha Nussbaum argues that novels provide important tools for considering the question of 'how to live.' Indeed, she considers novels more productive tools for exploring ethical dilemmas than philosophical examples. Schematic ethical case studies used in bioethics textbooks, Nussbaum argues, are overdetermined in terms of possible interpretations: 'much of the ethical work is already done, the result "cooked"' (Nussbaum 1990: 47). In contrast, literature is open-ended, ambiguous, and complex. Nussbaum argues that due to the particularity, indeterminacy, and emotive appeal of literary fiction novels 'engender in the reader a type of ethical work more appropriate for life' (47). According to Nussbaum, novels engender a form of experiential learning in their readers (44). In other words, literature provides not only a representation of ethical concerns, but evokes processes in the reader that may be considered a form of ethical deliberation in their own right.

In *Uses of Literature* Rita Felski provides a similar account of the type of learning that fictional narratives promote: 'As a form of context-sensitive knowledge conveyed to readers it is more akin to *connaître* rather than *savoir*, "seeing as" rather than "seeing that," learning by habituation and acquaintance rather than by instruction' (Felski 2008: 93). Indeed, literature's ability to make readers see something in terms of something else, using metaphor and mimesis to make readers see things *differently*, is considered one of its most valuable attributes in the medical humanities (see Charon 2006, Jones 2014). At the same time, most commentators argue that the 'knowledge' or 'learning' that literature promotes is elusive and hard to formulate in discourses other than its particular aesthetic instantiation (see Felski 2008, Nussbaum 1990, Wood 2005). Getting a handle on how novels inform and transform their readers—by providing access into the storyworld's social phenomenology[12] and the protagonists' minds, but also through the use of literary devices, content, and structure—requires close narratological analysis.

Lisa Genova's *Still Alice* (2007) and Margaret Forster's *Have the Men Had Enough?* (1989) make their readers in Rosenblatt's terms 'live through' fictional lives affected by dementia, and thereby invite those readers to think through bioethical questions concerning quality of life and end-of-life decisions. I include here a discussion of the film version of *Still Alice* in order to address how medial representations influence the exploration of bioethical questions in fictional narratives. The comparison underscores how each specific narrative environment creates a particular value system in the context of which the reader's or viewer's emotional and ethical responses will emerge.

Before turning to this task of ethico-aesthetic analysis, let me clarify however that 'living through' does not necessarily entail a process of (empathetic) identification in the reader; rather, as Rosenblatt stipulates, it concerns the aesthetic experience of a literary work. (She argues that while others might satisfactorily summarise a newspaper article for us, they cannot summarise a poem: 'If there is indeed to be a poem and not simply literal statement,' she writes 'the reader must experience, must "live through" what is being created during the reading' (1995: 33).) Similarly, I focus here on what aesthetic experiences dementia narratives create and how those experiences pertain, in turn, to larger questions about quality of life in dementia. I explore the *ethos* or narrative ethics the novel or film projects, while emphasising that the social or ethical effect in the reader, that is the 'reconstruction' of a narrative ethics, depends primarily on the reader's interpretative stance. In other words, novels suggest certain moral attitudes or (un)ethical solutions to caregiving dilemmas. They rarely, however, offer pat solutions to the reader. Due to the complexity and ambiguity of literary works and the diversity of their readers, these texts function as a moral laboratory rather than a moralistic treatise. That said, since 'the implied moral attitudes and unvoiced systems of social values are reinforced by the persuasiveness of art,' as Rosenblatt points out, the systems of beliefs and values that a text projects merit 'careful scrutiny' (Rosenblatt 1995: 8). Indeed, careful analysis might elucidate both the 'social' and 'narrative unconscious' that underpin our interpretation of the world (Meretoja 2018). It is here that the detailed analysis provided by literary critics (and in the case of medical education the teacher's explication) may play a particular role in exploring bioethics in and through literary fiction.

Still Alice: (precedent) autonomy and suicide in dementia

As noted in Chapter 2, in *Still Alice* (2007) Lisa Genova tells the story of a Harvard professor of cognitive psychology with early-onset Alzheimer's. Perhaps unsurprisingly—given the author's background as a pharmacy consultant with a neuroscience degree from Harvard herself—this novel largely endorses the neuroscientific understanding of dementia. Indeed, Genova's novel is aimed at supporting the Alzheimer's advocacy movement and its call for sustained research into the neuropathology of the disease. The novel does not therefore question the validity of the Alzheimer's disease category. Furthermore, in her choice of protagonist, Genova can be seen to celebrate the common 'virtues' of contemporary Western societies: autonomy, self-reliance, cognitive capacity, and a strong drive to achieve. The eponymous heroine Alice identifies herself with her academic persona, and struggles to find a new sense of self as her cognitive capacities slowly disintegrate. Even Alice's most intimate relationship, with her husband John, is based on her mental prowess and is therefore fundamentally threatened by the onset of the disease.

Still Alice, then, does not represent a straightforward counter-narrative to the dominant discourse of biomedicine or, indeed, to the cultural norms of hypercognitive Western societies. What it offers is a reflection on how cognitivist values play out in the life course of an individual character affected by Alzheimer's disease who, in this case, virtually embodies these values. However, in its narrative logic the novel also offers a subtle critique of the value-system it endorses. The novel highlights the shortcomings of cognitive skills-based tests to measure quality of life and concomitantly determine the end of a meaningful life. It suggests that despite cognitive impairment, people with dementia have the capacity to enjoy life. By depicting Alice's development from the inside and her changing perception of the world, the novel raises serious doubt about whether a person with dementia can adequately project herself into her future self. It thereby challenges, albeit without explicitly addressing this topic, the practical and ethical applicability of so-called 'precedent autonomy' and the use of living wills or advance directives to determine treatment options in case of mental incompetence.[13]

The narrative logic of *Still Alice* is highly pertinent to bioethical discussions about end-of-life decisions. In tracking the development and (failed) execution of Alice's suicide plan, the novel raises complex issues surrounding suicide and euthanasia in dementia.[14] In particular, the novel stimulates an imaginative exploration of the question whether advance directives still hold in the context of neurodegenerative disease and whether they should be considered legally and morally binding. Answers to these questions frequently centre on whether a person with dementia remains the same over the course of the disease. If not, changes to the affected person raise the question whether the pre-morbid self, or 'then-self,' can legitimately make choices that affect the 'now-self' in later stages of the disease (Francis 2001). As previously noted, Ronald Dworkin (1993) has famously argued that the 'critical interests' that shaped the life course and values of the per-morbid self take precedence over the 'experiential interests' of the person with dementia later in the disease. *Still Alice*, however, undermines this argument. Since the entire novel is focalised through Alice, the reader sees how her perception of the world changes over the course of the disease. The narrative tracks this change specifically in relation to Alice's suicide plans. Alice's previous attitude towards the value of a life with cognitive impairment is contrasted with her continuing enjoyment in life,[15] despite significant cognitive disability. So, for instance, the novel emphasises her continuing emotional capacity and her ability to maintain relationships with others, even when she can no longer remember the exact nature of these relationships. More importantly, the novel suggests that the criteria Alice chooses to determine whether her life is still meaningful—and whether to set in motion a suicide plan—are ill-suited to their purpose.

Mode, medium, and the suicide plot

Immediately after receiving her diagnosis, Alice is struck by thoughts of suicide. However, she soon realises that there are still many things worth living for and that the cut-off point for a meaningful life has not yet been reached. In order to determine this cut-off point, she develops a test involving five questions about her life. Failure to be able to answer any of the questions will set a suicide plan in motion. Her suicide plan is hatched during a moment of simple enjoyment—eating ice cream on an unexpectedly sunny spring day—and it is therefore linked to the *carpe diem* motif that runs through the entire novel. In response to her recent visit to a nursing home, Alice decides that 'she didn't want to be here ... when the burdens, both emotional and financial, grossly *outweighed* any *benefit* of sticking around' (116; my emphasis). Notice how Alice's reasoning represents a cost-benefit analysis and draws heavily on economic language. Her decision is influenced by an economic rationale, which weighs the literal 'fortune' of keeping her 'alive and safe' (116) against the metaphorical or emotional value of her life and person. Alice thinks that when she can no longer recognise her husband, and is 'in the most important ways' (116) no longer recognisable to him, her husband's (financial) obligation to her should cease to exist. Or rather, her reasoning suggests that honouring this financial obligation constitutes a waste of resources. Alice clearly subscribes to a notion of love relationships as forms of exchange. The novel then exemplifies Lucy Burke's point that the way popular discourse about love and relationships is permeated by the language (and logic) of economics has pernicious effects on care relationships:

> ... the idea that we must "get something back" from our love object or else move on to a more "profitable" partnership ... has significant implications for attitudes towards care and responsibility for others who are unable to reciprocate according to the logic of this "contract."
> (Burke 2015: 20)

Alice envisions a future in which she will not be able to fulfil her side of the 'contract,' to give 'something back,' and she therefore sees no reason for her family members to be obliged to support her—emotionally or financially.

In fact, *Still Alice* might be considered 'symptomatic'[16] of the trend to view caring as 'somehow *discontinuous* with normative familial relations and ... an impediment to the flourishing of those around the person with dementia' (Burke 2015: 25; original emphasis). As Burke points out, this view leads to caregiving itself being perceived 'as a form of suffering but crucially one that is often deemed to eclipse that of the disabled or ill person' (28). At this stage in the novel, Alice endorses such a view of caregiving as a 'burden' while devaluing the person receiving care. Over the course of her disease, however, the novel develops a different stance. Since the narrative is largely focalised through Alice, her experiences (her thoughts, feelings, and responses to a situation) overshadow those of her caregivers. Importantly, as Alice slowly loses her cognitive abilities, they also seem to matter less. Instead, the narrative stresses her capacity to 'seize the day,' to enjoy whatever pleasure comes her way. Her husband John, though, continues to adhere to their previously joint cognitivist value system. He seems unaware of the extent to which Alice can still enjoy her life, or what matters to her. The couple clashes over the extent to which John will accommodate Alice's needs in his life, and the value accorded to each separate life course.

It is worth considering how a novel that is otherwise so consonant with dominant Western discourses on the value of human life may invite its readers to reconsider some of the implications of these values. Alice's entire self-worth is linked to her IQ. Nonetheless, when she contemplates her future, she realises that the things she considers worth living for (holding her grandchild, seeing her children thrive and fall in love, and spending one more sabbatical year with her husband) do not require 'intellectual brilliance' (119). Indeed, she expresses her wish for simple pleasures, such as 'more sunny, seventy-degree days and ice cream cones' (118). In view of these life priorities, the questions she generates in order to determine whether this cut-off line to a meaningful life has been crossed are relatively ill-suited. The questions rely entirely on long-term declarative memory pertaining to biographical 'facts' rather than experiences: 'What month is it? ... Where do you live? ... Where is your office? ... When is Anna's birthday? ... How many children do you have?' (119). Such facts represent major coordinates of one's life. Nonetheless, this information resembles semantic memory. Semantic memory tests, like the Mini-Mental State Exam, are out of touch with the real-life concerns and important functional capacities of people with dementia. What, one may ask, does it matter whether one knows the name of the current prime minister or president? Such questions call attention to gaps in semantic memory but do not reveal a person's continuing capacity or incapacity in other areas equally (or more) relevant to everyday life. In defence of such tests, they are not used in order to determine whether the life of the person is still worth living. In *Still Alice*, however, they are. As the novel later highlights, these questions are woefully inadequate as a means of assessing whether Alice can enjoy the presence of her grandchild or the pleasure of an ice cream.

The temporal nature of narrative, in its ability to depict change and to juxtapose contrasting scenes with each other, plays a crucial role in making the reader consider the shortcomings of cognitivist notions of personhood and to see things differently. In a crucial scene, John and Alice return to their favourite ice cream parlour. While John is distressed that Alice can no longer remember what flavour ice cream she likes, Alice is seemingly indifferent to this change. She is enjoying her ice cream, the warmth of the sun, and the feel of her husband's hand in hers. According to her life priorities, even at the stage of making her suicide plan, her life is still worth living. However, when John asks her a number of questions from her list, it becomes apparent that she can no longer answer them. (She does make a convincing case that knowing the location of her office is of no practical relevance to her.) It is unclear, here, whether John has discovered her suicide plan or whether he is intuitively using similar questions in order to assess her 'quality of life.' In any case, the narrative suggests that he is trying to assess whether Alice has reached a point where she no longer wants to be alive: 'Alice, do you still want to be here?' (267), he asks in a noticeably serious tone. Alice takes this question literally. However, like his question her answer takes on a double meaning: 'Yes. I like sitting here with you. And I'm not done yet' (268). Since the latter can be seen to refer to her ice cream as well as her life, Alice unwittingly answers his question with a confident 'yes.' Within the logic of the narrative in which enjoying an ice cream was made *the* criterion for assessing quality of life, this answer is doubly significant. In contrast to Alice's formerly held world view, this scene represents a serious challenge to the notion that cognitive capacity is the be-all and end-all of human life.

I am taking some time over describing the development of this 'suicide plot' to suggest how readers, in the 'living through' of a certain aesthetic experience, may come to see things from various angles—particularly since this element of the narrative is so strikingly different in the film version of *Still Alice*. The *carpe diem* ice cream moment shared with John in the book is immediately followed by the chapter in which Alice, by chance, stumbles over her suicide instructions. Although she has serious problems carrying out the instructions, her plan ultimately fails only because the sleeping pills she relied on are no longer in their designated place. The reader is left to wonder whether John, having found her suicide plan (or simply the pills), and having no strong evidence to suggest that Alice no longer wants to live, has quietly removed the pills. In the film, this sequence of events is inverted. The failed suicide attempt comes first and blends into the scene in the ice cream parlour. Further, the emotional undertones and the atmosphere of both scenes differs significantly. In the book, the preceding scene primes readers to believe that suicide at this stage would not in fact be in her best interest. In the film, Alice finds the pills and is only prevented from taking them because a professional caregiver enters the house at that very moment and the sudden noise causes Alice to drop the pills [1:25:00]. There is a steady build-up in tension-creating music until the moment that she finds the pills [1: 24:00]. As the pills are scattered on the floor the image blends with the image of similarly fragmentary morsels of ice cream toppings. In contrast to her portrayal in the book, Alice in the film is shown clinging to John. While he does not seem fazed by her inability to remember her favourite ice cream flavour, she is uncertain and in need of emotional and physical reassurance. Alice's confident sense of enjoyment, which predominates in the novel, is absent in the film. The setting is also markedly different. John and Alice eat their ice cream indoors, in a decidedly cold, almost clinical environment. There is no sense of warmth or enjoyment. There are no geese that prompt Alice to giggle, no pink and white blossoms spread all around, which in contrast evoke such a positive mood in the novel.

Interestingly, in the film the ensuing conversation is less close to the questions Alice devised for her suicide plan. Instead, the conversation highlights her distance from her previous role as successful researcher and teacher. When John asks, 'Ali do you still want to be here?' his facial expressions and his fixed gaze on Alice and tone of voice (as in the book) suggest the intent of this question. As in the novel, Alice fails to understand the question.

However, in contrast to her confident answer in the book ('Yes I like sitting here with you.'), Alice is instead perplexed by John's seemingly abrupt suggestion to leave and responds with a troubled 'I'm not done yet, do we need to go?' [1:26:15]. The camera focuses on John's face as he continues to gaze at Alice, herself intent on her ice cream. Tears well up in his eyes as he seems to realise that the moment has passed in which he might be able to have a conversation with his wife about her wishes concerning end-of-life decisions. He also seems to realise that although Alice might not want to live anymore (as suggested by the previous scene of her failed suicide attempt), there is now no way out.

These gaps in the film, as well as the sequencing of events, are important. We do not know whether the caregiver or John discovered the pills scattered on the floor, but might presume that one of them did. What is the viewer then led to think or feel? While I cannot determine what any given viewer will feel, I believe that the film suggests that her failed suicide attempt is 'tragic.' The film presents a much less confident view that her life is in fact still enjoyable to herself. The film also represents her physical deterioration to a much starker degree than the novel. Indeed, the representation of Alice is close to that of a 'mindless zombie' as regards her shuffling walk, unfocused gaze, and lack of interaction with others.[17] In the novel, on the contrary, Alice 'in the most important ways' (and in contrast to Alice's earlier view cognitive capacity is not paramount) is still functioning emotionally and socially and is 'still' herself—as the title of the novel suggests. She enjoys the music of a street musician, the company of her daughters (despite not knowing their names) and of her grandchildren. One might argue that the novel represents Alzheimer's in a superficial manner here. The impact of the disease goes beyond losing the names of things or people, and as accounts by caregivers suggest, such qualities as caring about children or animals might be drastically altered by dementia.

But if the novel is unrealistically hopeful, the film is perhaps stereotypically pessimistic. What is remarkable is how, despite their inclusion of similar or even identical narrative elements, these two representations differ significantly in their narrative *ethos*. Not only the sequencing of events—and the emotional reactions that the differing narrational choices elicit—but the 'sense of an ending,' the closure each narrative provides, may lead readers and viewers to inhabit substantially different stances towards Alzheimer's and the question of suicide in dementia.[18] Both novel and film engage readers and viewers in thinking through bioethical questions by making them 'live through' an aesthetic experience. While the novel seems to question the predominant view that a person with dementia has the moral authority to decide her future life, or rather the end of her life, the film by contrast suggests that this moral authority extends into the future.[19] Indeed, the film suggests that the 'tragedy' of Alzheimer's lies in the affected person's inability to assert her right to self-determination and her inability to live out her life according to previously held values. As these narratives bear out, ethics and aesthetics are inextricably intertwined and the aesthetic has a role to play in both moral and political spheres.

Have the Men Had Enough? *Gender and the economies of care*

Margaret Forster's *Have the Men Had Enough?* (1989) is one of the earliest English-language novels which focuses on a character with dementia and the problem of caring for her. The novel's publication coincides with the rise of the Alzheimer's disease movement and the biomedicalisation of dementia. Further, as Lucy Burke points out, it appeared during the 'high point of Thatcherism and the particular form of individualism [Thatcher's politics] fostered' (Burke 2015: 37). Accordingly, Burke reads the novel as symptomatic of the effects of the biomedicalisation of dementia and of neoliberal politics on 'the concept of family' and in particular 'notions of familial obligation, personal choice, and the meaning of care' (Burke 2015: 25). I extend Burke's critique by focusing more squarely on the question of gender. In her aim to counter neoliberal conceptualisations of caregiving, Burke perhaps underplays the important contribution this novel makes to challenging pervasive gender imbalances in the context of both familial and professional caregiving (see also Kittay 1999).

Forster's novel suggests that caring for a declining family member necessarily constitutes an unbearable burden.[20] This view is common in both fictional and non-fictional representations of dementia. The caregiving son in *Scar Tissue*, for instance, rationalises placing his mother in a nursing home by suggesting that at some point 'you have to choose between sacrificing yourself and sacrificing somebody else' (Ignatieff 1993: 97). The decision to institutionalise a family member with dementia therefore resembles an assessment of whose life matters more: the caregiver's or the life of the person with dementia. In *Have the Men Had Enough?* this value judgment is played out through the perceptions of two family care partners: Grandma's daughter-in-law, Jenny, and Jenny's own daughter, Hannah. Their narratives provide alternating points of view on Grandma's[21] increasing care needs and the relative involvement of different family members in meeting those needs. So, for instance, Hannah repeatedly questions why it is that she, but not her brother, is expected to be involved in her grandmother's care and she challenges her mother's tendency to shield the male family members, including Hannah's father, from becoming involved in 'hands-on' care (see also Burke 2015: 35). Indeed, Grandma's adult son Stuart entirely washes his hands of his mother and Jenny's husband Charlie is only persuaded to manage the financial side of his mother's care because his wife acts as his moral conscience. Significantly, although he doesn't carry the main 'burden' of caregiving, Charlie is the driving force behind his mother's temporary stay in a care home which precipitates her rapid decline, and which in turn leads to her admission into a closed psychiatric ward—represented in the novel as an abject form of purgatory. All this happens in the absence of

Grandma's primary caregiver, her daughter Bridget, whose desire to care for her mother at home, but inability to do this without the support of the wider family, is represented as the main conflict within the novel. Importantly, neither Grandma's own perspective nor that of her primary caregiver is voiced directly. The quality of Grandma's life and the value of caregiving are all viewed from the daughter-in-law's and granddaughter's point of view.

The novel confronts the questions of Who should care? How and how long should we care? And, to a lesser degree, Why should we care for people with dementia? With regard to the first question, Hannah's thoughts about the value of life in dementia are couched, from the start, within a discussion of gender roles in relation to caregiving. Forster's novel is not alone in mirroring, and arguably compounding, widespread views (and anxieties) about male caregiving. The husband in *Still Alice* abandons his wife to the care of his daughters. In the film version of *Still Alice*, he somewhat ironically comments on his guilt at leaving his wife by telling his daughter, 'You are a better man than I am' [1:27:48]. In *Scar Tissue* the son's devotion to his mother unravels his own life, suggesting that a male caregiver cannot retain a sense of self. In contrast, in *The Story of Forgetting* (Block 2008) neither the narrator-son nor his father seems to visit the mother much after admission into a home. In Andrés Barba's *Ahora Tocad Música de Baile* (2004) the adult son nearly beats his dementing mother to death, and shortly afterwards causes her to get run over by a car (see Zimmermann 2010). And in Franzen's dystopian analysis of 21st-century American family life *The Corrections* (2001), it is the oldest son who pressurises his mother to contemplate admission into a nursing home. The only daughter in the family, in contrast, briefly figures as a potential primary caregiver. That she does not in fact have to take on this role is depicted as a narrow escape from the supposed drudgery and deadening burden of caregiving.[22]

What do these novels then suggest about who should care? And do they not enforce stereotypes about uncaring males and dutiful daughters and wives? Forster's novel challenges the fact that women are expected to and continue to undertake the largest bulk of 'hands-on' care work. That said, nowadays, male family care partners are no longer as unusual as they once were (Russell 2001). Cultural gender stereotypes, as Russell argues, frequently make male care work doubly invisible within society. Literary representations, such as those discussed here, may then compound the view of caring as 'naturally' female activity and act out societal anxieties and gender stereotypes about 'uncaring' males, even as they challenge the unjust distribution of care work.

Forster's novel also addresses the question of how, and how long, one should care for people with dementia. It explores what different characters consider the 'cut-off line' at which home care should end, or, to paraphrase *Still Alice*, the point at which the burdens, both emotional and financial, outweigh the benefits (for Grandma and others) of keeping Grandma at home—or, indeed, alive. At the outset of the novel Grandma is mildly confused, but still a largely functioning and contented person. The novel then follows a tragic downward spiral as Grandma's dementia rapidly progresses, and all the precarious and temporary caregiving arrangements fall apart. Her daughter-in-law Jenny is significantly involved in managing Grandma's day-to-day care. Unlike Bridget, she is not motivated as much by love as by a sense of duty. Nonetheless, she experiences satisfaction and even pride in looking after her mother-in-law, and she clearly voices an ethics of home care. Jenny also sees herself as repaying her mother-in-law for the debt of bringing up children, Jenny's husband among them, and she tries to compensate for her mother-in-law's hard life out of a sense of female solidarity. Jenny realises that institutionalising Grandma would deprive her of all the loving attention and 'all that was meaningful' to her, and she is therefore racked by guilt at the prospect: 'How can we "put her away," as she would call it? *How can we?*' (125; emphasis original). When her husband states that he has 'had enough,' her scruples prevent him, at least for a while, from placing Grandma in institutional care.

Despite Jenny's conviction that nursing home care would speed up her mother-in-law's decline, the latter's increasing care needs eventually cause a 'care crisis' in the family. The novel depicts Jenny's growing stress and emotional anxiety, and to a lesser extent her daughter's. Hannah's narrative, since she is at one removed from the responsibility of caring, represents a more detached and at times critical perspective on the family's views and actions. She also challenges the hypocrisy inherent in an idealised ethics of home care, including her own. In these cases, and others, Hannah succinctly pinpoints in lists of (rhetorical) questions the problems and dilemmas that dementia raises. Early in the narrative, Hannah begins to contemplate the question of suicide and euthanasia in dementia:

What I want to know is:
Why don't more old people kill themselves when they get old?
Why do relatives not kill old people more?
What is the point of keeping old people alive anyway?
Haven't the women had enough, as well as the men?

(13–4)

Since the questions are left unanswered it is up to readers to develop a response based on the events in the storyworld as well as on their own life experiences and convictions. While some readers might be categorically against suicide, or euthanasia, others may find themselves contemplating these questions, perhaps for the first time. It is significant that these questions are raised immediately after Hannah's benign description of Sunday lunch dinner, which highlights the ways in which Grandma still enjoys life. At this stage, Hannah's provocative questions seem premature. Or rather, the contrast between Grandma's apparent sense of enjoyment and the callous suggestion to murder family members based only on their advanced age may provoke a sense of outrage in the reader. Nevertheless, derogatory views of old age predominate in contemporary Western societies, and readers may perhaps find that their views chime with Hannah's at times. The expression of such stark views then confronts readers with their own attitudes and may lead them to ask: Do I share this evaluation of old age? Is euthanasia, assisted suicide or murder, an acceptable moral stance towards vulnerable dependents? On reflection, is seeing life with dementia as valueless the only way to look at things? The novel sets up such bioethical thought processes by drawing readers into the complexity of caregiving, as evoked by the storyworld, and by contrasting opposing, at times shocking points of view.

Indeed, the question of euthanasia represents one of the main themes of the narrative and is reframed in the context of Grandma's continuing decline and the increasing pressure this puts on the family. As Nussbaum states,

> the novel ... is a morally controversial form, expressing in its very shape and style, in its modes of interaction with its readers, a normative sense of life. It tells its readers to notice this and not this, to be active in these and not other ways. It leads them into certain postures of the mind and heart and not others.
>
> (Nussbaum 1995: 2)

Here, the reader is invited to see the question of care from the point of view of two female family caregivers of different generations. We are asked to note the seeming impossibility of providing home care throughout dementia. Furthermore, Hannah consistently challenges the ethics of caregiving as a natural female duty—a point I elaborate on below. While calling for female empowerment, Hannah also, however, represents the form of consumer-orientated individualism that, according to Burke (2015), neoliberal economies foster. Indeed, in line with Burke's recognition that care relationships are imbued with economic rationalising, the value of the person with dementia, as weighed against the 'costs' of caregiving for family members, is what is at issue in this novel.

Hannah eventually draws up such a cost-benefit analysis in order to assess Grandma's quality of life and concomitantly the question of whether one should end her life. She enumerates the pains and pleasures in her grandmother's life while weighing them against each other and the 'damage' to other people's life (emotional, financial, and other) (144–5). Only as an afterthought does it occur to Hannah to detail what Grandma 'returns for what she gets' (146), a revealing list in itself. Entirely within this economic logic, Grandma's daughter Bridget then emerges as the person who both gives and receives most from her mother and who, subsequently, is the most invested in keeping her alive ('*Who gives most to Grandma?* Bridget. *Who gets most from Grandma?* Bridget. *Who would never, ever kill Grandma?* Bridget' (146)). Importantly, Bridget is also the one character who resists seeing her mother as a financial and emotional pit. When Grandma finally dies, offering an end—if not a constructive 'solution'—to the family's care crisis, Bridget is the only family member to truly mourn her. To Grandma's daughter-in-law, and to a certain extent to her granddaughter, Grandma's death represents a release from the anxiety and responsibility of caregiving. Indeed, by withholding the severity of Grandma's condition from her sister-in-law, who 'would have had her pumped full with antibiotics' rather than letting nature 'take its course,' Jenny can be seen to be part responsible for her mother-in-law's death (234). Accordingly, she wants her sister-in-law to experience her mother's demise as release too, to reap some gain from her passing. Bridget, however, staunchly refuses: 'no, no gain,' she asserts 'only loss' (249).

The novel closes with Hannah's thoughts about her own and her family's reaction to her grandmother's death. If she feels irked by her mother's expression of relief and even happiness, she nevertheless expresses an equal relief that, now, with no 'old person in our family ... There's no more of that hideous disintegration to watch' (251). A significant part of her narrative indirectly quotes her mother's complex reaction to the ethical issues raised by Grandma's death. If Jenny felt called to look after her mother-in-law out of a sense of familial obligation, her sense of moral duty does not extend to those outside the family circle. Or rather, her guilt at ignoring the needs of others testifies that she may feel a moral duty but does not act on it:

> Mum says ... that she feels lucky and glad and relieved now Grandma is dead. But she says she also feels a coward too because now Grandma is dead she can ignore the problem of all the other Grandmas and she shouldn't, she should be inspired to do something and she knows she isn't going to. She is going to dodge the issue now. ... She isn't an activist and she can't help it. But somebody, somewhere, will have to do something soon. They'll have to.
> (250)

If this passage evokes the urgent need to address the challenges that dementia raises, it is also significant—and depressing—that the solution Jenny suggests is to embrace the practice of euthanasia:

> We've tinkered around enough with the start of life, we've interfered with all kinds of natural sequences, and now we'll have to tinker with the end. Mum says, "Your generation, Hannah, will have to have pro-death marches, you'll have to stop being scared to kill the old." Will we?
> (250)

Note that, as usual, Hannah challenges her mother's view. The two words 'Will we?' open up the question of whether this approach is ethical and whether there may not be other, better solutions. Nonetheless, Hannah does not develop any in the remaining space of her narrative. As such, one could argue that, in Meretoja's (2018) terms, the narrative diminishes the possibilities of future action. In particular, it closes down rather than opening up possibilities of an ethical response to the challenges dementia care poses. The novel's close centres on the desirability of terminating one's life rather than experiencing the 'hideous disintegration' dementia entails— while underscoring the seeming impossibility of such self-determination in dementia:

> When my time comes I'm not going to allow it.
> When my time comes I won't trust to mystery.
> When my time comes I will say I have had enough and go.
> That is, if my time comes like Grandma's time, if it is the same sort of time. But if it is, I won't be able to, will I?
>
> (251)

The novel then returns us to the difficulty of developing and executing a suicide plan in dementia, as explored in *Still Alice*. However, within the ethics and logic of *Have the Men Had Enough?* the impossibility of self-determination and individual agency is clearly considered tragic.[23] Burke argues that the closure the novel provides through Grandma's death 'simply removes the origin of the problem' but does not 'provide any kind of imaginary resolution' (2015: 39). In her view, 'the novel cannot move beyond the cognitive/cultural limits of the model of aging, dependency, and dementia that it—at times—appears to critique' (39). No doubt, the novel does not represent a straightforward counter-narrative to the dominant conceptualisation of dementia. It clearly offers material for a symptomatic reading of the neo-liberalist and cognitivist tendencies of its time. As Hannah's disgust at her grandmother's decline or Jenny's dehumanising discourse in relation to the dementia patients in the psychiatric ward highlight (see also Burke 2015: 36), the narrative is suffused with dehumanising tropes of dementia and a valorisation, primarily, of the lives of cognitively functioning individuals. In Meretoja's terms, it can be considered an ethically problematic narrative because it reinforces 'harmful cultural strereotypes' as well as 'fatalistic beliefs that present lives as predestined to follow a certain, inevitable trajectory' (2018: 97). In this case, the narrative buys into the culturally dominant narrative of dementia as a tragic downward spiral, with little or no chance of a meaningful life, continued well-being, or opportunities to contribute to society.

And yet, I wonder whether the novel is indeed stuck within its own paradigm. It is an interesting question whether Forster, or if one prefers, the implied author, here or elsewhere, consistently endorses Jenny's or Hannah's views. Within the novel, Hannah's narrative already acts as a counter-discourse to the narrative her mother tells (and wants to tell) about Grandma's decline and death. But her own view is not left unchallenged either. Indeed, as I suggested above, by making Hannah express at times

Making readers care: bioethics and novel 219

drastic and disturbing attitudes towards dementia (and contrasting these with the quality of life that her grandmother actually seems to experience at different stages), Forster may be deliberately confronting and destabilising her readers' received attitudes. As Nussbaum puts it,

> good literature is disturbing in a way that history and social science writing frequently are not. Because it summons powerful emotions, it disconcerts and puzzles. It inspires distrust of conventional pieties and exacts a frequently painful confrontation with one's own thoughts and intentions. ... Literary works [require] us to see and to respond to many things difficult to confront—and they make this process palatable by giving us pleasure in the very act of confrontation.
> (Nussbaum 1995: 5–6)

If the use of multiple first-person narrative perspectives, according to Burke, 'is indicative of a loss of shared values' (Burke 2015: 38), I consider the use of differing narrators one of the advantages of this particular novel. It multiplies opportunities for inspiring 'distrust in conventional pieties,' in Nussbaum's words, as well as for confrontations with one's own attitudes and beliefs.

The comments on the dust jacket of the novel suggest that it is 'not a comfortable novel, but a mighty powerful one.' Or, as another reviewer puts it, the novel 'ends as it begins, with questions ... that spill out over the covers' (Forster 1989). Rather than expressing a stable, shared belief system, this novel, like Johnson's, represents a multiplicity of discourses and allows the reader to linger over uncomfortable questions. It offers a 'pedagogy of discomfort' without offering pat solutions to these difficult questions (Wear and Aultman 2005: 1056, qtd. in Jones 2014: 36). But if the novel is powerful, then in what way? Of what is it trying to persuade the reader? Due to the complexity of the two narrative perspectives, which in themselves incorporate a number of inconsistencies, there may be no simple answer to this question. But the text does highlight the pressing need to address dementia care, voicing this need from a distinctly feminist perspective. While the commercialisation of care is certainly regrettable, the continuing pressure on women to provide care—to the detriment of their own health and well-being and with little appreciation and insufficient remuneration—urgently needs to be addressed.

Conclusion

Fiction may both counter and conform to dominant discourses about dementia, fiction may disturb its readers without this disturbance necessarily acting as a moral good, and fiction may act as a moral laboratory to assess questions of end-of-life care in dementia. In situating my discussion of dementia fiction within the debate about the role of medical humanities research in health-care practices, I am not proposing that such an approach to narrative supersedes current ones nor that it offers an exhaustive account of the complex interaction between illness narratives, biomedical and popular culture, and the well-being of individuals and communities. Instead, I have aimed to outline, in an exploratory fashion, some ways narratives may work on readers and may thereby contribute to the debate and delivery of dementia care. My aim was to extend the scope of literary reading from the locus of medical training, where Charon (2006) and others situate narrative medicine, to include a wider spectrum of readers. Further, I argue that the discussion of the effects of literary reading in medical humanities should go beyond the question of whether fiction induces empathy. Fiction may act as a source of (elusive) knowledge (Felski 2008, Nussbaum 1990, Wood 2005), as a means of experiential learning and quasi-Socratic thinking about how to live life (Nussbaum 1990, 1995), and as a challenge to dominant discourses. Through the processes of metaphor, mimesis and narrative rhetoric fiction may further engender in its readers new ways of seeing, understanding, and enacting care (Charon 2006).

And yet, fiction is neither morally good nor ethically unproblematic. Fictional dementia narratives may enforce dominant stereotypes, perpetuate harmful myths about dementia, and foreclose possibilities of envisioning other modes of acting and being in the world. Fiction's dangerous rhetoric might be put to deeply unethical ends; for instance, by persuading readers that life with dementia is not worth living, the person with dementia is no longer fully human, and he or she is better off dead than alive. As dementia activist Kate Swaffer has pointed out, believing that there is no meaningful or valuable life beyond a diagnosis of dementia also entails that little effort will be put into supporting people with dementia to lead the best life possible. In considering dementia narratives, we need to consider the narrative *ethos* these texts develop and whether they 'expand or diminish our sense of the possible' (Meretoja 2018: 89).

What this chapter has shown is that stories act as a space to approach and 'live through' (Rosenblatt 1995) certain dilemmas without having to take action oneself. Indeed, the counterfactual nature of these scenarios allows novels to probe the boundaries and limits of contemporary understandings of dementia or to follow certain conceptualisations of what it means to be human to their logical conclusion. In accepting reductionist conceptualisations of personhood, rather than necessarily challenging them, they may perpetuate harmful views of dementia as 'death before death.' However, by re-representing dominant negative discourse on dementia, these fictions may thereby also confront readers with their own implicit views, and raise, as Anne Whitehead puts it, 'uncomfortable questions' (Whitehead 2011: 58). I suggest that, in line with Whitehead's argument, rather than solving or resolving these ethical dilemmas for the reader, the particular value of certain literary representations of dementia may lie in their ability to 'open up, *and to hold open*, central ethical questions of responsiveness, interpretation, responsibility, complicity and care' (59; original emphasis). Indeed, the value of much contemporary literature resides in the way it provides a space for the reader to *be with* uncomfortable questions. Both the process of identification with the non-demented others in fictional worlds (usually the family care partner) and the process of 'empathic unsettlement' (LaCapra 2001: 41–2, qtd. in Whitehead 2011: 58) with regard to the character *with* dementia play out in the reader's appreciation, understanding of, and response to the bioethical dilemmas of end-of-life dementia care.

Since these difficult questions are aesthetically mediated, novels have the potential to focus their readers' attention on issues that they might otherwise be inclined to avoid. While most people do not seek out first-hand accounts about dementia care, dementia films and fiction reach wide audiences. It may be that literary fiction is less likely to cause 'empathic distress' in its readers (Keen 2007) than newspaper reports—which, in turn, can lead to a turning away from the issue at hand. The aesthetic mediation of counterfactual scenarios—that we nevertheless bring to bear on our own lives—may then confront us with ethical dilemmas we otherwise tend to ignore until acutely faced with a similar problem. Reading fiction, in its capacity to both 'delight and instruct,' to subvert and challenge, to simulate and evoke feelings, to draw in as well as shock, has the potential to make readers care: about fictional worlds, about questions of how we live and die, and about what it means to be human.

Bioethical decision-making concerning end-of-life treatment in dementia cannot be replaced by reading fictional narratives in which similar scenarios play out, in part because these narratives themselves develop an *ethos* that may be opposed to ethical action in the real world. However, reading such narratives stimulates and simulates bioethical thinking. By emotionally engaging readers, these narratives may move readers to consider previously unthinkable responses and solutions. The counterfactual scenarios may help expand the categories used for bioethical decision-making, and provide a kind of training field or moral laboratory for contemplating the diverse situational, personal, emotional, and financial aspects involved in making difficult care decisions. These narratives do not necessarily present 'ideal' solutions. Indeed, they may employ narrative rhetoric and dehumanising imagery to condone practices of euthanasia or indeed manslaughter of family members with advance dementia (see Zimmermann 2010). As Burke suggests vis-à-vis *Have the Men Had Enough?* and as I have indicated in my reading of *Still Alice*, these narratives may be trapped within the predominant logic of neoliberal and also cognitivist notions of the value of human life, promoting ways of thinking about vulnerability and interdependency that may in effect be counter to a responsive and responsible ethics of care which acknowledges the interdependency of human life. If such narratives are therefore to be used as tools within an ethically driven medical humanities agenda, they must themselves be opened up to ethical scrutiny through critical reading strategies.

How do these arguments relate, then, to broader medical humanities agendas and the role of literary critics within them? Theresa Jones argues that much like fiction, the humanities help us see things differently by 're-presenting, re-describing and re-contextualizing' (Jones 2014: 28). Jones, furthermore, points out how the humanities are frequently viewed as a 'democratizing force' and a means of challenging the status quo of biomedical practices (28). The traditional mode of 'critique' in the humanities is crucial here. I have suggested that while aspects of some fictional accounts act as forms of critique of current dementia care practices, careful literary analysis cautions us against assuming any unilateral democratising or ethical effect of literary fiction. It is here that I locate the need for literary scholars and narrative theorists to engage in debates about the role of narrative in the medical or health humanities. Literary scholars can offer a more complex account of how narratives work on their readers. And more generally, the tools of literary and cultural criticism can help train readers to become critical 'readers' or interpreters of culture and cultural productions in their own right. Further, these same modes of critical thinking can be turned on the humanities' own modes and techniques of producing knowledge. If good fiction 'opens up and keeps open' difficult questions about our responsibility to others, then critical thinking about fiction can extend that process of coduction between text and reader to engage wider audiences in a debate about the value of life, end-of-life care practices, and how we produce knowledge and protocols in these areas.

A number of problems nevertheless arise in the context of considering literary fiction and literary criticism in the context of the health humanities. For instance, Michael Wood suggests that if we consider critique of hard science the only role of literary critics (a bit like the opposition in politics), then we are selling short what literary critics do, as well as the value of the 'knowledge' or 'understanding' produced via the study of literary texts (Wood 2005). I have suggested instead that literary analysis offers tools to read fictional narratives, films, and other forms of cultural expression critically for the effects they may have on their readers. Yet even in Wood's account of scholarly knowledge, 'understanding' remains problematically linked to the individual reader or interpreter. How can this understanding be communicable or relevant to others? Perhaps the product of careful literary analysis may communicate understanding between readers. Scholarly publications and conferences in themselves function as forms of coduction, extending beyond the context of medical humanities teaching. However, the crucial question remains how insights from medical humanities research of all kinds, whether literary, anthropological, or other, may be communicated to the relevant actors in health care. Just as doctors may not have the time or inclination to read cutting-edge medical humanities publications, so policymakers, bioethicists, or care home designers are unlikely to turn to recent outputs of such journals as *Literature and Medicine* to inform their policies or decision-making.

Guillory warns against exaggerated expectations about the effects of critical ethical readings in the 'real world.' In a similar vein, I suggest that further thinking is necessary to translate insights from literary health humanities into policy and practice. Public engagement, reading groups, and consultancy work may offer the beginnings of an attempt to make the reading of dementia narratives relevant to future dementia care. At the very least, I hope to have widened the scope of critical reading of fiction in the medical humanities in emphasising literary criticism's ability to make us reflect on the social climate we live in, reconsider the modes of knowledge production we use to justify certain treatment measures, and challenge the structures of desire that are aroused by representing dementia as the ultimate tragedy, shattering not only projects of self-fulfilment but 'the self' as such.

Notes

1 Medical humanities have recently also been described as 'a series of intersections, exchanges and entanglements between the biomedical sciences, the arts and humanities, and the social sciences' (Whitehead and Woods 2016: 1).
2 Despite differing from the primary aims and methods expressed in *Narrative Medicine* (2006), my approach shares certain concerns with Charon's more recent work on ethics, see Irvine and Charon (2017). The latter as well as previous contributions (Charon and Montello 2002), however, focus more on the circumscribed domain of medical ethics and are primarily addressed to clinicians, health professionals, and ethics consultants rather than being concerned with the general public.
3 Compare also Morris (2002) on 'thinking *with* stories' (196; my emphasis).
4 See Korthals Altes (2005) for an overview of the 'ethical turn' in the humanities. For further discussion of the relation between ethics and literature or storytelling see Korthals Altes (2006, 2013, 2014) and Meretoja (2018).
5 See Hakemulder (2000) for empirical studies examining the effects of reading.
6 Compare Davis (2004), who criticises the demand placed on family caregivers to maintain the identity of the person with dementia.
7 See also Hawkins (1993) for a critical reflection on the self-help myth of 'healthy-mindedness,' which represents a dominant model for illness narratives in the US.
8 Aquilina and Hughes (2006: 149) critically reflect on the fact that medical staff often bypass the person with dementia and speak only to caregivers, thereby denying them their status as authorities of their own experience and even denying their personhood. Caregivers' memoirs and autopathographies alike suggest that it is a common occurrence that the person with dementia is bypassed in such interactions.
9 For a related debate see Selberg (2015).
10 The novel here develops a notion of embodied selfhood akin to Kontos's approach, as discussed in Chapter 1.
11 Hughes (2011), for instance, calls to replace 'dementia' with 'acquired diffuse neurocognitive dysfunction.'
12 Felski (2008) argues that the novel 'unfolds a social phenomenology, a rendering of the qualities of a life-world, that is formally distinct from either non-fiction or theoretical argument' (89). The novel does not only represent social norms, actions, and judgments, but 'enfolds readers through the inculcation of countless examples, into an experiential familiarity with the logic of such judgments'

(92). While I agree that this experiential familiarity is one of the effects of novel reading, one must not underestimate that readers do not entirely suspend their own values, norms, and experiences and may therefore vary significantly in their response to the social phenomenology rendered in a novel.

13 See Davis (2009) on the problems pertaining to 'Precedent Autonomy, Advance Directives, and End-of-Life Care.'
14 For some thought-provoking discussions on this topic see Davis (2009), Dresser (1995), and Hertogh et al. (2007).
15 Simple enjoyment and the absence of pain are usually classed 'welfare' interests in contrast to 'investment' interests such as personal dignity or religious commitment (Davis 2009: 350). These categories seem largely coterminous with Dworkin's distinction between 'critical' and 'experiential' interests.
16 According to Abbott, 'symptomatic reading' refers to the reading strategy of 'decoding a text as symptomatic of the author's unconscious or unacknowledged state of mind, or of unacknowledged cultural conditions' (2008: 242).
17 This description pertains to the penultimate scene of the film. As in the novel, the final scene by contrast highlights Alice's continuing capacity to engage with her daughter.
18 Laura Pritchett's *Stars Go Blue* (2014), for instance, develops an entirely different narrative ethos in which the murder-suicide of the character with dementia to avenge his daughter's murder is seemingly lauded as heroic as well as a logical and 'useful' conclusion to his life with dementia—as the character thereby avoids becoming a 'burden' to his family.
19 Referred to as the 'extension view' in discussions about advance directives (see Davis 2009: 354).
20 For a similar view, see the Japanese novel *The Twilight Years* ([1972] 1984) by Sawako Ariyoshi. This novel bears out Innes's point that the cultural expectation that female family members will care for the elderly is 'backed up by the absence of care alternatives provided by health and social care services' (Innes 2009: 48). This situation, she argues, places women who are juggling 'paid work and existing family responsibilities with the new caregiving role' under 'considerable pressure' (48).
21 The protagonist is referred to as 'Grandma' throughout by the narrators and as Mrs McKay by professional caregivers. This lack of individualisation compounds the external view on dementia in which Grandma's existence and care needs are primarily a 'problem' for the family. Although the narrators are concerned about her well-being and are frequently empathetic, Grandma's perspective is not represented—that is, Foster does not focalise events through her or employ other stylistic devices to communicate her thoughts, feelings, or attitude.
22 By contrast, recent children's and young adult fiction about dementia, such as Lindsay Eagar's *Hour of the Bees* (2016), Jenny Downham's *Unbecoming* (2015), Ruth Eastham's *The Memory Cage* (2011), and Ranjit Lal's *Our Nana was a Nutcase* (2015), to varying degrees portray the second generation—that is, the grandchildren of the protagonist with dementia—as much more willing to take on the role of caregiver than their parents. In the latter two cases the entire plot revolves around the grandchildren trying to keep their grandparent from being institutionalised and to protect them from the seemingly heartless, or at least unempathetic stance of their parents.
23 Hartung (2016: 202–3) reads this novel as promoting euthanasia. However, rather than advocating such a practice, the novel plays out conflicting points of views against each other in such a way as to challenge the reader to contemplate the problem of euthanasia.

Dementia narratives and beyond

In this study, my goal has been to show how both narrative and narrative studies are relevant to the exploration of the phenomenology of dementia, to reconsidering the question of selfhood in dementia, and to the development of dementia care. I have delineated the potential and limitations of narrative, and narrative identity, in relation to challenging the current dementia construct and developing new ways of seeing, acting towards, and caring for people with dementia. I contend that narrative remains both a crucial sense-making device and a significant form of representation relevant to medical humanities research and health-care practices. At the same time, I have aimed to contextualise and correct unilateral arguments about the use of narrative in the medical humanities by paying close attention to how different modes, media, and genres inflect the various functions narrative may play in the context of dementia studies and dementia care. In particular, I challenge the notion that illness narratives function straightforwardly as counter-narratives, that narrative empathy unproblematically translates to benefits for people with dementia, and that the ethical effect or value of literature can be boiled down to moral education. In all cases, narrative mode, medium, and genre, as well as readers' attitudes, historical context, and cultural narrative subconscious shape the meaning and function of a given dementia narrative.

As will have become apparent, my study shares certain preoccupations both with first-wave medical humanities methods and agendas, and with recent developments in second-wave or critical medical humanities. Turning to the phenomenology of dementia and the question of how illness narratives can further our understanding of a given condition resonates with first-wave medical humanities' concern to make the patient's voice and illness experience heard. Given the dearth of first-person accounts of dementia, by comparison with outside representations of the disease, I felt compelled to include and re-represent the majority of first-hand accounts currently available. Further, although the training of health-care professionals has not been the focus of this book, reading dementia narratives may be beneficial to health-care practitioners and their patients. A sustained engagement with the life world of a person with dementia may provide a more holistic view of the patient and her situation and may open up alternative therapeutic possibilities—beyond the limited scope of currently available drug treatments. Dementia narratives may contribute, together with other social forces, to a growing awareness of dementia, especially of the prevalence of early-onset forms, which in turn may speed up what is still often a circuitous and drawn-out process of (mis)diagnosis. Narratives that place persons with dementia centre stage, focusing on their intimate experiences of the disease as well as their continuing selfhood, may act as a reminder to take the person with dementia seriously—to meet her with respect and include her in clinical and social encounters. However, such an effect cannot be predicted for an engagement with any given dementia narrative, nor can it be measured quantitatively. As reader-response criticism highlights, narrative texts offer particular opportunities of engagement for the reader, but each individual 'flesh-and-blood' reader will nonetheless respond differently to these opportunities, based on his or her psychological make-up, social characteristics, and place in time.

In line, also, with first-wave medical humanities concerns, my discussion of illness narratives represents, to a certain extent, a criticism of the neurological approach to dementia and of current medical and care practices. And yet, the intent of this study has not been primarily to write against biomedicine, but to explore avenues of understanding dementia which complement forms of biomedical practice that have, as yet, little to offer to people with dementia and their care partners. While the notion of criticising biomedicine prevails in mainstream medical humanities, my study also activates the notion of the critical and of 'critique' in other ways. I purport a critical need to (1) reassess the current masterplot of dementia and the way master narrative and counter-narratives are entangled; (2) to recognise selfhood in people with dementia in its many instantiations (embodied, relational, and narrative); and (3) to explore the limits and possibilities of the implications of these views of selfhood for people with dementia. In addition, if a central element of critical medical humanities has been the turn away from the 'primal scene' of doctor-patient encounters to 'new scenes and sites' (Whitehead and Woods 2016: 2), I have extended the scope of medical humanities, by turning to literary narratives and the public spheres of care—an area that has become increasingly professionalised, but remains enmeshed with private life.

Taking my lead from Keen (2007), I have moreover questioned the notion that empathy leads to pro-social action as well as the notion that literature is necessarily a good in itself, or acts for 'the good' when harnessed to a medical humanities agenda. Among other problems, empathy expended on fictional characters may divert our attention from the needs of real-life others (Keen 2007). Indeed, while narrative empathy has been heralded as a means to extend the moral circle, Keen suggests that empathy might equally lead to the incitement of hatred. For example, the empathy aroused for a character with whom the reader identifies, and who has been harmed by a character who is perceived not to belong to the reader's 'in-group,' may incite that reader to a hateful attitude vis-à-vis the target group in question. Given these and other problems, I proposed to shift the focus beyond empathy to other ways in which fictional texts may act in the field of the health humanities. I suggested how literature, and literary critics, may contribute to the thinking through of dementia care. At the same time, I stressed the need to investigate whether the arts and humanities are necessarily 'supportive' of a humanist agenda or 'benign' in the first place (Whitehead and Woods 2016: 2). Instead, I suggested that fictional and non-fictional narratives shape the way we live in a manner that may at times also be detrimental to individuals or groups within society. Narrativist approaches to medical humanities need to be developed and refined by using the tools of narrative studies and by paying attention to the ways different storytelling environments shape how we come to see and understand things—and ultimately act in the world.

Finally, my work also activates a crucial meaning of the word 'critical' as it pertains to the notion of urgency or 'critical mass' (Whitehead and Woods 2016: 14). Given current demographic and political developments, we urgently need to address the ways we, as society, want to lead and end our lives. Dementia care, in the community and in institutions, represents a topic currently under-represented in medical humanities research, perhaps because nursing constitutes a separate field. I would venture to maintain that this established discipline could benefit from some of the critical (re) thinking that animates the medical humanities, and in this study I have outlined some practical ways in which my own literary strand of medical humanities research might contribute to the development of dementia care.

Work in the field of literary approaches to dementia is just beginning. The continuing boom of dementia narratives opens up ever new sites of inquiry that raise questions of the sort addressed in this book—questions that might be approached through the approach (or approaches) that I have sketched here. Nor does this study represent an exhaustive account of already extant dementia narratives, some of which might suggest both different questions and different preliminary answers to those proposed in my account. One important area to explore, for instance, is how children's literature[1] and young adult fiction represent the experience of dementia. Given the pedagogical intent of these narratives, what ways of seeing and relating to people with dementia do the narratives suggest to their child or teenaged readers? And what particular affordances and constraints do children's picture books on dementia share, for instance, with (adult) graphic narratives? What is more, I acknowledge that many of the questions raised in this book may also be broached through creative forms of expression other than narrative. The exploration of other artistic and literary engagements with and representations of dementia merits closer attention in its own right.

Thus, dementia poetry, written by affected family members, professional carers, and by people with dementia,[2] still needs to be explored in detail. A number of relevant questions arise in this context: how do collaborative poetry projects, such as John Killick's (Killick 1997, 2008, 2010; Killick and Cordonnier 2000), differ from collaborative life writing projects, as discussed in this study? Compared with life writing, does poetry open up other, less linear, more metaphoric means of representing the phenomenology of dementia (see also Aadlandsvik 2008) or co-constructing selfhood? What are the ethical implications of refashioning the words of vulnerable subjects into poetry? And does the figurative and often enigmatic language and structure of poetry enhance or deter the reader's engagement with the subjectivity of people with dementia? Also, what potential is there for poetry interventions in dementia care (Petrescu, MacFarlane, and Ranzijn 2014, Swinnen 2016) as compared, for instance, with storytelling interventions (Basting 2001, 2003b) or interventions that draw on the visual arts (see, among others Huebner 2011), or indeed music and dance? In short, there is a need to explore more thoroughly how aesthetic experience and creative practice may actively enhance the well-being of people with dementia and their caregivers (Basting 2009).

Drama and opera—narrative genres not explored in this book—raise new aesthetic questions due to their multimodal and performative aspects. The possibility of autobiographical performance or verbatim theatre involving people with dementia in particular, such as in the production *To Whom I May Concern*, represents an as yet under-explored area of practice and research (see Basting 2009, Gibson 2018). Moreover, the performance arts may open up the possibility of more interdisciplinary and participatory research methods. For instance, the performance of dementia plays could be paired with pre- and post-performance questionnaires, post-performance discussions, lectures, or any number of public engagement activities. People with dementia might be asked to respond to artistic representations of dementia, or might, as in the case of verbatim theatre, even participate in their design and production.

Integrating social science research methods with a literary approach to dementia studies could yield more diverse and empirically sound results on the interaction, for instance, between aesthetic experience and ethical reflection. At the same time, finding ways to quantify health humanities research will help translate insights from this research in such a way that it might be adopted in mainstream health-care settings. An approach that integrates participatory and empirical research methods could also be developed vis-à-vis reading groups with people with dementia and their care partners, and by taking one's cue from the participants in these groups, literary dementia scholars might unearth altogether new research questions in relation to dementia generally, and dementia narratives in particular. The problem remains that even if literary medical humanities scholars find ways to collaborate with the social and medical sciences and to make their research more quantifiable, such research will always be gauged with regard to how time and cost-effective any implementations it suggests are. Finally, while

I welcome a move towards interdisciplinary, participatory, and empirical modes of exploring dementia and dementia narratives, I must equally assert that attempts to turn qualitative into quantitative research will always risk short-changing the value or particular contribution of such research in the first place.

If new research methods present one area to be explored, so do ever-new forms of storytelling. New media are opening up new spaces for dementia narratives to be told. While blogs only found their way into this study once they were published in book form, dementia blogs, by people with dementia and by family care partners, present powerful tools of advocacy. Blogs function both as 'memory device' for the writer and as a forum to create a global community. Further research needs to address how dementia blogs shape the cultural and political discourse about dementia. The use of blogs, twitter, and other social media also allows for forms of narrative self-presentation that offer particular affordances for people with dementia. In their day-to-day immediateness, lack of narrative arc, and by offering opportunities for short interactions and the sharing of small stories, they allow people with dementia to continue to share their experiences in writing, beyond a stage where the writing of a journal article or memoir might be possible.

Another new medium and format for telling dementia stories that to my knowledge has not yet received any critical attention are 'dementia diaries.'[3] These are audio diaries by people with dementia about their everyday experiences. Like Cary Henderson, who used of a tape recorder to put together his Alzheimer's journal, some people may find it less challenging to record themselves than to put down their experience in writing. Also the website offers a forum that can be more easily accessed than the publishing market. This format may then extend the opportunities for self-representation and autobiographical storytelling, as well as allowing listeners insight into the everyday challenges of living with dementia. At the same time, audio diaries raise new questions with regard to their form and content as well as their ethical and political dimension. With ever-emerging forms of dementia life writing and the current boom in cultural representations of dementia, much research remains to be done in literary dementia studies.

In this book, I hope to have outlined a framework for a narrativist approach to issues in the health humanities which apart from being applied to current and future dementia narratives might be adapted to other contexts and contents. Questions of identity and the problems of care arise in connection with any serious illness. I suggest that these issues might be approached through a literary medical humanities methodology that draws on the tools and insight of contemporary narrative studies. Simultaneously, critical literary medical humanities delineate not only the potential but also the limitations of narrative in the context of an ethically driven health humanities agenda. Narratives are neither the be-all and end-all of identity construction, or the creation of empathic relations, nor are they simply tools of evil, dehumanising, neo-liberal agendas. However, dementia narratives are entangled with wider cultural narratives about empathy, identity, and care—how we come to care, who we care for, and why we care. As such, they have much to tell us about what it means to be human, that is, interdependent beings who live in relationships of care.

Notes

1 For a first exploration of children's literature and dementia see Chapter 5 in Falcus and Sako (2019).
2 See, among others, the blog http://alzpoetry.blogspot.co.uk/.
3 See the project website https://dementiadiaries.org/.

Bibliography

Aadlandsvik, Ragna. 2008. 'The Second Sight: Learning About and With Dementia by Means of Poetry.' *Dementia* 7 (3): 321–39.
Abbott, H. Porter. 2008. *The Cambridge Introduction to Narrative.* Cambridge: Cambridge University Press.
Akpınar, Burcu, Özlem Küçükgüçlü, and Görsev Yener. 2011. 'Effects of Gender on Burden among Caregivers of Alzheimer's Patients.' *Journal of Nursing Scholarship* 43: 248–54.
Alber, Jan. 2013. 'Unnatural Spaces and Narrative Worlds.' In *A Poetics of Unnatural Narrative*, edited by Jan Alber, Henrik Skov Nielsen, and Brian Richardson, 45–66. Columbus: Ohio State University Press.
———. 2014. 'Unnatural Narrative.' In *The Living Handbook of Narratology*, edited by Peter Hühn, John Pier, Wolf Schmid, and Jörg Schönert. Hamburg: Hamburg University Press. www.lhn.uni-hamburg.de/article/unnatural-narrative.
Albert, Trevor, and James Keach. 2014. *Glen Campbell: I'll Be Me.* United States: PCH Films.
Alterra, Aaron. 1999. *The Caregiver: A Life with Alzheimer's.* South Royalton: Steerforth Press.
Alzheimer's Disease International. 2009. *World Alzheimer Report 2009.* Alzheimer's Disease International.
———. 2010. *World Alzheimer Report 2010: The Global Economic Impact of Dementia.* Alzheimer's Disease International.
Appignanesi, Lisa. 1999. *Losing the Dead.* London: Chatto & Windus.
Aquilina, Carmelo, and Julian C. Hughes. 2006. 'The Return of the Living Dead: Agency Lost and Found?' In *Dementia: Mind, Meaning and the Person*, edited by Julian C. Hughes, Stephen J. Louw, and Steven R. Sabat, 143–61. Oxford: Oxford University Press.
Ariyoshi, Sawako. 1984. *The Twilight Years.* [*Kōkotsu no hito.*] Translated by Mildred Tahara. London: Peter Owen. Original edition, 1972.
Asai, Atsushi, Yuka Sato, and Miki Fukuyama. 2009. 'An Ethical and Social Examination of Dementia as Depicted in Japanese Film.' *Medical Humanities* 35 (1): 39–42.
Avrahami, Einat. 2007. *The Invading Body: Reading Illness Autobiographies.* Charlottesville: University of Virginia Press.
Ballenger, Jesse F. 2006. *Self, Senility, and Alzheimer's Disease in Modern America: A History.* Baltimore: Johns Hopkins University Press.
Bamberg, Michael. 1997. 'Positioning between Structure and Performance.' *Journal of Narrative and Life History* 7: 335–42.

———. 2004. 'Considering Counter Narratives.' In *Considering Counter-Narratives: Narrating, Resisting, Making Sense*, edited by Michael Bamberg and Molly Andrews, 351–71. Amsterdam: John Benjamins.

Bamberg, Michael, and Molly Andrews, eds. 2004. *Considering Counter-Narratives: Narrating, Resisting, Making Sense*. Amsterdam: John Benjamins.

Barba, Andrés. 2004. *Ahora Tocad Música de Baile*. Barcelona: Editorial Anagrama.

Basting, Anne Davis. 2001. '"God is a Talking Horse": Dementia and the Performance of Self.' *The Drama Review* 45 (3): 78–94.

———. 2003a. 'Looking Back from Loss: Views of the Self in Alzheimer's Disease.' *Journal of Aging Studies* 17: 87–99.

———. 2003b. 'Reading the Story behind the Story: Context and Content in Stories by People with Dementia.' *Generations* 3: 25–9.

———. 2009. *Forget Memory: Creating Better Lives for People With Dementia*. Baltimore: The Johns Hopkins University Press.

Basting, Anne Davis, and John Killick. 2003. *The Arts and Dementia Care: A Resource Guide*. New York: The National Center for Creative Aging.

Battersby, James L. 2006. 'Narrativity, Self, and Self-Representation.' *Narrative* 14 (1): 27–44.

Bayley, John. 1999. *Elegy for Iris*. New York: Picador.

Behuniak, Susan M. 2011. 'The Living Dead? The Construction of People with Alzheimer's Disease as Zombies.' *Ageing and Society* 31 (1): 70–92.

Bell, Chris. 2010. 'Is Disability Studies Actually White Disability Studies?' In *The Disability Studies Reader*, edited by Lennard J. Davis, 374–82. New York: Routledge.

Berliner, Alan. 2012. *First Cousin Once Removed*. United States: HBO.

Bernaerts, Lars. 2014. 'Minds at Play: Narrative Games and Fictional Minds in B.S. Johnson's *House Mother Normal*.' *Style* 48 (3): 294–312.

Bernlef, J. 1988. *Out of Mind*. Translated by Adrienne Dixon. London: Faber and Faber. Original edition, *Hersenshimmen* 1984.

Bitenc, Rebecca A. 2012. 'Representations of Dementia in Narrative Fiction.' In *Knowledge and Pain*, edited by Esther Cohen, Leona Toker, Manuela Consonni, and Otniel E. Dror, 305–29. Amsterdam: Rodopi.

———. 2018. '"No Narrative, No Self"? Reconsidering Dementia Counter-Narratives in *Tell Mrs Mill Her Husband Is Still Dead*.' *Subjectivity* 11: 128–43.

Block, Stefan Merrill. 2008. *The Story of Forgetting*. London: Faber and Faber.

Bolaki, Stella. 2016. *Illness as Many Narratives: Arts, Medicine and Culture*. Edinburgh: Edinburgh University Press.

Booth, Wayne C. 1988. *The Company We Keep: An Ethics of Fiction*. Berkeley: University of California Press.

Brecht, Bertold. 1964. 'Alienation Effects in Chinese Acting.' In *Brecht on Theatre: The Development of an Aesthetic*, edited by John Willett, 91–9. New York: Hill and Wang.

Brockmeier, Jens. 2015. *Beyond the Archive: Memory, Narrative, and the Autobiographical Process*. Oxford: Oxford University Press.

Brody, Elaine M., Morton H. Kleban, M. Powell Lawton, and Herbert A. Silverman. 1971. 'Excess Disabilities of Mentally Impaired Aged: Impact of Individualized Treatment.' *The Gerontologist* 11 (2): 124–33.

Brody, Howard. 2011. 'Defining the Medical Humanities: Three Conceptions and Three Narratives.' *Journal of Medical Humanities* 32: 1–7.

Bruner, Jerome. 1991. 'The Narrative Construction of Reality.' *Critical Inquiry* 18: 1–21.

———. 2003. *Making Stories: Law, Literature, Life*. Cambridge, MA: Harvard University Press.

———. 2004. 'Life as Narrative.' *Social Research* 71 (3): 691–710.

Bryden, Christine [formerly Boden]. 1998. *Who Will I Be When I Die?* East Melbourne: Harper Collins Religious.

———. 2005. *Dancing with Dementia: My Story of Living Positively with Dementia*. London: Jessica Kingsley.

———. 2015. *Nothing about Us without Us! 20 Years of Dementia Advocacy*. London: Jessica Kingsley.

———. 2018. *Will I Still Be Me? Finding a Continuing Sense of Self in the Lived Experience of Dementia*. London: Jessica Kingsley.

Buber, Martin. 1958. *I and Thou*. Translated by Ronald Gregor Smith. Second edition. Edinburgh: T&T Clark. Original edition, 1923.

Burke, Lucy. 2007a. Alzheimer's Disease: Personhood and First Person Testimony. In *CDSRN Cultural Disability Studies Research Network*. www.cdsrn.org.uk/ICP.html.

———. 2007b. 'The Poetry of Dementia: Art, Ethics, and Alzheimer's Disease in Tony Harrison's *Black Daisies for the Bride*.' *Journal of Literary Disability* 1 (1): 61–73.

———. 2008. '"The Country of My Disease": Genes and Genealogy in Alzheimer's Life-writing.' *Journal of Disability* 2 (1): 63–74.

———. 2014. 'Oneself as Another: Intersubjectivity and Ethics in Alzheimer's Illness Narratives.' *Narrative Works* 4: 28–47.

———. 2015. 'The Locus of Our Dis-ease: Narratives of Family Life in the Age of Alzheimer's.' In *Popularizing Dementia: Public Expressions and Representations of Forgetfulness*, edited by Aagje Swinnen and Mark Schweda, 23–41. Bielefeld: Transcript Verlag.

———. 2016. 'On (not) Caring: Tracing the Meanings of Care in the Imaginative Literature of the "Alzheimer's Epidemic."' In *The Edinburgh Companion to the Critical Medical Humanities*, edited by Anne Whitehead and Angela Woods, 596–610. Edinburgh: Edinburgh University Press.

———. 2017. 'Imagining a Future without Dementia: Fictions of Regeneration and the Crises of Work and Sustainability.' *Palgrave Communications* 3 (52): 2–9.

———. 2018. 'Missing Pieces: Trauma, Dementia, and the Ethics of Reading in *Elizabeth Is Missing*.' In *Dementia and Literature: Interdisciplinary Perspectives*, edited by Tess Maginess, 88–102. New York: Routledge.

Capstick, Andrea, John Chatwin, and Katherine Ludwin. 2015. 'Challenging Representations of Dementia in Contemporary Western Fiction Film: From Epistemic Injustice to Social Participation.' In *Popularizing Dementia: Public Expressions and Representations of Forgetfulness*, edited by Aagje Swinnen and Mark Schweda, 229–52. Bielefeld: Transcript Verlag.

Carel, Havi. 2008. *Illness: The Cry of the Flesh*. Stocksfield: Acumen.

Cassavetes, Nick. 2004. *The Notebook*. United States: New Line Cinema.

Cavanagh, Paul. 2015. *Missing Steps*. London, Ontario: Not That London.

Chappell, Neena L., Carren Dujela, and André Smith. 2015. 'Caregiver Well-Being: Intersections of Relationship and Gender.' *Research on Aging* 37 (6): 623–45.

Charon, Rita. 2006. *Narrative Medicine*. Oxford: Oxford University Press.

Charon, Rita, and Martha Montello. 2002. *Stories Matter: The Role of Narrative in Medical Ethics*. New York: Routledge.

Chast, Roz. 2014. *Can't We Talk About Something More Pleasant? A Memoir*. New York: Bloomsbury.
Chiche, Bruno. 2010. *Small World*. France and Germany: Majestic Filmverleih.
Chute, Hilary. 2007. 'Book review of *Our Cancer Year, Janet and Me: An Illustrated Story of Love and Loss, Cancer Vixen: A True Story, Mom's Cancer, Blue Pills: A Positive Love Story, Epileptic*, and *Black Hole*.' *Literature and Medicine* 26 (2): 413–29.
Clark, Andy, and David Chalmers. 1998. 'The Extended Mind.' *Analysis* 58 (1): 7–19.
Clegg, David. 2010. *Tell Mrs Mill Her Husband Is Still Dead*. No place: The Trebus Project.
Cohen, David, and Carl Eisdorfer. 1986. *The Loss of Self: A Family Resource for the Care of Alzheimer's Disease and Related Disorders*. New York: W.W. Norton.
Cohen, Lawrence. 1998. *No Ageing in India: Alzheimer's, The Bad Family, and Other Modern Things*. Berkeley: University of California Press.
Cohn, Dorrit. 1978. *Transparent Minds: Narrative Modes for Presenting Consciousness in Fiction*. Princeton: Princeton University Press.
Coleman, Rowan. 2014. *The Memory Book*. London: Ebury Press.
Conway, Kathlyn. 2007. *Beyond Words: Illness and the Limits of Expression*. Albuquerque: University of New Mexico Press.
Cooney, Eleanor. 2003. *Death in Slow Motion: A Memoir of a Daughter, Her Mother, and the Beast Called Alzheimer's*. New York: Harper Perennial.
Couser, G. Thomas. 1991. 'Autopathography: Women, Illness, and Lifewriting.' *a/b: Auto/Biography Studies* 6 (1): 65–75.
———. 1997. *Recovering Bodies: Illness, Disability, and Life Writing*. Madison: The University of Wisconsin Press.
———. 2004. *Vulnerable Subjects: Ethics and Life Writing*. Ithaca: Cornell University Press.
———. 2005. "Paradigms' Cost: Representing Vulnerable Subjects.' *Literature and Medicine* 24 (1): 19–30.
———. 2009. 'Memoir and (Lack of) Memory: Filial Narratives of Paternal Dementia.' In *New Essays on Life Writing and the Body*, edited by Christopher Stuart and Stephanie Todd, 223–40. Newcastle upon Tyne: Cambridge Scholars.
———. 2012. *Memoir: An Introduction*. Oxford: Oxford University Press.
Couturier, Claude. 2004. *Puzzle. Journal d'une Alzheimer*. Paris: Josette Lyon.
Crawford, Paul, Brian Brown, Victoria Tischler, and Charley Baker. 2010. 'Health Humanities: The Future of Medical Humanities?' *Mental Health Review* 15 (3): 4–10.
Crisp, Jane. 1995. 'Making Sense of the Stories that People with Alzheimer's Tell: A Journey with My Mother.' *Journal of Narrative and Life History* 2 (3): 133–40.
Damasio, Antonio R. 1994. *Descartes' Error*. London: Vintage.
———. 2000. *The Feeling of What Happens: Body and Emotion in the Making of Consciousness*. London: W. Heinemann.
———. 2010. *Self Comes to Mind: Constructing the Conscious Brain*. New York: Pantheon Books.
Davis, Daniel H. J. 2004. 'Dementia: Sociological and Philosophical Constructions.' *Social Science & Medicine* 58 (2): 369–78.
Davis, John K. 2009. 'Precedent Autonomy, Advance Directives, and End-of-Life Care.' In *The Oxford Handbook of Bioethics*, edited by Bonnie Steinbock. Oxford: Oxford University Press. DOI: 10.1093/oxfordhb/9780199562411.003.0016.

Davis, Robert. 1989. *My Journey into Alzheimer's Disease: Helpful Insights for Family and Friends*. Carol Stream, IL: Tyndale House Publishers.
Dawson, Paul. 2013. *The Return of the Omniscient Narrator: Authorship and Authority in Twenty-First Century Fiction*. Columbus: Ohio State University Press.
DeBaggio, Thomas. 2002. *Losing My Mind: An Intimate Look at Life with Alzheimer's*. New York: The Free Press.
———. 2003. *When It Gets Dark: An Enlightened Reflection on Life with Alzheimer's*. New York: Free Press.
Demetris, Alex. 2016. *Dad's Not All There Any More*. London: Singing Dragon.
Dennett, Daniel Clement. 1993. *Consciousness Explained*. London: Penguin Books.
Dickens, Charles. 1854. *Hard Times*. London: Thomas Nelson and Sons.
Donohue, Mike. 2009. *From AA to AD, a Wistful Travelogue*. Seattle: CreateSpace.
Downham, Jenny. 2015. *Unbecoming*. Oxford: David Fickling Books.
Downs, Murna. 2000. 'A World without Dementia? What Do We Need To Do?' *Dementia in Scotland: Newsletter of Alzheimer's Scotland - Action on Dementia*, March 6.
Dresser, Rebecca. 1995. 'Dworkin on Dementia: Elegant Theory, Questionable Policy.' *The Hastings Center Report* 25 (6): 32–8.
Dworkin, Ronald. 1993. *Life's Dominion: An Argument about Abortion, Euthanasia, and Individual Freedom*. New York: Alfred A. Knopf.
Eagar, Lindsay. 2016. *Hour of the Bees*. Somerville, MA: Candlewick Press.
Eakin, Paul John. 1992. *Touching the World: Reference in Autobiography*. Princeton: Princeton University Press.
———. 1998. 'Relational Selves, Relational Lives: The Story of the Story.' In *True Relations: Essays on Autobiography and the Postmodern*, edited by G. Thomas Couser and Joseph Fichtelberg, 63–82. Westport: Greenwood.
———. 1999. *How Our Lives Become Stories: Making Selves*. Ithaca: Cornell University Press.
———. 2001. 'Breaking Rules: The Consequences of Self-Narration.' *Biography* 24: 113–27.
———. 2006. 'Narrative Identity and Narrative Imperialism: A Response to Galen Strawson and James Phelan.' *Narrative* 14 (2): 180–7.
———. 2008. *Living Autobiographically: How We Create Identity in Narrative*. Ithaca: Cornell University Press.
Eastham, Ruth. 2011. *The Memory Cage*. Sheffield: Shrine Bell.
Eisner, Will. 2008. *Comics and Sequential Art: Principles and Practices from the Legendary Cartoonist*. New York: W. W. Norton.
Erll, Astrid. 2008. 'Naïve, Repetitive, or Cultural: Options of an Ethical Narratology.' *Amsterdam International Electronic Journal for Cultural Narratology* 5.
Ernaux, Annie. 1987. *Une Femme*. Paris: Gallimard.
———. 1999. *I Remain in Darkness*. Translated by Tanya Leslie. New York: Seven Stories Press. Original edition, 1997.
Evans, Fiona. 2012. *Geordie Sinatra*. Newcastle upon Tyne: New Writing North.
Eyre, Richard. 2001. *Iris*. United Kingdom and United States: Miramax Films.
Falcus, Sarah, and Katsura Sako. 2019. *Contemporary Narratives of Dementia: Ethics, Ageing, Politics*. New York: Routledge.
Farmer, Joyce. 2010. *Special Exits: A Graphic Memoir*. Seattle: Fantagraphics.
Faulkner, William. 1929. *The Sound and the Fury*. New York: Jonathan Cape and Harrison Smith.

Feil, Naomi. 1989. 'Validation: An Empathetic Approach to the Care of Dementia.' *Clinical Gerontologist* 8 (3): 89–94.
———. 1992. 'Validation Therapy.' *Geriatric Nursing* 13 (3): 129–33.
Feil, Naomi, and Rita Altman. 2004. 'Validation Theory and the Myth of the Therapeutic Lie.' *American Journal of Alzheimer's Disease and Other Dementias* 19 (2): 77–8.
Felski, Rita. 2008. *Uses of Literature*. Oxford: Blackwell.
Fernyhough, Charles. 2012. *Pieces of Light: The New Science of Memory*. London: Profile.
Fludernik, Monika. 1993. *The Fictions of Language and the Languages of Fiction: The Linguistic Representation of Speech and Consciousness*. London: Routledge.
———. 1996. *Towards a 'Natural' Narratology*. New York: Routledge.
Fontana, Andrea, and Ronald W. Smith. 1989. 'Alzheimer's Disease Victims: The "Unbecoming" of Self and the Normalization of Competence.' *Sociological Perspectives* 32 (1): 35–46.
Forster, Margaret. 1989. *Have the Men Had Enough?* London: Penguin Books.
Fox, Judith. 2009. *I Still Do: Loving and Living with Alzheimer's*. New York: Power House Books.
Fox, Patrick. 1989. 'From Senility to Alzheimer's Disease: The Rise of the Alzheimer's Disease Movement.' *Millbank Quarterly* 1: 58–102.
Francis, Leslie Pickering. 2001. 'Decisionmaking at the End of Life: Patients with Alzheimer's or Other Dementias.' *Georgia Law Review* 35 (2): 539–92.
Frank, Arthur W. 1995. *The Wounded Storyteller: Body, Illness, and Ethics*. Chicago: University of Chicago Press.
Franzen, Jonathan. 2001. *The Corrections*. New York: Picador.
———. 2002. 'My Father's Brain.' In *How to Be Alone*, authored and edited by Jonathan Franzen, 7–38. New York: Picador.
Freeman, Mark. 2007. 'Autobiographical Understanding and Narrative Inquiry.' In *Handbook of Narrative Inquiry: Mapping a Methodology*, edited by D. Jean Clandinin, 120–45. Thousand Oaks: Sage.
Fricker, Miranda. 2007. *Epistemic Injustice: Power and the Ethics of Knowing*. Oxford: Oxford University Press.
Friedman, Susan Stanford. 1988. 'Women's Autobiographical Selves: Theory and Practice.' In *The Private Self: Theory and Practice of Women's Autobiographical Writings*, edited by Shari Benstock, 34–62. Chapel Hill: University of North Carolina Press.
Gallagher, Shaun, and Dan Zahavi. 2008. *The Phenomenological Mind: An Introduction to Philosophy of Mind and Cognitive Science*. London: Routledge.
Garden, Rebecca Elizabeth. 2007. 'The Problem of Empathy: Medicine and the Humanities.' *New Literary History* 38 (3): 551–67.
Gardner, Jared. 2008. 'Autography's Biography, 1972–2007.' *Biography* 31 (1): 1–26.
Genette, Gérard. 1980. *Narrative Discourse: An Essay in Method*. Translated by Jane E. Lewin. Ithaca: Cornell University Press. Original edition, 1972.
Genova, Lisa. 2007. *Still Alice*. London: Simon and Schuster.
Gerrig, Richard J. 1993. *Experiencing Narrative Worlds*. New Haven: Yale University Press.
Gibson, Janet Louise. 2018. '"Talking Back, Talking Out, Talking Otherwise": Dementia, Access and Autobiographical Performance.' *Research in Drama Education: The Journal of Applied Theatre and Performance* 23 (3): 340–54.

Gillies, Andrea. 2010. *Keeper: A Book about Memory, Identity, Isolation, Wordsworth and Cake*. London: Short. Original edition, 2009.
Glatzer, Richard, and Wash Westmoreland. 2014. *Still Alice*. United States: Sony Pictures Classics.
Goffman, Erving. 1963. *Stigma: Notes on the Management of Spoiled Identity*. Englewood Cliffs: Prentice-Hall Inc.
———. 1981. *Forms of Talk*. Philadelphia: University of Pennsylvania Press.
Gordon, Mary. 2007. *Circling My Mother: A Memoir*. New York: Anchor Books.
Graboys, Thomas, and Peter Zheutlin. 2008. *Life in the Balance. A Physician's Memoir of Life, Love, and Loss with Parkinson's Disease and Dementia*. New York: Sterling Publishing.
Graham, Peter. 1997. 'Metapathography: Three Unruly Texts.' *Literature and Medicine* 16 (1): 70–87.
Grant, Linda. 1998. *Remind Me Who I Am, Again*. London: Granta Books.
Green, Melanie C. 2004. 'Transportation into Narrative Worlds: The Roles of Prior Knowledge and Perceived Realism.' *Discourse Processes* 38 (2): 247–66.
Green, Melanie C., and Timothy C. Brock. 2000. 'The Role of Transportation in the Persuasiveness of Public Narratives.' *Journal of Personality and Social Psychology* 79 (5): 701–21.
Green, Melanie C., Jennifer Garst, and Timothy C. Brock. 2004. 'The Power of Fiction: Determinants and Boundaries.' In *The Psychology of Entertainment Media: Blurring the Lines between Entertainment and Persuasion*, edited by L. J. Shrum, 161–76. Mahwah: Lawrence Erlbaum Associates Publishers.
Greenhalgh, Trisha, and Brian Hurwitz. 1999. 'Why Study Narrative?' *BMJ* 318: 48–50.
Gubrium, Jaber F. 1986. *Oldtimers and Alzheimer's: The Descriptive Organization of Senility*. Greenwich: JAI Press.
Guillory, John. 2000. 'The Ethical Practice of Modernity: The Example of Reading.' In *The Turn to Ethics*, edited by Marjorie Garber, Beatrice Hanssen, and Rebecca L. Walkowitz, 29–46. New York: Routledge.
Gusdorf, Georges. 1980. 'Conditions and Limits of Autobiography.' In *Autobiography: Essays Theoretical and Critical*, edited by James Olney, 28–48. Princeton: Princeton University Press. Original edition, 1956.
Hacking, Ian. 1999a. *Mad Travellers: Reflections on the Reality of Transient Mental Illnesses*. London: Free Association Books.
———. 1999b. *The Social Construction of What?* Cambridge, MA: Harvard University Press.
Hadas, Rachel. 2011. *Strange Relation: A Memoir of Marriage, Dementia, and Poetry*. Philadelphia: Paul Dry Books.
Hakemulder, Jèmeljan. 2000. *The Moral Laboratory: Experiments Examining the Effects of Reading Literature on Social Perception and Moral Self-Concept*. Amsterdam: John Benjamins.
Harrison, Tony. 1993. *Black Daisies for the Bride*. London: Faber and Faber.
Hartung, Heike. 2016. *Ageing, Gender and Illness in Anglophone Literature: Narrating Age in the Bildungsroman*. New York: Routledge.
Haugse, John. 1998. *Heavy Snow: My Father's Disappearance into Alzheimer's*. Deerfield Beach: Health Communications.
Hawkins, Anne Hunsaker. 1993. *Reconstructing Illness: Studies in Pathography*. West Lafayette: Purdue University Press.

Hayes, Jeanne, Craig Boylstein, and Mary K. Zimmerman. 2009. 'Living and Loving with Dementia: Negotiating Spousal and Caregiver Identity Through Narrative.' *Journal of Aging Studies* 23: 48–59.

Healey, Emma. 2014. *Elizabeth is Missing*. St Ives: Penguin Books.

Heidegger, Martin. 1962. *Being and Time*. Translated by John Macquarrie and Edward Robinson. Oxford: Blackwell.

Henderson, Cary. 1998. *Partial View: An Alzheimer's Journal*. Dallas: Southern Methodist University Press.

Henry, Peaches. 2006. 'A Revised Approach to Relationality in Women's Autobiography: The Case of Eliza Linton's *The Autobiography of Christopher Kirkland*.' *a/b: Auto/Biography Studies* 20 (1): 18–37.

Herman, David. 2011. *The Emergence of Mind: Representations of Consciousness in Narrative Discourse in English*. Lincoln: University of Nebraska Press.

———. 2013. *Storytelling and the Sciences of Mind*. Cambridge, MA: The MIT Press.

Herman, Luc, and Bart Vervaeck. 2005. *Handbook of Narrative Analysis*. Lincoln: University of Nebraska Press.

Herskovits, Elizabeth. 1995. 'Struggling over Subjectivity: Debates About the "Self" and Alzheimer's Disease.' *Medical Anthropology Quarterly* 9 (2): 146–64.

Hertogh, Cees M. P. M., Marike E. de Boer, Rose-Marie Dröes, and Jan A. Eefstinga. 2007. 'Would We Rather Lose Our Life Than Lose Our Self? Lessons from the Dutch Debate on Euthanasia for Patients with Dementia.' *The American Journal of Bioethics* 7 (4): 48–56.

Hester, Rebecca. 2016. 'Culture in Medicine: An Argument against Competence.' In *The Edinburgh Companion to the Critical Medical Humanities*, edited by Anne Whitehead and Angela Woods, 463–80. Edinburgh: Edinburgh University Press.

Heywood, Bernard. 1994. *Caring for Maria: An Experience of Coping Successfully with Alzheimer's Disease*. Shaftesbury: Element.

Hoffmann, Deborah. 1994. *Complaints of a Dutiful Daughter*. United States: No distributor.

Holstein, Martha. 1997. 'Alzheimer's Disease and Senile Dementia, 1885–1920: An Interpretive History of Disease Negotiation.' *Journal of Aging Studies* 11 (1): 1–13.

———. 2000. 'Aging, Culture, and the Framing of Alzheimer's Disease.' In *Concepts of Alzheimer Disease: Biological, Clinical, and Cultural Perspectives*, edited by Peter J. Whitehouse, Konrad Maurer, and Jesse F. Ballenger, 158–80. Baltimore: John Hopkins University Press.

Huebner, Berna G. 2011. *I Remember Better When I Paint – Art and Alzheimer's: Opening Doors, Making Connections*. Glen Echo: Bethesda Communications Group and New Publishing Partners.

Hughes, Julian C. 2011. *Thinking through Dementia*. Oxford: Oxford University Press.

Hughes, Julian C., Stephen J. Louw, and Steven R. Sabat, eds. 2006. *Dementia: Mind, Meaning, and the Person*. Oxford: Oxford University Press.

Husband, Tony. 2014. *Take Care Son: The Story of My Dad and His Dementia*. London: Robinson.

Hussein, Faten. 2018. 'Representations of Dementia in Arabic Literature.' In *Dementia and Literature: Interdisciplinary Perspectives*, edited by Tess Maginess, 71–87. New York: Routledge.

Hutto, Daniel D. 2007a. *Folk Psychological Narratives: The Sociocultural Basis of Understanding Reasons*. Cambridge, MA: MIT Press.

———. 2007b. 'The Narrative Practice Hypothesis: Origins and Applications of Folk Psychology.' In *Narrative and Understanding Persons*, edited by Daniel D. Hutto, 43–68. Cambridge: Cambridge University Press.

Hydén, Lars-Christer. 2010. 'Identity, Self, Narrative.' In *Beyond Narrative Coherence*, edited by Matti Hyvärinen, Lars-Christer Hydén, Marja Saarenheimo, and Maria Tamboukou, 33–48. Amsterdam: John Benjamins.

———. 2011. 'Narrative Collaboration and Scaffolding in Dementia.' *Journal of Aging Studies* 25: 339–47.

———. 2018. *Entangled Narratives: Collaborative Storytelling and the Re-Imagining of Dementia*. Oxford: Oxford University Press.

Hydén, Lars-Christer, and Jens Brockmeier, eds. 2008. *Health, Illness and Culture: Broken Narratives*. New York: Routledge.

Hydén, Lars-Christer, and Linda Örulv. 2009. 'Narrative and Identity in Alzheimer's Disease: A Case Study.' *Journal of Aging Studies* 23 (4): 205–14.

Hyvärinen, Matti, Lars-Christer Hydén, Marja Saarenheimo, and Maria Tamboukou, eds. 2010. *Beyond Narrative Coherence*. Amsterdam: John Benjamins.

Iacoboni, Marco. 2008. *Mirroring People: The New Science of How We Connect with Others*. New York: Farrar, Straus and Giroux.

Ignatieff, Michael. 1993. *Scar Tissue*. London: Vintage.

———. 1994. 'All in the Mind.' *BBC Radio* 4.

Innes, Anthea. 2009. *Dementia Studies: A Social Science Perspective*. Los Angeles: Sage.

Irvine, Craig, and Rita Charon. 2017. 'Deliver Us from Certainty: Training for Narrative Ethics.' In *The Principles and Practice of Narrative Medicine*, edited by Rita Charon et al., 110–29. Oxford: Oxford University Press.

Ishiguro, Kazuo. 1995. *The Unconsoled*. London: Faber and Faber.

Iversen, Stefan. 2013. 'Unnatural Minds.' In *A Poetics of Unnatural Narrative*, edited by Jan Aber, Henrik Skov Nielsen, and Brian Richardson, 94–112. Columbus: Ohio State University Press.

Jens, Tilman. 2009. *Demenz: Abschied von meinem Vater*. Gütersloh: Gütersloher Verlagshaus.

Johnson, B.S. 2013. *House Mother Normal*. Basingstoke: Picador. Original edition, 1971.

Johnstone, Megan-Jane. 2011. 'Metaphors, Stigma and the 'Alzheimerization' of the Euthanasia Debate.' *Dementia* 12 (4): 377–93.

———. 2013. *Alzheimer's Disease, Media Representation, and the Politics of Euthanasia: Constructing Risk and Selling Death in an Ageing Society*. London: Routledge.

Jones, Rebecca. 2004. '"That's Very Rude, I Shouldn't Be Telling You That": Older Women Talking about Sex.' In *Considering Counter-Narratives: Narrating, Resisting, Making Sense*, edited by Michael Bamberg and Molly Andrews, 169–89. Amsterdam: John Benjamins.

Jones, Therese. 2014. '"Oh, the Humanit(ies)!" Dissent, Democracy, and Danger.' In *Medicine, Health and the Arts: Approaches to the Medical Humanities*, edited by Victoria Bates, Alan Bleakley, and Sam Goodman, 27–38. New York: Routledge.

Kaufman, Sharon R. 2006. 'Dementia-Near-Death and "Life Itself."' In *Thinking about Dementia: Culture, Loss, and the Anthropology of Senility*, edited by Annette Leibing and Lawrence Cohen, 23–42. New Brunswick: Rutgers University Press.

Keen, Suzanne. 2007. *Empathy and the Novel*. Oxford: Oxford University Press.

Killick, John. 1997. *You Are Words: Dementia Poems*. London: Hawker Publications.
———. 2008. *Dementia Diary: Poems and Prose*. London: Hawker Publications.
———, ed. 2010. *The Elephant in the Room: Poems by People with Memory Loss in Cambridgeshire*. Cambridge: Cambridgeshire County Council.
Killick, John, and Kate Allan. 2001. *Communication and the Care of People with Dementia*. Buckingham: Open University Press.
Killick, John, and Carl Cordonnier. 2000. *Openings: Dementia Poems and Photographs*. London: Hawker Publications.
Kittay, Eva Feder. 1999. *Love's Labor: Essays on Women, Equality and Dependency*. New York: Routledge.
Kitwood, Tom. 1990. 'The Dialectics of Dementia: With Particular Reference to Alzheimer's Disease.' *Ageing and Society* 10: 177–96.
———. 1997. *Dementia Reconsidered: The Person Comes First*. Philadelphia: Open University Press.
Kitwood, Tom, and Kathleen Bredin. 1992. 'Towards a Theory of Dementia Care: Personhood and Well-being.' *Ageing and Society* 12: 269–87.
Klein, Kitty. 2003. 'Narrative Construction, Cognitive Processing, and Health.' In *Narrative Theory and the Cognitive Sciences*, edited by David Herman, 56–84. Stanford: CSLI Publications.
Kleinman, Arthur. 1988. *The Illness Narratives: Suffering, Healing, and the Human Condition*. New York: Basic Books.
Kölbl, Carlos. 2004. 'Blame it on Psychology?' In *Considering Counter-Narratives: Narrating, Resisting, Making Sense*, edited by Michael Bamberg and Molly Andrews, 27–32. Amsterdam: John Benjamins.
Kokanović, Renata, and Jacinthe Flore. 2017. 'Subjectivity and Illness Narratives.' *Subjectivity* 10 (4): 329–39.
Konek, Carol Wolfe. 1991. *Daddyboy: A Family's Struggle with Alzheimer's*. Saint Paul: Graywolf Press.
Kontos, Pia C. 2003. '"The Painterly Hand": Embodied Consciousness and Alzheimer's Disease.' *Journal of Aging Studies* 17: 151–70.
———. 2004. 'Ethnographic Reflections on Selfhood, Embodiment and Alzheimer's Disease.' *Ageing and Society* 24 (6): 829–49.
———. 2005. 'Embodied Selfhood in Alzheimer's Disease.' *Dementia* 4 (4): 553–70.
Korthals Altes, Liesbeth. 2005. 'Ethical Turn.' In *Routledge Encyclopedia of Narrative Theory*, edited by David Herman, Manfred Jahn, and Marie-Laure Ryan, 142–6. New York: Routledge.
———. 2006. 'Some Dilemmas of an Ethics of Literature.' In *Theology and Literature: Rethinking Reader Responsibility*, edited by Gaye Williams Ortiz and Clara A.B. Joseph, 15–31. Basingstoke: Palgrave Macmillan.
———. 2013. 'Narratology, Ethical Turns, Circularities, and a Meta-Ethical Way Out.' In *Narrative Ethics*, edited by Jakob Lothe, Jeremy Hawthorn, and Leonidas Donskis, 25–40. Amsterdam: Rodopi.
———. 2014. *Ethos and Narrative Interpretation: The Negotiation of Values in Fiction*. Lincoln: University of Nebraska Press.
Krause, Allison M., Lynda D. Grant, and Bonita C. Long. 1999. 'Sources of Stress Reported by Daughters of Nursing Home Residents.' *Journal of Aging Studies* 13 (3): 349–64.
Krüger, Naomi. 2018. *May*. Bridgend: Seren Books.

Krüger-Fürhoff, Irmela Marei. 2015. 'Narrating the Limits of Narration: Alzheimer's Disease in Contemporary Literary Texts.' In *Popularizing Dementia: Public Expressions and Representations of Forgetfulness*, edited by Aagje Swinnen and Mark Schweda, 89–108. Bielefeld: Transcript Verlag.

LaCapra, Dominick. 2001. *Writing History, Writing Trauma*. Baltimore: Johns Hopkins University Press.

Lakoff, George, and Mark Johnson. 2003. *Metaphors We Live By*. Chicago: University of Chicago Press.

Lal, Ranjit. 2015. *Our Nana Was A Nutcase*. New Delhi: Red Turtle Rupa.

LaPlante, Alice. 2011. *Turn of Mind*. London: Harvill Secker.

Leavitt, Sarah. 2010. *Tangles: A Story About Alzheimer's, My Mother and Me*. London: Jonathan Cape.

Lee, Jeanne L. 2003. *Just Love Me: My Life Turned Upside-Down by Alzheimer's*. West Lafayette: Purdue University Press.

Leibing, Annette. 2002. 'Flexible Hips? On Alzheimer's Disease and Aging in Brasil.' *Journal of Cross-Cultural Gerontology* 17: 213–32.

Leibing, Annette, and Lawrence Cohen. 2006. *Thinking about Dementia: Culture, Loss, and the Anthropology of Senility*. New Brunswick: Rutgers University Press.

Lejeune, Philippe. 1988. *On Autobiography*. Minneapolis: University of Minnesota Press.

Lévinas, Emmanuel. 1961. *Totalité et Infini: Essai sur l'Extériorité*. The Hague: Martinus Nijhof.

———. 1979. *Le Temps et L'Autre*. Paris: Fata Morgana.

Levine, Judith. 2004. *Do You Remember Me? A Father, a Daughter, and a Search for the Self*. New York: Free Press.

Lloyd, Phyllida. 2011. *The Iron Lady*. United States: 20th Century Fox.

Lyman, Karen A. 1989. 'Bringing the Social Back in: A Critique of the Biomedicalization of Dementia.' *The Gerontologist* 29 (5): 597–605.

———. 1998. 'Living with Alzheimer's Disease: The Creation of Meaning Among Persons with Dementia.' *The Journal of Clinical Ethics* 9 (1): 49–57.

MacIntyre, Alasdair. 1981. *After Virtue*. Notre Dame: University of Notre Dame Press.

MacRae, Hazel. 2010. 'Managing Identity While Living with Alzheimer's Disease.' *Qualitative Health Research* 20 (3): 293–305.

Maginess, Tess. 2018. *Dementia and Literature: Interdisciplinary Perspectives*. New York: Routledge.

Magnusson, Sally. 2014. *Where Memories Go: Why Dementia Changes Everything*. London: Two Roads.

Margolin, Uri. 1999. 'Of What Is Past, Is Passing, or to Come: Temporality, Aspectuality, Modality, and the Nature of Literary Narrative.' In *Narratologies: New Perspectives on Narrative Analysis*, edited by David Herman, 142–66. Columbus: Ohio State University Press.

Marx, Marcia S., J. Cohen-Mansfield, Natalie G. Regier, Maha Dakheel-Ali, Ashok Srihari, and Khin Thein. 2010. 'The Impact of Different Dog-Related Stimuli on Engagement of Persons with Dementia.' *American Journal of Alzheimer's Disease and Other Dementias* 25 (1): 37–45.

Mason, Mary. 1980. 'The Other Voice: Autobiographies of Women Writers.' In *Autobiography: Essays Theoretical and Critical*, edited by James Olney, 207–35. Princeton: Princeton University Press.

Mattingly, Cheryl. 1998. *Healing Dramas and Clinical Plots: The Narrative Structure of Experience*. Cambridge: Cambridge University Press.
Maxwell, Glyn, and Elena Langer. 2010. *The Lion's Face*. London: Oberon Books.
McCloud, Scott. 1994. *Understanding Comics: The Invisible Art*. New York: Harper Perennial.
McGowin, Diane Friel. 1994. *Living in the Labyrinth: A Personal Journey through the Maze of Alzheimer's*. New York: Delta. Original edition, 1993.
McLean, Athena Helen. 2006. 'Coherence without Facticity in Dementia: The Case of Mrs. Fine.' In *Thinking about Dementia: Culture, Loss, and the Anthropology of Senility*, edited by Annette Leibing and Lawrence Cohen, 157–79. New Brunswick: Rutgers University Press.
Medina, Raquel. 2018. *Cinematic Representations of Alzheimer's Disease*. New York: Palgrave Macmillan.
Medved, Maria I., and Jens Brockmeier. 2010. 'Weird Stories: Brain, Mind and Self.' In *Beyond Narrative Coherence*, edited by Matti Hyvärinen, Lars-Christer Hydén, Marja Saarenheimo, and Maria Tamboukou, 17–32. Amsterdam: John Benjamins.
Meretoja, Hanna. 2018. *The Ethics of Storytelling: Narrative Hermeneutics, History, and the Possible*. Oxford: Oxford University Press.
Miller, Nancy K. 1994. 'Representing Others: Gender and the Subjects of Autobiography.' *Differences: A Journal of Feminist Cultural Studies* 6 (1): 1–27.
———. 1996. *Bequest and Betrayal: Memoirs of a Parent's Death*. New York: Oxford University Press.
Miller, Sue. 2003. *The Story of My Father*. London: Bloomsbury.
Millett, Stephan. 2011. 'Self and Embodiment: A Bio-Phenomenological Approach to Dementia.' *Dementia* 10 (4): 509–22.
Mitchell, David, and Sharon Snyder. 2001. *Narrative Prosthesis: Disability and the Dependencies of Discourse*. Ann Arbor: University of Michigan Press.
Mitchell, Wendy. 2018. *Somebody I Used to Know*. London: Bloomsbury.
Mobley, Tracy. 2007. *Young Hope. The Broken Road*. Denver: Outskirts Press.
Montgomery Hunter, Kathlyn. 1993. *Doctors' Stories: The Narrative Structure of Medical Knowledge*. Princeton: Princeton University Press.
Morgan, Abi. 2011. *27*. London: Oberon Books.
Morris, David B. 1998. *Illness and Culture in the Postmodern Age*. Berkeley: University of California Press.
———. 2002. 'Narrative, Ethics, and Pain: Thinking with Stories.' In *Stories Matter: The Role of Narrative in Medical Ethics*, edited by Rita Charon and Martha Montello, 196–218. New York: Routledge.
Mukadam, Rukiya. 2016. 'Time to Break the Taboo.' In *People with Dementia Speak Out*, edited by Lucy Whitman, 234–41. London: Jessica Kingsley.
Murphy, Tom. 2009. 'Bailegangaire.' In *The Methuen Drama Anthology of Irish Plays*, edited by Patrick Lonergan, 111–85. London: Methuen.
Nagel, Thomas. 1974. 'What Is It Like to Be a Bat?' *The Philosophical Review* 83 (4): 435–50.
Nayar, Pramod K. 2018. 'Dementia in Recent Indian Fiction in English.' In *Dementia and Literature: Interdisciplinary Perspectives*, edited by Tess Maginess, 148–59. New York: Routledge.
Nielsen, Henrik Skov. 2004. 'The Impersonal Voice in First-Person Narrative Fiction.' *Narrative* 12 (2): 133–50.
Noyes, Brigg B., Robert D. Hill, Bret L. Hicken, Marilyn Luptak, Randall Rupper, Nancy K. Dailey, and Byron D. Bair. 2010. 'Review: The Role of Grief in

Dementia Caregiving.' *American Journal of Alzheimer's Disease and Other Dementia* 25 (1): 9–17.
Nussbaum, Martha Craven. 1990. *Love's Knowledge: Essays on Philosophy and Literature.* Oxford: Oxford University Press.
———. 1995. *Poetic Justice: The Literary Imagination and Public Life.* Boston: Beacon Press.
———. 1997. *Cultivating Humanity: A Classical Defense of Reform in Liberal Education.* Cambridge, MA: Harvard University Press.
Ochs, Elinor, and Lisa Capps. 2001. *Living Narrative: Creating Lives in Everyday Storytelling.* Cambridge, MA: Harvard University Press.
Oksenberg Rorty, Amélie. 2000. 'Characters, Persons, Selves, Individuals.' In *Theory of the Novel: A Historical Approach*, edited by Michael McKeon, 537–53. Baltimore: Johns Hopkins University Press.
Örulv, Linda, and Lars-Christer Hydén. 2006. 'Confabulation: Sense-Making, Self-Making and World-Making in Dementia.' *Discourse Studies* 8 (5): 647–73.
Palmer, Alan. 2004. *Fictional Minds.* Lincoln: University of Nebraska Press.
Parker, David. 2004. 'Narratives of Autonomy and Narratives of Relationality in Auto/Biography.' *a/b: Auto/Biography Studies* 1 (2): 137–55.
Peterson, Linda. 1993. 'Institutionalizing Women's Autobiography: Nineteenth-Century Editors and the Shaping of an Autobiographical Tradition.' In *The Culture of Autobiography: Constructions of Self-Representation*, edited by Robert Folkenflik, 80–103. Stanford: Stanford University Press.
Petrescu, Ioana, Kit MacFarlane, and Robert Ranzijn. 2014. 'Psychological Effects of Poetry Workshops with People with Early Stage Dementia: An Exploratory Study.' *Dementia* 13 (2): 207–15.
Phelan, James. 2003. 'Dual Focalization, Retrospective Fictional Autobiography, and the Ethics of *Lolita*.' In *Narrative and Consciousness: Literature, Psychology and the Brain*, edited by Gary D. Fireman, Ted E. McVay, and Owen J. Flanagan, 129–45. Oxford: Oxford University Press.
Phinney, Alison. 2002. 'Fluctuating Awareness and the Breakdown of the Illness Narrative in Dementia.' *Dementia* 1 (3): 329–44.
Pier, John. 2013. 'Metalepsis.' In *The Living Handbook of Narratology*, edited by Peter Hühn, John Pier, Wolf Schmid, and Jörg Schönert. Hamburg: Hamburg University Press. www.lhn.uni-hamburg.de/article/unnatural-narrative.
Pitt, Brice. 1993. 'Psychiatry and the Media: Black Marks for Black Daisies' *Psychiatric Bulletin* 17: 672–3.
Polley, Sarah. 2006. *Away from Her.* Canada: Lionsgate Films.
Post, Stephen G. 2000. *The Moral Challenge of Alzheimer Disease: Ethical Issues from Diagnosis to Dying.* Baltimore: Johns Hopkins University Press.
Pratchett, Terry, and Charlie Russell. 2009. *Terry Pratchett: Living with Alzheimer's.* Produced by Craig Hunter. BBC Two.
Pritchett, Laura. 2014. *Stars Go Blue.* Berkeley: Counterpoint.
Radden, Jennifer, and Joan M. Fordyce. 2006. 'Into the Darkness: Losing Identity with Dementia.' In *Dementia: Mind, Meaning, and the Person*, edited by Julian C. Hughes, Stephen Louw, and Steven R. Sabat, 71–88. Oxford: Oxford University Press.
Ratcliffe, Matthew. 2007. *Rethinking Commonsense Psychology: A Critique of Folk Psychology, Theory of Mind, and Simulation.* New York: Palgrave Macmillan.
———. 2008. *Feelings of Being: Phenomenology, Psychiatry, and the Sense of Reality.* Oxford: Oxford University Press.

Rees, Geoffrey. 2010. 'The Ethical Imperative of Medical Humanities.' *Journal of Medical Humanities* 31: 267–77.
Richardson, Brian. 2007. 'Drama and Narrative.' In *The Cambridge Companion to Narrative*, edited by David Herman, 142–55. Cambridge: Cambridge University Press.
Richler, Mordechai. 1997. *Barney's Version*. Toronto: Knopf Canada.
Ricœur, Paul. 1991a. 'Life in Quest of Narrative.' In *On Paul Ricœur: Narrative and Interpretation*, edited by David Wood, 20–33. New York: Routledge.
———. 1991b. 'Narrative Identity.' In *On Paul Ricœur: Narrative and Interpretation*, edited by David Wood, 188–99. New York: Routledge.
Rill, Eric. 2015. *An Absent Mind*. Seattle: Lake Union Publishing.
Ringkamp, Daniela, Sara Strauß, and Leonie Süwolto, eds. 2017. *Dementia and Subjectivity: Aesthetic, Literary and Philosophical Perspectives*. Frankfurt: Lang.
Ritivoi, Andreea Deciu. 2009. 'Explaining People: Narrative and the Study of Identity.' *Storyworlds: A Journal of Narrative Studies* 1: 25–41.
———. 2016. 'Reading Stories, Reading (Others') Lives: Empathy, Intersubjectivity, and Narrative Understanding.' *Storyworlds: A Journal of Narrative Studies* 8 (1): 51–75.
Roca, Paco. 2007. *Wrinkles*. Translated from the French by Nora Goldberg. London: Knockabout.
Rohra, Helga. 2011. *Aus dem Schatten treten. Warum ich mich für unsere Rechte als Demenzbetroffene einsetze*. Frankfurt am Main: Mabuse-Verlag.
Rose, Larry. 1996. *Show Me the Way to Go Home*. Forest Knolls: Elder Books.
———. 2003. *Larry's Way: Another Look at Alzheimer's from the Inside*. New York: iUniverse.
Rosenblatt, Louise. 1995. *Literature as Exploration*. New York: The Modern Language Association. Original edition, 1938.
Rossato-Bennett, Michael. 2014. *Alive Inside*. United States: Projector Media.
Roth, Philip. 1991. *Patrimony: A True Story*. New York: Simon and Schuster.
Roy, Wendy. 2009. 'The Word is Colander: Language Loss and Narrative Voice in Fictional Canadian Alzheimer's Narratives.' *Canadian Literature* 203: 41–61.
Russell, Richard. 2001. 'In Sickness and in Health: A Qualitative Study of Elderly Men Who Care for Wives with Dementia.' *Journal of Aging Studies* 15 (4): 351–67.
Ryan, Ellen Bouchard, Karen A. Bannister, and Ann P. Anas. 2009. 'The Dementia Narrative: Writing to Reclaim Social Identity.' *Journal of Aging Studies* 23 (3): 145–57.
Ryan, Marie-Laure. 2005. 'Mode.' In *The Routledge Encyclopedia of Narrative Theory*, edited by David Herman, Manfred Jahn, and Marie-Laure Ryan, 315–6. New York: Routledge.
Sabat, Steven R., and Rom Harré. 1992. 'The Construction and Deconstruction of Self in Alzheimer's Disease.' *Ageing and Society* 12 (4): 443–61.
———. 1994. 'The Alzheimer's Disease Sufferer as a Semiotic Subject.' *Philosophy, Psychology, Psychiatry* 1 (3): 145–60.
Sacks, Oliver. 2015. *The Man Who Mistook His Wife for a Hat*. London: Picador Classic. Original edition, 1985.
Samson, Séverine, Sylvain Clément, Pauline Narme, Loris Schiaratura, and Nathalie Ehrlé. 2015. 'Efficacy of Musical Interventions in Dementia: Methodological Requirements of Nonpharmacological Trials.' *Annals of the New York Academy of Sciences* 1337 (1): 249–55.

Sartre, Jean-Paul. 1943. *L'Être et le Néant*. Paris: Tel Gallimard.
Sartwell, Crispin. 2000. *End of Story: Toward an Annihilation of Language and History*. Albany: State University of New York Press.
Schechtman, Marya. 1996. *The Constitution of Selves*. Ithaca: Cornell University Press.
———. 2007. 'Stories, Lives, and Basic Survival: A Refinement and Defense of the Narrative View.' In *Narrative and Understanding Persons*, edited by Daniel D. Hutto, 155–78. Cambridge: Cambridge University Press.
Schneider, Charles. 2006. *Don't Bury Me, It Ain't Over Yet!* Bloomington: Author House.
Schreier, Jake. 2012. *Robot and Frank*. United States: Momentum Pictures.
Selberg, Scott. 2015. 'Dementia on the Canvas: Art and the Biopolitics of Creativity.' In *Popularizing Dementia: Public Expressions and Representations of Forgetfulness*, edited by Aagje Swinnen and Mark Schweda, 137–62. Bielefeld: Transcript Verlag.
Shenk, David. 2001. *The Forgetting: Understanding Alzheimer's: A Biography of a Disease*. London: Harper Collins.
Sicveking, David. 2012. *Vergiss Mein Nicht*. Germany: Farbfilm home entertainment.
Skelton, John. 2003. 'Death and Dying in Literature.' *Advances in Psychiatric Treatment* 9: 211–20.
Small, Helen. 2007. *The Long Life*. Oxford: Oxford University Press.
Small, Jeff A., Kathy Geldart, Gloria Gutman, and Mary Ann Clarke Scott. 1998. 'The Discourse of Self in Dementia.' *Ageing and Society* 18: 291–316.
Smith, Sidonie, and Julia Watson. 2009. 'New Genres, New Subjects: Women, Gender and Autobiography after 2000.' *Revista Canaria de Estudios Ingleses* 58: 13–40.
———. 2010. *Reading Autobiography: A Guide for Interpreting Life Narratives*. Minneapolis: University of Minnesota Press.
Snowdon, David A. 1997. 'Aging and Alzheimer's Disease: Lessons from the Nun Study.' *The Gerontologist* 37 (2): 150–6.
Snyder, Lisa. 1999. *Speaking Our Minds: Personal Reflections from Individuals with Alzheimer's*. New York: W. H. Freeman.
Sontag, Susan. 1979. *Illness as Metaphor*. New York: Vintage.
———. 1989. *AIDS and Its Metaphors*. New York: Farrar, Straus and Giroux.
Spiegel, Maura. 2012. 'Rita Felski *Uses of Literature*: Book Review.' *Literature and Medicine* 30 (1): 203–7.
Stokes, Graham. 2010. *And Still the Music Plays: Stories of People with Dementia*. London: Hawker Publications. Original edition, 2008.
Stokes, Graham, and Fiona Goudie. 2002. *The Essential Dementia Care Handbook: A Good Practice Guide*. Bicester: Speechmark.
Strawson, Galen. 2004. 'Against Narrativity.' *Ratio* 17: 428–52.
Suter, Martin. 1997. *Small World*. Zürich: Diogenes Verlag.
Swaffer, Kate. 2016. *What the Hell Happened to My Brain? Living Beyond Dementia*. London: Jessica Kingsley.
Swinnen, Aagje. 2012. 'Dementia in Documentary Film: *Mum* by Adelheid Roosen.' *The Gerontologist* 53 (1): 113–22.
———. 2016. 'Healing Words: A Study of Poetry Interventions in Dementia Care.' *Dementia* 15 (6): 1377–404.
Swinnen, Aagje, and Mark Schweda, eds. 2015. *Popularizing Dementia: Public Expressions and Representations of Forgetfulness*. Bielefeld: Transcript.

Taylor, Richard. 2007. *Alzheimer's from the Inside Out*. Baltimore: Health Professions Press.
Thane, Pat. 2005. *A History of Old Age*. Oxford: Oxford University Press.
Thomas, Lewis. 1983. *Late Night Thoughts on Listening to Mahler's Ninth Symphony*. New York: Viking.
Thorndike, John. 2009. *The Last of His Mind: A Year in the Shadow of Alzheimer's*. Athens, Ohio: Swallow Press.
Toker, Leona. 1993. *Eloquent Reticence: Withholding Information in Fictional Narrative*. Lexington: University Press of Kentucky.
Traphagan, John. 2006. 'Being a Good *Rōjin*: Senility, Power, and Self-Actualization in Japan.' In *Thinking about Dementia: Culture, Loss, and the Anthropology of Senility*, edited by Annette Leibing and Lawrence Cohen, 269–87. Piscataway, NJ: Rutgers University Press.
Truscott, Marilyn. 2003. 'Life in the Slow Lane.' *Alzheimer's Care Quarterly* 4 (1): 11–7.
———. 2004a. 'Adapting Leisure and Creative Activities for People with Early Stage Dementias.' *Alzheimer's Care Quarterly* 5 (2): 92–102.
———. 2004b. 'Looks Can Be Deceiving: Dementia, the Invisible Disease.' *Alzheimer's Care Quarterly* 5 (4): 274–7.
Usita, Paula M., Ira E. Hyman, and Keith C. Herman. 1998. 'Narrative Intentions: Listening to Life Stories in Alzheimer's Disease.' *Journal of Aging Studies* 12 (2): 185–97.
Vassilas, Christopher A. 2003. 'Dementia and Literature.' *Advances in Psychiatric Treatment* 9: 439–45.
Vickers, Neil. 2016. 'Illness Narratives.' In *A History of English Autobiography*, edited by Adam Smyth, 388–401. Cambridge: Cambridge University Press.
Viney, William, Felicity Callard, and Angela Woods. 2015. 'Critical Medical Humanities: Embracing Entanglement, Taking Risks.' *Medical Humanities* 41: 2–7.
Waugh, Patricia. 2013. 'The Naturalistic Turn, the Syndrome, and the Rise of the Neo-Phenomenological Novel.' In *Diseases and Disorder in Contemporary Fiction: The Syndrome Syndrome*, edited by T.J. Lustig and James Peacock, 17–34. New York: Routledge.
Wear, Delese, and Julie M. Aultman. 2005. 'The Limits of Narrative: Medical Student Resistance to Confronting Inequality and Oppression in Literature and Beyond.' *Medical Education* 39: 1056–65.
Wennberg, Alexandra, Cheryl Dye, Blaiz Streetman-Loy, and Hiep Pham. 2015. 'Alzheimer's Patient Familial Caregivers: A Review of Burden and Interventions.' *Health & Social Work* 40 (4): 162–9.
Wetzstein, Verena. 2005. *Diagnose Alzheimer: Grundlagen einer Ethik der Demenz*. Frankfurt a.M.: Campus Verlag.
Whitehead, Anne. 2011. 'Writing with Care: Kazuo Ishiguro's *Never Let Me Go*.' *Contemporary Literature* 52 (1): 54–83.
———. 2014. 'The Medical Humanities: A Literary Perspective.' In *Medicine, Health and the Arts: Approaches to the Medical Humanities*, edited by Victoria Bates, Alan Bleakley, and Sam Goodman, 107–27. London: Routledge.
———. 2017. *Medicine and Empathy in Contemporary British Fiction: An Intervention in Medical Humanities*. Edinburgh: Edinburgh University Press.
Whitehead, Anne, and Angela Woods, with Sarah Atkinson, Jane Macnaughton and Jennifer Richards, eds. 2016. *The Edinburgh Companion to the Critical Medical Humanities*. Edinburgh: Edinburgh University Press.

Whitehouse, Peter J. 2008. *The Myth of Alzheimer's: What You Aren't Being Told about Today's Most Dreaded Diagnosis*. New York: Macmillan.
Whitehouse, Peter J., Konrad Maurer, and Jesse F. Ballenger, eds. 2000. *Concepts of Alzheimer Disease: Biological, Clinical, and Cultural Perspectives*. Baltimore: Johns Hopkins University Press.
Whitlatch, Carol J., Katherine Judge, Steven H. Zarit, and Elia Femia. 2006. 'Dyadic Intervention for Family Caregivers and Care Receivers in Early Stage Dementia.' *Gerontologist*. 46: 688–94.
Whitman, Lucy, ed. 2016. *People with Dementia Speak Out*. London: Jessica Kingsley.
Wiltshire, John. 2000. 'Biography, Pathography, and the Recovery of Meaning.' *The Cambridge Quarterly* 29 (4): 409–22.
Wood, Michael. 2005. *Literature and the Taste of Knowledge*. Cambridge: Cambridge University Press.
Woods, Angela. 2011. 'The Limits of Narrative: Provocations for the Medical Humanities.' *Medical Humanities* 37: 73–8.
World Health Organization. 2012. *Dementia: A Public Health Priority*. Geneva: World Health Organization.
Zahavi, Dan. 2007. 'Self and Other: The Limits of Narrative Understanding.' In *Narrative and Understanding Persons*, edited by Daniel D. Hutto, 179–201. Cambridge: Cambridge University Press.
Zeilig, Hannah. 2013. 'Dementia as a Cultural Metaphor.' *The Gerontologist* 54 (2): 258–67.
Zimmermann, Martina. 2010. 'Deliver Us from Evil: Carer Burden in Alzheimer's Disease.' *Medical Humanities* 36 (2): 101–07.
———. 2017. *The Poetics and Politics of Alzheimer's Disease Life-Writing*. London: Palgrave Macmillan.

Index

Note: Page numbers followed by "n" denote endnotes.

abuse 2, 105, 130, 147, 188n13, 203, 205; *see also* neglect
An Absent Mind see Rill, Eric
account: autobiographical 25, 30, 32, 39; caregivers' 129, 148, 152, 162, 166, 171, 186, 188n13, 212, 225; fictional 64, 202, 222, 188n13; first-person 1, 4, 25, 30–5, 40, 44, 58, 99–100, 105–14; *see also* autopathography
advance directives 14, 147–8, 164, 208; *see also* end-of-life
advice literature 30, 129, 133, 138, 142, 168, 185–6
advocacy 45, 107, 116; (dementia) advocacy movement 13, 30, 61n8, 93, 107–8, 114, 125, 133–4, 142, 155n1, 183–7, 188n14, 207, 229
advocate 108, 124, 131, 143, 161, 187
agency 45, 81, 89, 108, 110, 120, 124, 126, 127n12, 162, 218
Alive Inside 178–9
Alzheimer's disease 8, 10, 51, 102, 135, 148–9, 154, 207; early-onset 30, 65, 207; *see also* early-onset dementia
Alzheimer's Disease International 12
Alzheimer's disease movement 15, 76, 213; *see also* advocacy movement
Alzheimer's from the Inside Out 30
Andrews, Molly 16, 100, 104
Andrews, Nancy 4, 38, 39; *see also* photography
apology 133; *see also* genre
appropriation 7, 64, 91, 93, 131–2, 202
Ariyoshi, Sawako 224n20
assisted suicide 3, 10, 216; *see also* end-of life; euthanasia;
authenticity 35, 78, 111, 112–13
authority 60, 115, 141, 212

autobiographical writing 3, 35, 43, 58, 63, 99, 104–5, 108, 150, 193
autobiography 3, 15, 21n4, 105–6, 111, 117, 129, 132, 149, 155; *see also* autographics; autopathography; graphic memoir
autographics 149, 150, 158n24, 158n25
autopathography 4, 21n4, 35, 40, 42, 52, 59–60, 99, 104, 106, 108, 110–11, 113, 123–4; *see also* first-person account; pathography
autonomy 10, 15, 111, 126, 142, 147, 163–4, 167, 174, 174, 190, 207–8; loss of 14, 70, 121

Bamberg, Michael 16, 100, 104, 113
Barney's Version see Richler, Mordechai
Basting, Anne Davis 10, 61n12, 108, 111, 113–14, 179–80, 228
Battersby, James L. 100, 101
Bayley, John 55, 156n4, 157n22
Bernlef, J. 18, 65, 72–6, 82, 85, 89, 94n6
bildungsroman 106, 133, 138, 156n10
bioethical: decision-making 20, 192, 216, 221; dilemmas 192, 221; principles 147; questions and issues 190, 192, 206, 208, 212
bioethics 190, 191, 205–7
biomedicine 8–9, 17, 25, 92, 103–4, 138, 191–3, 195, 197, 207, 226
Black Daisies for the Bride see Harrison, Toni
blog 30, 35, 42, 61n8, 107, 111–2, 126n5, 135, 229; *see also* journal; diary
Bruner, Jerome 6, 100–1
Bryden, Christine 32, 39, 41, 44, 46, 48, 49, 61n9, 106, 124
Buber, Martin 152

Burke, Lucy 2, 3, 9, 13, 15, 34, 105, 108, 11–3, 136–7, 147, 156n7, 157n15, 168, 186–7, 188n13, 188n15, 193–4, 205, 209, 213, 216, 218–9

Can't We Talk About Something More Pleasant see Chast, Roz
care: crisis 3, 215, 217; environment/setting 11, 105, 115, 120, 147, 180; home 27, 76–7, 85, 115, 120–1, 171, 173, 201, 203, 205, 213, 222; institutional 20, 162, 183; intimate/personal 152, 154, 162–3, 168–70; scandal 2, 105; staff 115, 122, 183
care partner 19, 20, 25, 113, 128, 137, 155n1, 161–2, 213–4, 221, 226, 228–9; *see also* caregiver
care-receiver 46, 55, 76, 144, 150, 152, 155n1, 161, 165, 167, 185, 187n4, 204
care-writing 19, 136, 161, 171, 185
caregiver: familial 2, 3, 161, 183; primary 2, 50, 52, 128, 142, 214; professional 2, 55, 146, 183; secondary 128, 155; spousal 145–6, 155, 156n8, 157n22
caregivers' memoir 46, 51, 59, 76, 128–57, 161–89; filial 19, 46, 128, 130, 134, 149
caregiving: burden 2, 29, 46, 58–9, 147–8, 161, 173, 187n2, 188n14, 209, 213–4, 224n18; dilemma 15, 20, 147, 162–8, 171–4, 207; duty 2, 31, 164, 215, 217
Carel, Havi 5, 25, 38, 45, 58, 88
carer *see* caregiver; care partner
Cavanagh, Paul 94n7
chaos narrative 200; *see also* Frank, Arthur
Charon, Rita 7, 16, 43, 60, 64, 190, 191, 193, 206, 220; *see also* narrative medicine
chart: parallel 95n12; patient 77–8, 80, 95n12
Chast, Roz 136, 150–1, 158
childhood 69, 76, 85, 119, 122, 146; second 139–140, 146
children's literature 224n22, 227, 230n1
Circling My Mother: A Memoir see Gordon, Mary
Clegg, David 5, 19, 78, 85, 99, 100, 104, 114–22, 125
closure 65, 106, 107, 133, 168, 200, 212, 218
coercion 14–5, 162–3, 163–8; *see also* paternalism

coherence 19, 51, 79, 99, 102, 107, 113, 114–20, 123, 127n9, 177, 199, 200; *see also* incoherent
Coleman, Rowan 94n7, 95n11
comic plot 105–6
comics 149, 150, 154; *see also* graphic narrative
communication: embodied 18, 25–6, 29, 50, 53–4, 58–9, 63; non-verbal 25, 37, 50, 54, 123
confabulation 117–8, 120, 174, 175–8
confessional writing 134
conversational storytelling 5, 19, 51, 102, 105, 114–5
conversion narrative/tale 106, 133
Cooney, Eleanor 135, 171, 188n14
cost: of care 12, 13; cost-benefit analysis 190, 209, 216; emotional 173
counter-narrative 4, 12, 16, 19, 20, 35, 93, 99, 100, 103–6, 114–7, 120–6, 145, 191, 196–8, 201, 207, 218, 225–6
Couser, G. Thomas 9, 16, 19, 30, 51, 94, 100, 105–7, 125, 127n15, 128–31, 133–4, 136, 141–2, 146, 155, 157n19, 186, 187
creativity 20, 36, 195, 228
crime story 94n7
Crisp, Jane 118–9, 178

Damasio, Antonio R. 41, 61n5, 95n8
Dancing with Dementia see Bryden, Christine
Death in Slow Motion: A Memoir of a Daughter, Her Mother, and the Beast Called Alzheimer's see Cooney, Eleanor
death sentence 40; *see also* metaphor
DeBaggio, Thomas 36, 40–3, 45, 48, 61n9, 108–10, 113, 124
defamiliarisation 71, 84, 91
dementia: early-onset 19, 30–1, 35, 45, 65, 68, 69, 94n7, 100, 107, 126n7, 132, 157n22, 207; frontotemporal 8, 61; Lewy-Body 8, 61n7, 106; vascular/multi-infarct 8, 135n7 *see also* Husband, Toni
diagnosis 31, 35, 40, 51, 106, 111–3, 127n8, 174, 195, 197, 208, 226; post 42, 45, 46, 108, 220
diary 107, 129; audio 61n13, 229; *see also* journal
dignity 11, 15, 28, 131, 13, 171, 188n13
dilemma *see* caregiving dilemma

disability 12, 16, 90, 100–3, 115; approach 40; studies 15, 103, 113, 124, 135, 101, 199, 202
documentary film 3, 18, 25, 29, 49, 50–8, 59–60, 63, 131–2, 154, 163, 166–8, 178–9, 186
Downham, Jenny 95n11, 224n22
Do You Remember Me? A Father, a Daughter, and a Search for the Self see Levine, Judith
dramatic irony 66, 89
Dresser, Rebecca 147, 164
Dworkin, Ronald 147–8, 164, 208

Eagar, Lindsay 224n22
Eakin, Paul John 6, 100–3, 117, 129, 131–2, 136, 155
Eastham, Ruth 224n22
elegy 133
Elegy for Iris 156n4
Elizabeth is Missing see Healey, Emma
embodied self 18, 25, 26–9, 49, 50, 56–9; *see also* embodied communication
embodiment 6, 18, 25–7, 59, 74, 101, 195, 198
empathy 7–8, 51, 64, 67–8, 71, 82–3, 92, 167, 176, 184, 190, 204, 22; ambassadorial strategic empathy 69; broadcast strategic empathy 69, 92; empathy-altruism hypothesis 19, 64; *see also* narrative empathy
Empathy and the Novel see Keen, Suzanne
end-of life: care 219, 221–2, 224n13; decisions 14, 15, 107, 162, 191–2, 206, 208, 212; *see also* assisted suicide; euthanasia
epistemic injustice 107
essay 19, 41–2, 61n8, 106–8, 110–11, 128, 138–42, 155
ethics 7, 8, 15, 19, 50, 125, 130, 132, 133, 138, 141, 146–7, 155, 156n7, 156n8, 166, 186, 192, 201, 202, 212, 216, 221, 223n2, 223n4; *see also* bioethics
euthanasia 2, 3, 10, 13, 99, 105, 190, 208, 215–7, 221, 224n23; *see also* assisted suicide; end-of-life

Feil, Naomi 69, 176
Felski, Rita 7, 15, 63, 91–2, 206, 220, 223n12
film 7, 14–5, 18, 20, 21n8, 63–5, 67–8, 70–1, 88–9, 93, 130, 156n7, 163, 174, 186, 192, 206–7, 211–2, 214, 221–2; *see also* documentary film
flow 47–9, 62n18
focalisation 3, 21n8, 65–6, 75, 84, 94n3, 95n11, 208–9, 224n21
Forster, Margaret 1–3, 20, 192, 206, 213–14, 218–19, 221
fragmentation 35, 73–4, 77, 78, 79, 106, 118–19, 140
Frank, Arthur W. 16, 25, 99, 100–1, 130, 200
Franzen, Jonathan 19, 128, 131, 136–42, 146, 155, 157, 214

gender 19, 30, 83, 90, 104, 128, 134–9, 145, 147, 154–5, 157n17, 157n22, 187n5, 213–14; transgender 61n10
Genova, Lisa 18, 64, 66–70, 90–2, 206, 207–13, 214, 218, 221
genre 3–4, 8, 14–15, 18–19, 21n8, 35, 53, 59, 78, 85, 100–1, 105, 106, 111, 113–14, 128, 133–5, 137–8, 141, 149, 150–1, 154–5, 156n1, 158n11, 163, 186, 200, 225, 228; *see also* apology; autobiography; autographics; autopathography; *bildungsroman*; confessional writing; conversion narrative; crime writing; diary; documentary; elegy; essay; journal
Gillies, Andrea 133, 135, 156n2
Gordon, Mary 130, 135, 156n3, 188n17
Grant, Linda 135, 156n3, 157n12
graphic: memoir 14, 19, 59, 128, 135, 136, 148–54, 155, 157n20, 163, 168, 171, 174, 182; narrative 7, 153, 227; novel 158n24; *see also* autographics

Hacking, Ian 9
Hadas, Rachel 132, 157n22, 163, 173
Harrison, Toni 156n7
Hartung, Heike 3, 156n10, 224n23
Haugse, John 151, 157n20, 158n24
Have the Men Had Enough? see Forster, Margaret
Hawkins, Anne Hunsaker 16, 21n4, 141, 223n7
Healey, Emma 94n7
Heavy Snow: My Father's Disappearance into Alzheimer's see Haugse, John
Henderson, Cary 1, 3–4, 32–4, 36–9, 42–9, 51–2, 61n9, 108, 112–13, 229
Herman, David 5, 63, 127n14
hero 143; eponymous 202, 207
home see institution; care

Hour of the Bees see Eagar, Lindsay
House Mother Normal see Johnson, B.S.
Hughes, Julian C. 11, 36, 126n1, 223n8
Husband, Toni 158n24
Hydén, Lars-Christer 5, 6, 12, 78, 102–3, 105, 116–17, 119, 121, 123, 175, 177–8
hypercognitive 8, 10, 135, 142, 207

identification 64, 72, 90, 157n15, 162, 188n20
identity: co-construction of 102; constitution of 101, 103, 125; construction 6, 12, 18, 119, 135–6, 229; performance of 103, 113, 119, 123; relational 6, 19, 71, 128, 135–6, 137, 148, 154, 194, 196; *see also* narrative identity; positioning; self-making
Ignatieff, Michael 15, 20, 54, 75, 137, 191, 193–201, 213, 214
illness narrative 4, 5, 15–16, 18–19, 21, 60, 99, 103, 108, 124, 133, 141, 174, 195, 200, 220, 225, 226; *see also* pathography; autopathography
immersion 67, 72, 91, 96n22
incoherent 73, 75, 77, 78, 114, 116, 122, 123, 127n9
infantilisation 11, 70, 105, 116, 121, 127n12, 140, 145, 174
Innes, Anthea 31–2, 110, 128, 147, 184, 224n20
institutionalisation 20, 115, 142–3, 154, 162–3, 168, 171–4, 213, 215, 224n22; *see also* care home
intersubjectivity 7, 18, 25, 50, 54, 63, 89, 102, 114, 118, 123, 126, 137, 193, 194, 198
Ishiguro, Kazuo 19, 65, 83–8, 89, 90

Johnson, B.S. 18, 20, 65, 76–83, 89, 91, 95n14, 192, 201–5, 219
Johnstone, Megan-Jane 2, 10, 13
Jones, Rebecca 125
Jones, Therese 17, 20, 191, 206, 219, 222
journal 4, 32–4, 38–9, 45, 49, 107, 126n5, 129
Just Love Me: My Life Turned Upside-Down by Alzheimer's see Lee, Jeanne L.

Keen, Suzanne 7, 19, 64, 66–9, 71, 82, 89, 91–2, 185, 189n20, 201, 221, 226
Killick, John 25, 29, 42, 53–8, 153, 156n8, 187n1, 188n7, 228

Kitwood, Tom 11, 29, 45, 144–5, 148, 152
Kleinman, Arthur 16, 25
Kontos, Pia C. 25–8, 49, 57, 223n10
Korthals Altes, Liesbeth 193, 201, 223n4
Krüger, Naomi 78, 94n7
Krüger-Fürhoff, Irmela M. 95n9, 95n15, 157n16

Lal, Ranjit 224n22
Laplante, Alice 94n7
Leavitt, Sarah 128, 148–54, 155, 163, 168–73, 182, 188n12, 188n13
Lee, Jeanne L. 46, 61n9, 106
Leibing, Annette 21n7, 21n11, 21n12, 126n7
Lejeune, Philippe 117
Lévinas, Emmanuel 28, 92, 202
Levine, Judith 19, 128, 133, 137, 142–8, 155, 164
life world 5–7, 25, 57, 59, 60, 88, 145, 167, 192, 225
life writing: collaborative 5, 60, 78, 102, 114, 127n16, 135, 228; *see also* autobiographical writing; autobiography; autographics; graphic memoir; memoir
Living in the Labyrinth: A Personal Journey through the Maze of Alzheimer's see McGowin, Diane Friel
Losing My Mind: An Intimate Look at Life with Alzheimer's see DeBaggio, Thomas

McGowin, Diane Friel 35, 36, 40, 61n9, 111, 124
McLean, Athena Helen 118–19
Magnusson, Sally 133, 135, 163, 166, 177–84, 186–7, 188n16
master narrative 12, 16, 103–5, 110, 129, 195, 197–8
masterplot *see* master narrative
May see Krüger, Naomi
media: audiovisual 21n8, 59, 67, 174; cross-medial 5, 7; different 8, 9, 15, 18, 20, 26, 130, 133, 154–5, 163, 174, 187n10, 192, 206, 225; medium 3, 18, 35, 49, 51, 53, 59, 65, 128, 149, 150, 153–5, 162–3, 208, 225, 229; new 157n14, 229; social media 229; visual 3, 59; *see also* audio diary; film; graphic memoir

memoir *see* graphic memoir; caregivers' memoir
memory 113, 137, 138, 147, 142, 177, 196, 199; aid 33, 107, 229; autobiographical 43, 82; declarative 210; embodied 26, 57, 109, 145; episodic 32; loss 30, 32, 34, 44, 51, 116, 73, 85–6, 88, 100–1, 105, 108, 109, 136, 140, 148, 180–1; semantic 32, 210; procedural 26, 32, 33–4, 56–7
The Memory Cage see Eastham, Ruth
Meretoja, Hanna 7, 67, 90–1, 191–3, 201, 207, 218, 220, 223
metafiction 72
metalepsis 77, 202
metaphor: 10, 13, 14, 35, 36, 119, 195, 197–9, 206, 220; child 139; death before death, living death 4, 10, 11, 41, 100, 107, 109–10, 124, 157n18, 196, 199; dehumanising 41, 104, 124, 125; epidemic 3, 12; fading 39, 156n8; prisoner 80–1; renewal, spring 76; (empty) shell 10, 11, 39, 70, 74, 81, 105, 110, 144, 179; vegetable 11, 105, 110, 120, 196; visual 153, 154, 171, 199n12; zombie 10, 70, 110, 179, 180, 212
Miller, Nancy K. 6, 61n6, 130, 136, 141
Miller, Sue 69, 133, 157n18, 175–7
Millet, Stephan 6, 10, 26–9, 57
mind: embedded 78–9, 82, 91, 190; embodied 63, 79, 91; fictional 78–9, 82
Mini-Mental State Examination 68, 210
Missing Steps see Cavanagh, Paul
Mitchell, Wendy 33–8, 40, 45, 47, 49, 61n8, 61n9, 112
mode: 3, 8, 15, 21n8, 49, 60, 84, 91, 110, 138, 150, 153, 208, 225; experimental 71, 82–3, 89 imperative 73; lyrical 65; *see also* focalisation
monologue: interior 65, 77–8, 202
motif: *carpe diem* 44, 106, 205, 209; *memento mori* 134
murder mystery *see* crime story
music 48–9, 57, 74, 113, 145, 157n21, 174, 178–80, 184, 188n7, 188n16, 212; film music 50, 68, 167, 211
'My Father's Brain' *see* Franzen, Jonathan

narrative: broken 102, 114, 127n9; frame 77, 202; linear 35, 65, 74, 107, 199; retrospective 34, 42, 61n12, 72, 107, 117; scaffolding 103; sense-making 5, 91, 101, 119, 123, 127n14, 177, 178, 225; self-making 107, 119, 177–8; world-making 123, 178; *see also* coherence; counter-narrative; ethics; identity; master narrative; narrative medicine; triumph narrative; you-narrative
narrative coherence *see* coherence
narrative empathy 3, 7, 18, 19, 60, 64–7, 71–2, 88–94, 225–7; *see also* empathy
narrative ethics *see* ethics
narrative identity 4, 6, 7, 15, 19, 26, 35, 99, 100–3, 119, 122, 137, 225
narrative medicine 18, 190, 193
narrator/narration: autodiegetic 72, 83; concurrent or present tense 72–3, 76, 85; first-person 72–3, 83–4, 87, 94n7, 95n11, 95n17, 219; omniscient 83, 95n17; second-person 74, 177; third-person 65, 70, 73–4, 94n2, 95n7; unreliable 65, 73, 87, 89
neglect 2, 105, 174, 183; *see also* abuse
Nussbaum, Martha Craven 7, 64, 189n20, 192, 201, 205–6, 216, 219, 220

Our Nana was a Nutcase see Lal, Ranjit
Out of Mind see Bernlef, J.

Palmer, Alan 63, 75, 79
parallel experience 38, 65–7, 73, 86, 89, 92, 96n21
parent-child relationship 141, 146, 151, 152; reversal of 136, 144, 150, 163, 194
Partial View: An Alzheimer's Journal see Henderson, Cary
paternalism 14, 146, 174; *see also* coercion
pathography 16, 21n4
People with Dementia Speak Out see Bryden, Christine
personhood 10, 11, 15, 26–7, 29, 74, 92, 100, 101, 104–5, 108, 11, 113, 126n1, 134, 137–8, 142, 195, 210, 220, 223n8; movement 186
photography 4, 18, 38–9, 49, 130, 154, 156n8
physician-assisted suicide 3, 10, 216; *see also* euthanasia
placement 142, 153, 163, 171, 173, 213, 215; *see also* institutionalisation; home
poetics 133
politics 4, 15, 19, 50, 103, 128, 130, 134, 149, 188n14, 213
polyphony 90–1, 192, 201

positioning 11, 84, 103, 108, 123, 124
Post, Stephen G. 10, 142; *see also* hypercognitive
Pritchett, Laura 95n11, 224n18
privacy 51, 115–16, 130–1, 133, 141, 154, 156n7, 168, 170, 187, 188n13

quality of life 166, 190, 206–8, 210–11, 216, 219; *see also* end-of-life decisions
quest narrative 101, 106

Ratcliffe, Matthew 7, 29, 53, 62n14, 198
redemption 106, 200
referentiality 117–18, 123, 155, 185, 193
relational identity *see* identity
relationality 26, 136, 140, 148–9, 186, 200; *see also* relational identity
Remind Me Who I Am, Again see Grant, Linda
Richler, Mordechai 94n7
Rill, Eric 94n7, 95n11
Ritivoi, Andreea Deciu 91, 102
Roca, Paco 158n24
Rohra, Helga 35, 47, 61n9, 112, 126n8
Rose, Larry 61n9
Rosenblatt, Louise 15, 19, 162, 167, 174, 192, 206, 207, 220

Sabat, Steven R. 5, 11–12, 28, 70, 136
Scar Tissue see Ignatieff, Michael
Sieveking, David 18, 25, 49, 50–8, 59, 132, 163, 166–8, 188n7
Small World see Suter, Martin
Snyder, Lisa 10, 29, 31, 38, 45–6, 49
Somebody I Used to Know see Mitchell, Wendy
Sontag, Susan 9, 198–9
Stars Go Blue see Pritchett, Laura
stereotype: cultural 90; dominant/common 15, 70, 220; gender 157, 214; literary 78; negative 5, 35, 39, 93, 144, 154, 191
Still Alice: film 18, 20, 65, 67–8, 70–1, 89, 93, 206, 207, 211–13, 214, 218, 221; novel *see* Genova, Lisa
Stokes, Graham 52, 127n12, 189n17
The Story of My Father see Miller, Sue
Strange Relation: A Memoir of Marriage, Dementia, and Poetry see Hadas, Rachel
Strawson, Galen 6, 100–2, 109
stream of consciousness 65, 77, 82, 89, 95n9

suicide 3, 190, 200, 207–13, 215, 216, 218, 224n18; *see also* physician-assisted suicide
Suter, Martin 95n7
Swaffer, Kate 42, 47, 61n8, 61n9, 107–8, 220
Swinnen, Aagje 4, 14, 186, 228
sympathy 66–7, 70, 79, 83, 118, 189n20

Tangles: A Story about Alzheimer's, My Mother, and Me see Leavitt, Sarah
Taylor, Richard 30, 41, 44, 47, 61n8, 61n9, 106–7, 110–11, 126n5
Tell Mrs Mill her Husband is Still Dead see Clegg, David
testimony 30, 31, 112–13, 114, 133, 142
therapy: alternative 174, 188n7; animal-assisted 62n19; benefits 126n6, 184, 199; reminiscence 175; speech 179; scriptotherapy/writing 48, 107, 126n6, 129; therapeutic intervention 13, 25, 166, 175, 179, 180; validation 69, 176; *see also* music
Thorndike, John 136, 163–8
Toker, Leona 38, 65–7, 71, 89
transportation *see* immersion
Trebus project 121; *see also* Clegg, David
triumph narrative 105–6, 127n17
truth 35, 82, 110, 118, 122, 132–3, 173, 195, 198, 200, 203
Turn of Mind see LaPlante, Alice
The Twighlight Years see Ariyoshi, Sawako

Unbecoming see Downham, Jenny
The Unconsoled see Ishiguro, Kazuo

validation *see* validation therapy
Vergiss Mein Nicht (Forget-Me-Not) see Sieveking, David
verisimilitude 35, 78
victim 10, 20n2, 111, 143, 144
voyeurism 64, 93, 131, 133, 156n7, 156n8
vulnerability 93, 125, 130, 157n19, 180, 205, 221
vulnerable subjects 19, 51, 115, 130, 188n10 *see also* Couser, G. Thomas

Waugh, Patricia 7, 15, 18, 63, 93, 197
Wetzstein, Verena 7, 10–11, 13, 21n12
What the Hell Happened to My Brain? Living Beyond Dementia see Swaffer, Kate

When It Gets Dark: An Enlightened Reflection on Life with Alzheimer's see DeBaggio, Thomas
Where Memories Go: Why Dementia Changes Everything see Magnusson, Sally
Whitehead, Anne 7, 16–17, 21, 64, 92, 220–1, 223n1, 226–7
Whitman, Lucy 31, 60, 61n10, 157n22
Who Will I Be When I Die? see Bryden, Christine
Wiltshire, John 16, 199–200
Woods, Angela 4, 5, 7, 17, 21n3, 65, 113, 163, 223n1, 226–7

The Wounded Storyteller see Frank, Arthur
Wrinkles see Roca, Paco

you-narrative 35, 112; *see also* second-person narrator
young adult fiction 224n22

Zahavi, Dan 7, 11, 26, 29, 32, 54, 60n1, 92, 101–3
Zeilig, Hannah 12
Zimmermann, Martina 14, 35, 58, 106–8, 111, 127n8, 129, 133, 135, 155, 156n8, 167, 187n2, 214, 221
zombie *see* metaphor